Veterinary Nursing
(Formerly Jones's Animal Nursing 5th edition)

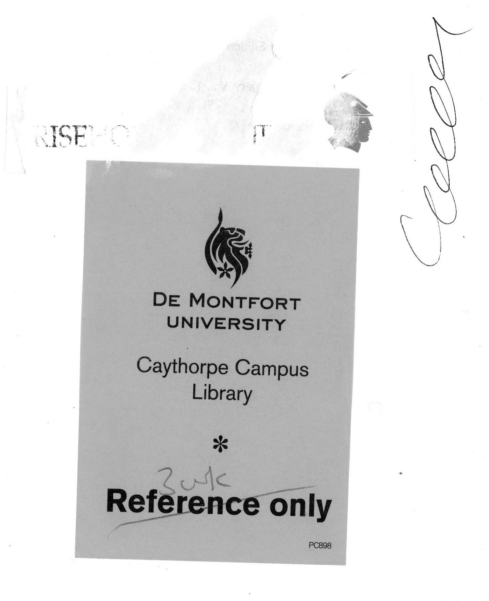

TITLES OF RELATED INTEREST FROM PERGAMON

Pergamon Veterinary Handbook Series

Series Editor: A. T. B. EDNEY

BROWN
Aquaculture for Veterinarians: Fish Husbandry and Medicine

ANDERSON & EDNEY
Practical Animal Handling

EMILY & PENMAN
Handbook of Small Animal Dentistry, 2nd Edition

GELATT & GELATT
Handbook of Small Animal Ophthalmic Surgery, Vol. 1: Extraocular Procedures

GORREL, PENMAN & EMILY
Handbook of Small Animal Oral Emergencies

MORIELLO & MASON
Handbook of Small Animal Dermatology

PENMAN, EMILY & GORREL
Handbook of Advanced Small Animal Dentistry

SHERIDAN & McCAFFERTY
The Business of Veterinary Practice

WILLS & WOLF
Handbook of Feline Medicine

Other books

BURGER
The Waltham Book of Companion Animal Nutrition

GOLDSCHMIDT & SHOFER
Skin Tumours of the Dog and Cat

IHRKE, MASON & WHITE
Advances in Veterinary Dermatology, Volume 2

ROBINSON
Genetics for Cat Breeders, 3rd Edition
Genetics for Dog Breeders, 2nd Edition

THORNE
The Waltham Book of Dog and Cat Behaviour

WILLS AND SIMPSON
The Waltham Book of Clinical Nutrition of the Dog and Cat

WOLDEHIWET & RISTIC
Rickettsial and Chlamydial Diseases of Domestic Animals

Journals

Veterinary Dermatology
The official journal of the European Society of Veterinary Dermatology and the American College of Veterinary Dermatology

Veterinary Nursing

(Formerly Jones's Animal Nursing, 5th edition)

Edited by

D. R. LANE

Leamington Spa, Warwickshire CV32 4EZ, UK

and

B. COOPER

College of Animal Welfare, Wood Green Animal Shelters,
Huntingdon PE18 8LJ, UK

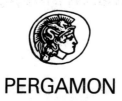

PERGAMON

U.K.   Elsevier Science Ltd., The Boulevard, Langford Lane,
            Kidlington, Oxford OX5 1GB, England

U.S.A.   Elsevier Science Inc., 660 White Plains Road, Tarrytown,
            New York 10591-5153, U.S.A.

JAPAN   Elsevier Science Japan, Tsunashima Building Annex, 3-20-12 Yushima,
            Bunkyo-ku, Tokyo 113, Japan

First edition 1994

Library of Congress Cataloging-in-Publication Data
Veterinary nursing: formerly Jones's animal nursing
edited by D. Lane and B. Cooper
p. cm.
Includes bibliographical and indexes.
1. Veterinary nursing.   2. Pets—Diseases.   I. Jones, Bruce V.
II. Lane, D. R.   III. Cooper, B.   IV. Jones's animal nursing.
SF774.5.V48   1994
636.089'073—dc20   94-22434

British Library Cataloguing in Publication Data
A catalogue record for this book is available from the British Library

ISBN 0-08-0422888 (Hardcover)
ISBN 0-08-0422896 (Flexicover)

DISCLAIMER
Whilst every effort is made by the Publishers to see that no inaccurate or misleading
data, opinion or statement appear in this book, they wish to make it clear that the
data and opinions appearing in the articles herein are the sole responsibility of the
contributor concerned. Accordingly, the Publishers and their employees, officers and
agents accept no responsibility or liability whatsoever for the consequences of any
such inaccurate or misleading data, opinion or statement.

Drug and Dosage Selection: The Authors have made every effort to ensure the
accuracy of the information herein, particularly with regard to drug selection and
dose. However, appropriate information sources should be consulted, especially for
new or unfamiliar drugs or procedures. It is the responsibility of every veterinarian to
evaluate the appropriateness of a particular opinion in the context of actual clinical
situations, and with due consideration to new developments.

Typeset by Cotswold Typesetting Limited
Printed in Great Britain by Redwood Books, Trowbridge

Preface

After many years of involvement by the senior editor in the training of veterinary nurses and since 1978 preparing previous editions of *Jones's Animal Nursing*, this is the first time that a book has been titled with the correct description of 'Veterinary Nursing'. The change in name for a book concerned with the nursing and care of small animals became possible once the title of veterinary nurse was confirmed as result of long and patient negotiations with organisations involved in the nursing world. The help of a joint editor is another welcome innovation for this new edition, representing the greater participation of veterinary nurses in their own training, examination system and maintenance of standards.

The reader will find many other changes since the 5th edition of *Jones's Animal Nursing* was produced. There are 17 new authors for this book, first prepared as a 6th edition of the well known and trusted book *Jones's*. New topics reflect the wider role of veterinary nurses in all animal-concerned areas, bereavement counselling and behavioural problems are obvious examples. The concern for health and safety and the expanding legislation in the everyday dealings of the veterinary nurse are other new areas for nurses to become familiar with and these topics are dealt with for the first time in this book.

Career opportunities have increased rapidly for veterinary nurses. The National Council for Vocational Qualifications established by the government in 1986 recognises too that skills gained in one occupation can be used to transfer into others. Veterinary nurses now work in the universities and for animal charities. They are also employed in the pharmaceutical industry, pet insurance, advertising, teaching, bereavement and health counselling and in business management. The scope of the nurse's training has increased in an attempt to meet the needs of the clients and the new challenges to the profession. The educational demands go far beyond the range of a single text book but this new edition sets out to cover the technical requirements of the veterinary nurse working in a practice. The student veterinary nurse requires knowledge not only in the basic sciences, animal nutrition, animal husbandry and hospital procedures, but also in surgical techniques, radiography, computers, etc. as well as in the general nursing care of animals.

Veterinary nurses have much to be proud of. Their role in practice has been further enhanced since the amendment to Schedule Three of the Veterinary Surgeons Act. Under the direction of the veterinary surgeon, veterinary nurses can now perform all medical and minor surgical procedures not involving entry into a body cavity of a companion animal. This places an increased responsibility on the veterinary nurses to ensure that they may have the training and expertise to carry out these new tasks. One cannot overemphasise the importance of continuing veterinary nurses' professional development in order to keep pace with all these new opportunities.

The veterinary nurse qualification is not an end result, it is a beginning. Veterinary nurses must remember to act in such a way as to ensure the well being of all animals entrusted to their care. Not only must they make certain that no action or omission is made that could be detrimental to the patient but they should acknowledge their own limitations and where necessary decline certain tasks until they have received further training. A veterinary nurse should take every opportunity to maintain and improve professional knowledge and competence, working in a collaborative and helpful manner with other colleagues.

There are now opportunities for surgical skills to be measured by the Diploma in Advanced Veterinary Nursing (Surgical). This book will cover the groundwork for such further studies but additional sources of information will be required. Discussions are currently under way regarding the development of other diplomas, possibly in medicine and in equine nursing. Further training in laboratory work is available to obtain qualifications in diagnostic techniques and diplomas studies in counselling skills may be developed in the near future.

Veterinary nurses have a responsibility for keeping pace with all these changes, not only for their own personal development, but also to assist their own staff with their training and for the further advancement of the profession of veterinary nursing.

B. Cooper
VN, Cert. Ed.

D. R. Lane
BSc, FRAgS, FRCVS

Acknowledgements

The illustrations on the front cover were drawn by Glynnis Wootton and adapted from her winning poster in the 1993 BSAVA Veterinary Nursing competition; they are reproduced with grateful thanks to Glynnis, the BSAVA and to Duphar and Cox Veterinary Division who sponsored the printing of the poster.

We would like to thank Seward medical for supplying the illustrations used in Chapter 26 (Theatre practice) and MDC Components for their help and permission to reproduce photographs of their equipment used in Chapter 1 (Handling and control).

Contents

List of Contributors

Dr P. Bloxham, MVB, MRCVS, 8 George Street, Teignmouth TQ14 8AH

Mr R. Butcher, MA, Vet MB, MRCVS, 196 Hall Lane, Upminster, Essex RM14 1TD

Ms S. Chandler, VN, Dip AVN (Surg), Cambridge Veterinary School, Madingley Road, Cambridge

Mr R. E. Clutton, BVSc, DVA, MRCVS, Dept. of Veterinary Clinical Studies, Royal (Dick) School of Veterinary Studies, Veterinary Field Station, Easter Bush, Roslin, Midlothian EH25 9RG

Miss B. Cooper, VN, Cert Ed, College of Animal Welfare, Wood Green Animal Shelters, King's Bush Farm, Godmanchester, Huntingdon PE18 8LJ

Professor J. Cooper, BSc, FRCVS, BVSC, DTVM, C Biol, F Biol, Cert LAS, MRC Path, Volcano Veterinary Centre, B.P. 105, Ruhengeri, Rwanda, Africa

Mrs R. Dennis, MA, Vet MB, DVR, MRCVS, Animal Health Trust, P.O. Box 5, Newmarket, Suffolk CB8 7DW

Dr J. Elliott, MA, Vet MB, Cert SAC, Royal Veterinary College, Royal College Street, London NW1 0TU

Dr G. England, B Vet Med, DVR, Cert VA, FRCVS, Department of Large Animal Medicine & Surgery, Royal Veterinary College, Hawkshead Lane, North Mymms, Hatfield, Herts. AL9 7TAD

Mrs M. Fisher, B Vet Med, MRCVS, Brentknoll Veterinary Centre, 152 Bath Road, Worcester WR5 3EP

Mrs S. Hiscock, B Vet Med, MRCVS, 16 Hill Place, Bursledon, Southampton, Hants. SO3 8AE

Ms J. Jowitt, BSc, 22 Fontainhall Road, Edinburgh EH9 2LW

Mr D. R. Lane, BSc, FRCVS, FRAgS, 47 Newbold Terrace, Leamington Spa, Warwickshire CV32 4EZ

Dr S. E. Long, BVMS, MRCVS, Department of Animal Husbandry, University of Bristol, Langford House, Langford, Bristol BS18 7DU

Dr C. May, MA Vet MB, Cert SAO, University of Liverpool, Small Animal Hospital, Crown Street, Liverpool, Merseyside L7 7EX

Ms D. McHugh, VN, Dip AVN (Surg), Animal Health Trust, Balaton Lodge, Snailwell Road, Newmarket, Suffolk

Mr D. S. Mills, BVSc, MRCVS, Lincs. College of Agriculture, Caythorpe Court, Caythorpe, Nr Grantham, Lincs. NG32 3EP

Mrs A. J. Pearson, BA, Vet MB, MRCVS, Whitegates, Button End, Harston, Cambridge CB2 5NX

Mr A. Porter, MA, DVM&S, 4 Savill Road, Lindfield, Haywards Heath, Sussex RG16 2NX

Ms J. Seymour, VN, Cert Ed, Staffordshire College of Agriculture, Rodbaston, Penkridge, Stafford ST19 5PH

Mr J. Simpson, Department of Veterinary Clinical Studies, Royal (Dick) School of Veterinary Studies, University of Edinburgh, Summerhall, Edinburgh EH9 1Q

Dr B. Tennant, BVSc, PhD, Cert VR, MRCVS, University of Liverpool, Small Animal Hospital, Crown Street, Liverpool, Merseyside L7 7EX

Mrs C. Van der Heiden, VN, Larabus Farm, Bridgend, Islay, Argyll PA44 7PL

Ms E. Welsh, BVMS, MRCVS, 38 Lunan Drive, Bishopbriggs, Glasgow, Lanarkshire G64 1AN

Ms J. White, VN Cert Ed, 10 Springfield Avenue, Harrogate, North Yorkshire HG1 2HR

Miss K. Wiggins, VN Dip AVN (Surg), 13 The Ridgeway, Flitwick, Bedfordshire NR45 1DH

Mrs E. Williams, VN, 3 Cae Haf, Northop Hall, Nr Mold, Clwyd CH7 6GB

Book 1

1
Handling and Control

E. M. WILLIAMS

Most nurses working with animals have some experience in handling certain species and breeds. It is essential to be familiar with the behaviour characteristics of various breeds but it is important to remember that patients in the surgery will be reacting under stressful conditions, encountering unfamiliar people and environments, as well as perhaps being in pain, and they may not exhibit their normal behaviour.

Each procedure requires a differing degree and type of restraint. The nurse should be able to assess the situation and act accordingly. As a rule the *minimum effective restraint* should be applied, to avoid excessive discomfort for the patient whilst bearing in mind the safety of all personnel.

Restraint at the Practice

Restraint of a patient's activity—by verbal, physical and pharmacological means—is necessary so that the animal is prevented from injuring itself or others. This chapter gives guidance on restraint of dogs and cats; Chapter 3 (First Aid) considers the problems of approaching, handling and controlling patients at the scene of an emergency; and Chapter 4 (Exotic Pets and Wildlife) describes the handling of species other than dogs and cats, including wildlife.

Indications for Restraint

- To allow diagnostic procedures to be carried out, e.g. physical examination, urinary catheterisation, venepuncture.
- To allow therapeutic procedures to be carried out, e.g. administration of oral, parenteral and topical preparations and the application of bandages.
- To prevent self-inflicted injury, e.g. attempting to scramble off an examination table because of fear.

Approach to Restraint

- Quickly assess the patient, bearing in mind the conditions it may be experiencing.
- Ask the client to describe the patient's normal behaviour.
- Assess whether the client will be of help or a hindrance in assisting with restraining their pet.

With non-emergency examination, always take time to gain the confidence of both the animal and its owner. Always approach a patient quietly but confidently. Use its name and talk in a reassuring tone of voice. Lowering yourself to the patient's level is often less threatening than towering over it. A few animals may be naturally gregarious and trusting, requiring little in the way of preliminary introductions, but do not assume this.

The patient's 'body language' response will show whether it has accepted a friendly approach (Fig. 1.1). If a dog relaxes, sniffs your hand and wags its tail, this favourable response indicates that restraint may be carried out. If the response to the initial

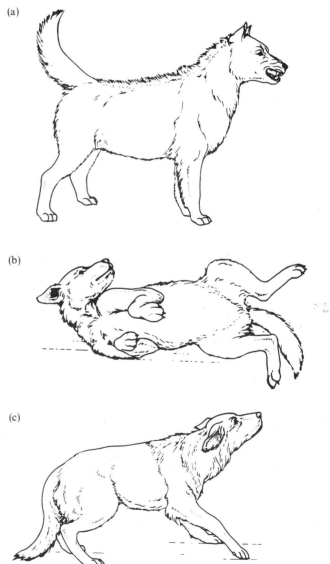

(a)

(b)

(c)

Fig. 1.1. The body language of a dog: (a) dominant, with hackles raised and teeth displayed; (b) submissive posture; (c) fearful and potentially aggressive, tail tucked in and avoiding eye contact.

approach is unfavourable, consider the options carefully. For example, the behaviour of some patients improves once the owner is out of sight. On the other hand, caution should always be exercised: often a patient reacts quite favourably for an initial examination with the owner present but becomes difficult when placed in a kennel or run.

A confident approach is required for cats allowing plenty of time to reassure the patient and make friends with it. Cats are often more apprehensive than dogs with strange people and in strange surroundings. Speak quietly to the cat and stroke it gently if it is approachable. If this friendly gesture is accepted, the cat can be lifted gently from its basket (Fig. 1.2). Cats should be handled with minimal restraint. It is not necessary to scruff a cat unless it is obviously aggressive or difficult.

Difficult or Aggressive Patients

Difficult or aggressive animals present a challenge for the nurse. As the safety of all personnel is of the utmost importance, and 'no chances' should be taken, which may allow the patient the opportunity to bite or escape. Once the nurse has decided that a patient will obviously not respond to gentle/firm handling, other measures must be adopted.

Transporting, Carrying and Lifting

Safety is of the utmost importance at all times during transport, in order to:

- prevent injury to patient and personnel;
- avoid making an injury worse;
- prevent a driving accident on the road;
- prevent escape.

Explain to owners who bring in cats and small dogs that the pet will feel more secure in closed quarters, e.g. a box or cage carrier. Cats are often quieter if the cage is covered with a blanket. The container must be a secure one and its use will also prevent altercations between pets in the waiting room and help to calm nervous cats while they wait to be examined.

WARNING

A cat that has been sedated or is recovering from anaesthesia should never be placed in a small enclosed carrier, in case its neck 'kinks' and thus obstructs the airway, causing asphyxiation, or there is unobserved fatal haemorrhaging.

Carrying Cats

Within the surgery, do not carry a cat from room to room in your arms as it may become frightened and bolt. If the cat is not particularly nervous, it should be carried with its hindquarters placed under the holder's elbow area and pressed securely to the holder's body with the forearm (Fig. 1.3). The cat should lie in a sternal position along the forearm, with its forelimbs secured by the hand and with one finger between them. In such a position the cat can

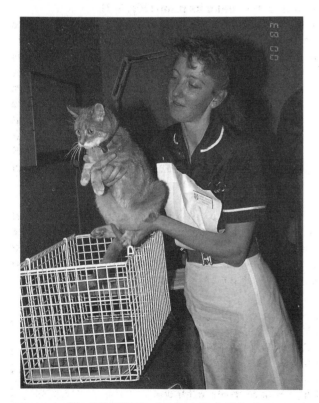

Fig. 1.2. Lifting a cat from its basket.

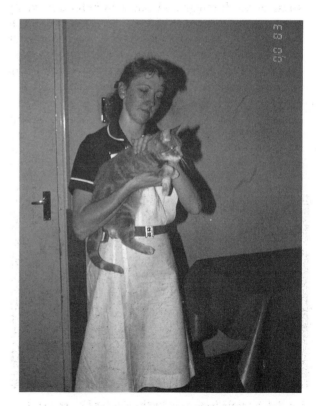

Fig. 1.3. Carrying a cat.

still use its hindlegs to injure the holder. Be prepared to hold the scruff of the cat's neck should it panic and become wild. As a last resort most cats can effectively be immobilised if they are held by the scruff and the hindlegs are grasped and extended (Fig. 1.4).

Carrying dogs

When carrying dogs (Fig. 1.5) or taking them from the owner, make sure that they are wearing a secure collar and lead or a **slip lead** and that the head cannot slip free from it. Slip leads must be fitted correctly; the principle is similar to the correct application of check chains (see Fig. 10.2).

Anaesthetised, recumbent or large dogs may be transported on trolleys or stretchers. They should always wear an identity collar, with a lead attached as an additional means of restraint. Make sure that there are sufficient personnel to prevent a patient from jumping off the trolley and escaping or injuring itself. Able-bodied patients will try to jump off and may also attempt to bite if nervous.

Lifting Dogs

Dogs are generally restrained for examination on non-slip tabletops. Care must be taken to avoid causing or aggravating pain or injury whilst the animal is lifted on to the table.

- **Small or medium-sized dogs** can be lifted by one person. Put one arm around the dog's neck in front of the forelegs and one arm behind its rump or under its abdomen. Then pull the arms towards the chest (Fig. 1.6). The arm around its neck should secure the dog's head so that it cannot turn and bite. If the dog is known to be aggressive or nervous, a muzzle should be applied before lifting.
- **Large dogs** can be very difficult to lift. Many are unaccustomed to being lifted, and may panic and struggle. Two people together can lift a dog: one places an arm around the animal's neck and under

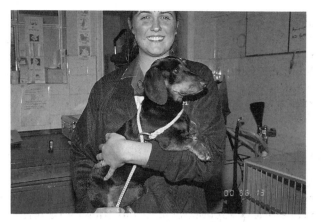

Fig. 1.5. Carrying a small or medium-sized dog.

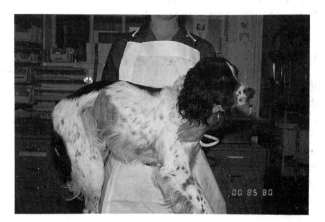

Fig. 1.6. Lifting a small or medium-sized dog.

its chest, while the other places an arm under its abdomen and under its rump (Fig. 1.7).
- **Giant breeds** are probably best examined on the floor in the abscence of a hydraulic lift.
- **Injured or sick animals** may pose more problems in lifting and more personnel may be needed. For example, it may be necessary to provide support for fractured limbs, or to avoid applying pressure to a painful abdomen. Lifting an injured patient requires skilled nursing assessment of the situation. The movement of animals with suspected fractures, especially of the spine, is described in Chapter 3 (First Aid).

The degree of restraint required whilst the animal is on the examination table depends on the procedure being carried out. It is always essential to restraint the forelimbs and hindlimbs at all times to prevent the dog from jumping or falling off.

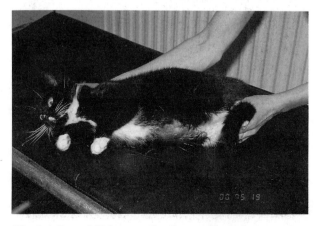

Fig. 1.4. Immobilising a cat by the scruff as a last resort.

> WARNING
> *Never* allow a dog to jump down from a tabletop, in case it slips and injures itself. A dog should be lifted down from the table, using the same method as was used to place it there.

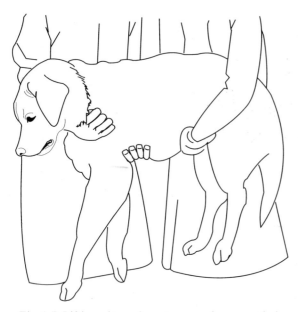

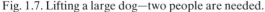

Fig. 1.7. Lifting a large dog—two people are needed.

Dogs

There are various techniques for handling aggressive dogs. If the dog is more manageable in the presence of its owner, then this should be used to advantage to prevent the situation becoming worse.

Muzzles

A capable owner can apply and secure a well-fitting nylon or box muzzle, or can be trusted to hold the dog while a muzzle is applied. Once muzzled and on a secure collar and lead, the dog can be restrained for examination or procedures.

> WARNING
> Because of the risk of vomiting or asphyxiation, a muzzled dog should never be left unattended.

A tape muzzle should be prepared in advance to minimise the time the nurse's hands need to be in close contact with the dog's mouth. To restrain the dog's head for muzzling, stand behind and astride the dog (if possible) and hold the scruff on either side of the ears (Fig. 1.8). Alternatively, loop the dog's lead through a ring attached to the wall and pull so that the dog is flattened against the wall.

Commercially produced muzzles (Fig. 1.9) are made in a variety of materials but can be difficult to adjust, so that a range of sizes is required. It is dangerous to use a poorly made or loosely applied muzzle which can easily be removed or broken by the dog.

A simple tape muzzle can be created from a length of 3/4 in (2 cm) wide cotton tape or gauze bandage, cut to a length of approximately 125 cm for a dog weighing 20–25 kg. Before approaching the dog,

form a loop as if beginning to tie a loose square knot (Fig. 1.10). Slip this loop over the dog's nose with th knot uppermost and quickly pull at the free ends to restrict the muzzle. Cross the free ends under the lower jaw to prevent slipping, then bring them under the dog's ears to the back of the head and tie them there in a quick-release bow (which must always be used, to allow for fast release in case the dog is asphyxiated or vomits).

It is difficult, or even impossible, to muzzle brachycephalic breeds (e.g. boxers). They should never be restrained by the scruff of the neck, as the eyes may prolapse. A useful method of restraint for a small brachycephalic breed is to wrap a rolled-up towel or blanket around the animal's neck, which prevents the dog from turning around to bite.

Dog-catchers

In the case of very aggressive dogs, or vicious patients which have decided to guard their kennel, it is usually necessary to lasso them with a slip lead or a dog-catcher to keep the head out of reach whilst a muzzle is applied or an injection administered.

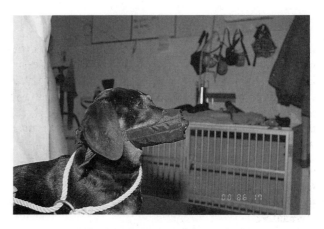

Fig. 1.8. Holding a dog for muzzling.

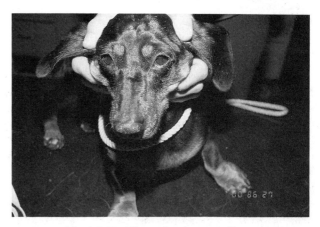

Fig. 1.9. A commercial muzzle.

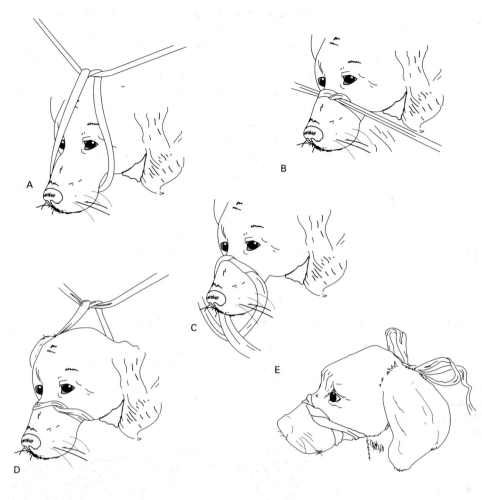

Fig. 1.10. Making a tape muzzle.

The dog-catcher (Fig. 1.11) is an implement with an adjustable loop of cable at the far end which is slipped over the dog's head. The cable passes through an aluminium handle that enables the handler to keep at a distance from the dog and to draw the loop manually so that the dog is captured. The loop can be locked in position by a single twist action. There is a small fixed loop at the handler's end of the tube and this can be hitched over a hook or other firm object so that the tool becomes a tether while a muzzle is applied. To avoid causing excess distress or choking the patient, the catcher should be removed once the muzzle has been applied.

Cats

In general, cats can be restrained as small dogs, but difficult or aggressive cats pose greater problems because not only do they bite but they also use their claws to their advantage. Chemical restraint is usually necessary with aggressive cats, as they only give one chance for physical restraint. The following techniques may help:

- Scruff and secure in a shoe bag.
- Roll in a towel (Fig. 1.12).
- Press down with a blanket in a box to administer a sedative.
- Use gauntlets.

Special equipment (Fig. 1.13) may be required in handling aggressive or feral cats:

- **Crush cages** allow for easy intramuscular injection or treatment of frightened or fractious cats (and toy breeds of dog). The moveable internal wall is eased across gently to hold the patient against the side of the cage, allowing injection between the bars or mesh.
- **Cat restraining bags** are zipped up around the cat's body so that only its head protrudes. A limb can be examined by unzipping a leg-hole so that the limb protrudes.
- **Cat muzzles** made of nylon fabric and secured on the cat by nylon webbing with quick-fit plastic catches are designed to subdue and calm the cat for treatment or grooming.
- **Cat grabbers** prevent close contact with very aggressive cats but should be used only as a last resort for seizure and restraint of feral cats in confined spaces.

Chemical Restraint

Chemical restraint (sedation) can be administered, using a suitable drug prescribed by the veterinary surgeon. Common products for the dog are acepromazine, medetomidine and xylazine. Cats can be given combinations of xylazine and ketamine, or midazolam and ketamine.

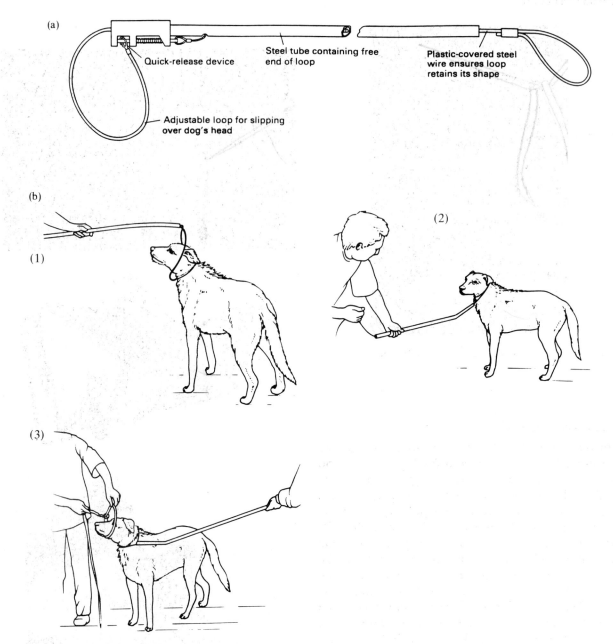

Fig. 1.11. The dog-catcher: (a) details of the catcher; (b) the catcher in use for a very aggressive animal.

Restraint for Various Procedures

Cats

Figures 1.14 to 1.21 give examples of restraint techniques for a variety of procedures. Particular attention should be paid to the positioning of the patient and the nurse's hands.

Dogs

Standing position

Place one arm under the dog's neck with the forearm securely holding the dog's head, this should be positioned so that it is virtually impossible for the animal to turn around and bite either the person restraining it or the person performing the procedure. The other arm should be placed underneath the dog's abdomen to prevent it from sitting down during the procedure and to keep the dog close to the holder's chest, limiting the dog's movement.

Sitting position

Place one arm under the dog's neck so that the forearm restrains the dog's head securely (Fig. 1.22). The other arm should be around the dog's hind-quarters to prevent it from standing up or lying down. The dog must be kept close to the holder's chest to limit movement.

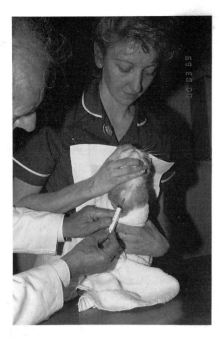

Fig. 1.12. Restraining a cat in a towel.

(a)

(b)

(c)

(d)

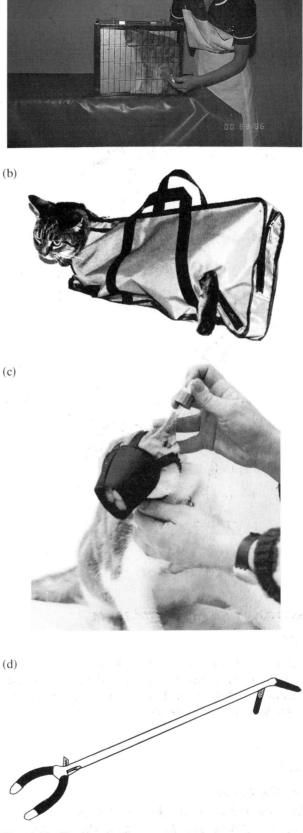

Lateral recumbency

With the dog in the standing position, reach across its back and take hold of both forelegs in one hand and both hindlegs in the other (Fig. 1.23). (Large breeds will required two people—one person holds the forelegs and the other the hindlegs.) Gradually lift the dog's legs off the table or floor and allow its body to slide gently and slowly against the restrainer's body into lateral recumbency. Use the forearm to restrain the dog's head by exerting pressure on the side of its neck to immobilise its head. The index finger of each hand should be placed between its two legs to ensure a good grip in case the dog tries to move. If possible, hold the dog's legs proximal to the carpus and tarsus for better restraint.

Restraint and positioning for venepuncture

Venepuncture for either blood sampling or administration requires secure restraint. The animal must not be allowed to move, as this is the commonest cause of haematomas which are both painful and unsightly. Hold the dog's elbow in the palm of the right hand and pass the thumb over its radius to compress the vein. Once the needle or canula has entered the vein, release pressure on the vein but still hold the leg securely to prevent movement. The position for collection from the **jugular vein** is shown in Fig. 1.24, and for **cephalic** collection in Fig. 1.25.

Further Reading

Anderson, R. S. and Edney, A. T. B. (1991) *Practical Animal Handling*. Pergamon, Oxford.

Fig. 1.13. Equipment for restraint of aggressive or feral cats: (a) crush cage; (b) restraining bag; (c) cat-calming muzzle; (d) cat-grabber.

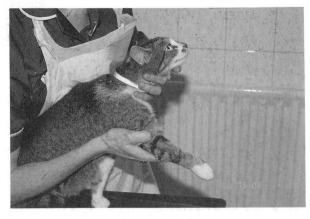

Fig. 1.14. Restraint for cephalic venepuncture.

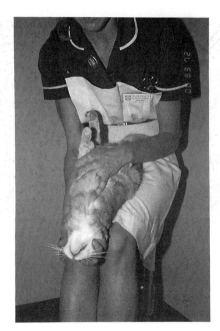

Fig. 1.17. Dorsal recumbency for jugular collection.

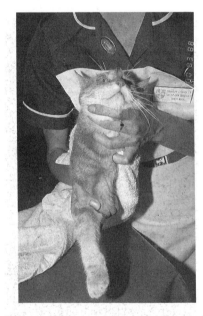

Fig. 1.15. Restraint in a towel for cephalic vein injection or blood sampling.

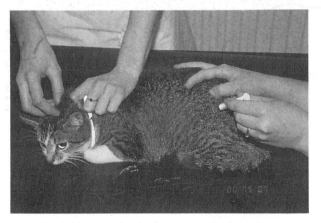

Fig. 1.18. Restraint for intramuscular injection.

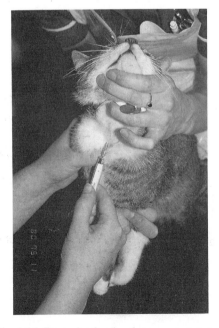

Fig. 1.16. Restraint for jugular venepuncture.

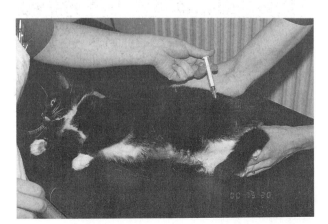

Fig. 1.19. 'Scruffing' restraint for intramuscular injection.

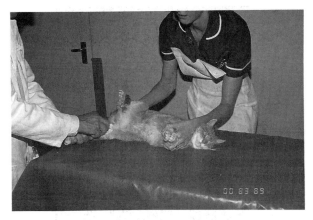

Fig. 1.20. Restraint for femoral injection.

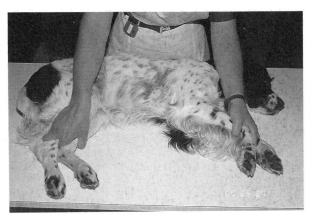

Fig. 1.23. Restraint in lateral recumbency.

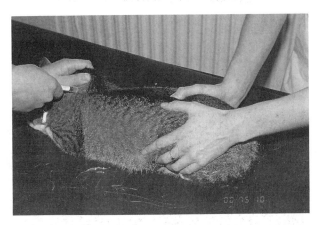

Fig. 1.21. Subcutaneous injection.

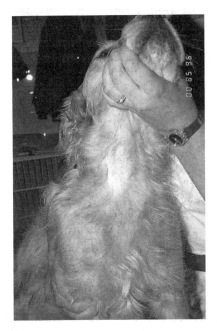

Fig. 1.24. Restraint for collection from the jugular vein.

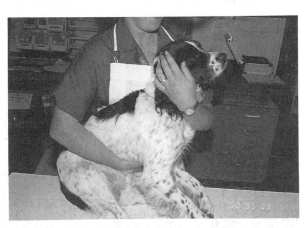

Fig. 1.22. Restraint in sitting position.

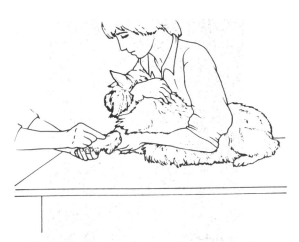

Fig. 1.25. Restraint for cephalic vein collection.

2
Observation and Care of the Patient

J. S. SEYMOUR

Observation

During the course of the working day the veterinary nurse will come into contact with a range of patients. They will have to deal with healthy animals of many species and temperaments and care for in-patients whose needs will vary from basic tender loving care to intensive treatment and nursing procedures. They must recognise the normal and abnormal appearance and behaviour patterns of those in their care and report all relevant information to the veterinary surgeon. The nurse's observations can give valuable input to the case history of the patient and may assist the veterinary surgeon's diagnosis and treatment. All observations should be noted and any abnormalities reported immediately.

Dogs and Cats in the Hospital Environment

It should be remembered that each patient is different. What would be considered normal for one patient may be abnormal for another. It is necessary, therefore, to become familiar with each animal and to recognise its normal appearance and behavioural patterns.

The veterinary hospital is not a normal environment for dogs or cats. They are surrounded by unfamiliar faces, smells and sounds and therefore may behave in an abnormal fashion. Normally placid animals may become nervous and exhibit signs of aggression or submission.

Fear and anxiety are not conducive to a smooth and speedy recovery. The veterinary nurse should do everything possible to alleviate stress in the hospitalised patient. The following are guidelines for stress reduction:

- Wherever possible, avoid placing animals in cages where they can see and be seen by other patients. If necessary, cover the cage with a blanket, but ensure that regular observation of the patient is maintained.
- Direct eye contact may be perceived by a dog as a challenging gesture and one that demands an aggressive response. It should be avoided.
- Noise levels should be kept to a minimum and any sudden loud noises should be avoided. Barking dogs should be isolated if practical and returned home as soon as possible.
- Ample provision should be made for urination and defecation. Animals easily become agitated if this

is not allowed and are often mortified if they soil their kennel. Outdoor cats confined to cages may be reluctant to use a litter tray and therefore become constipated.
- Male dogs can become extremely agitated if kennelled in close proximity to a bitch in season. It is therefore inadvisable to admit bitches in-oestrus to the veterinary hospital unless absolutely necessary.
- Ideally, each patient should be monitored and cared for by a specific nurse. This will provide continuity and allow mutual trust to develop.

Normal Appearance of the Dog and Cat

A normal, healthy dog or cat will exhibit the following signs:

- Keen reflexes with sharp reaction to stimuli.
- Clear, bright eyes that are free of discharge.
- Clear nasal orifices with no discharge.
- Clean and odour-free ears.
- Glossy coat with skin that is supple and free from wounds and parasites.
- Suitable weight for breed and size with no signs of obesity or muscle wastage.
- Free limb movement with no signs of stiffness or pain.
- Temperature, pulse and respiration within the normal range (although these may increase slightly under the stress of hospital conditions).
- Pink mucous membranes with a capillary refill time of 1–2 seconds (Fig. 2.1).
- Clear, yellow urine passed without pain or difficulty.
- Firm, brown faeces passed freely without undue straining or pain.
- Interest shown in food, if offered, with an ability to eat and drink comfortably.

Abnormal Appearance of the Dog and Cat

Any abnormality, however minor, will be significant to the case history of the patient and therefore to the veterinary surgeon in charge. It is vital that all abnormal signs are reported by the veterinary nurse as soon as possible. It is recommended that hospital charts are utilised for all patients and that vital signs are monitored and recorded routinely.

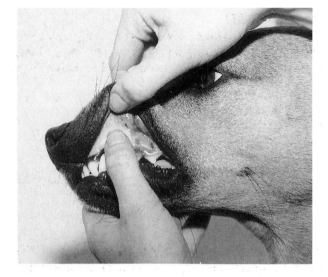

Fig. 2.1. Assessing capillary refill time by applying pressure to the mucous membranes of the gum. Photograph courtesy of Roy Hancocks and Rachel Meredith.

Abnormal Signs and their Possible Significance

Appetite changes

Many animals, especially cats, have a normal capricious appetite. However, alterations in feeding patterns may occur in the hospital as a result of a change in environment or diet.

Loss of appetite is often the first sign that an animal is unwell. This may be due to a number of factors, including:

- Mouth ulcers.
- Nasal congestion, causing impaired olfactory function.
- Infectious diseases and pyrexia.
- Metabolic diseases.

Voracious appetite with subsequent loss of weight and condition may be a symptom of pancreatic insufficiency or worms. **Pica** (craving for unnatural foodstuffs) may occur as a result of dietary imbalance, but is often merely an undesirable habit. **Coprophagia** (the eating of faeces) is an example of this condition.

Changes in urination patterns

Polyurea (increased urine production) and **polydipsia** (increased thirst) are symptoms of many diseases, including:

- Nephritis.
- Diabetes mellitus.
- Diabetes insipidus.
- Pyometra.

Dysuria (difficulty in passing urine), **anuria** (total inability to pass urine) and **haematuria** (presence of blood in the urine) are potentially emergency situations. They may be caused by:

- Cystic calculi.
- Feline urological syndrome.
- Prostatic enlargement.

All changes in urination patterns should be monitored, and water intake and urine output accurately measured. (The normal urine output for a dog is 2ml/kg/hour.) The colour, smell and consistency of the urine passed should be assessed and reported.

Unless otherwise instructed by the veterinary surgeon, clean, fresh water should be available to patients at all times.

Changes in defecation patterns

Constipation (the failure to evacuate faeces which may cause straining) may be caused by a number of factors, including:

- Ingestion of foreign material such as bones or fur balls.
- Tumours in the rectum or colon.
- Environmental factors such as soiled litter trays or confinement.
- Enlargement of the prostate gland.
- Dehydration.
- Key–Gaskell syndrome in cats.

Diarrhoea (the frequent evacuation of watery faeces from the bowel) may be caused by:

- Canine parvovirus.
- Bacterial infections.
- Distemper.
- Feline panleukopenia.
- Colitis.
- Tumours of the intestine.
- Intussusception.
- Endoparasites.
- Unsuitable diet.
- Ingestion of placental membranes by post-parturient bitch.

The volume and frequency of faecal material passed should be monitored and recorded. The faeces should be assessed for colour, smell and texture and examined for the presence of blood, mucus or parasitic worms. Microscopic examination may also be carried out.

Vomiting

This is the emission from the mouth of stomach contents and may be caused by:

- Ingestion of foreign material such as poisons, decaying food or small prey.
- Viral infections (hepatitis, canine parvovirus, feline panleukopenia, feline infectious peritonitis).
- Diabetes mellitus.

- Nephritis.
- Pancreatitis.
- Pyometra.
- Foreign body in digestive tract such as plastic, balls or stones.
- Endoparasites.

The volume and frequency of vomitus should be monitored and recorded and the specimen examined for blood, mucus or evidence of poisons. The incidence of vomiting related to feeding patterns is of great relevance and should be monitored, with recording of the times that sickness occurs.

The veterinary nurse should be able to recognise the various types of vomiting that may be seen in the cat and dog. These include:

- **Projectile vomit**—forceful vomiting of stomach contents, usually without retching.
- **Regurgitation**—the backflow of food from the oesophagus.
- **Stercoraceous vomit**—vomit containing faeces.
- **Haematemesis**—vomit containing blood.
- **Bilious vomit**—vomit containing bile.
- **Cyclic vomiting**—recurring acts of vomiting.
- **Retching**—ineffectual attempts to vomit. (This may be confused with coughing, especially in cats.)

Nasal discharge

This is commonly accompanied by sneezing and may be caused by:

- Foreign bodies such as grass seeds, tumours or polyps.
- Distemper.
- Feline calicivirus.
- Feline viral rhinotracheitis.

The nasal passages should be examined for any evidence of foreign bodies and the discharge examined for presence of blood or pus. Patients, especially cats, may be reluctant to eat when their nasal passages are congested, because the olfactory function is diminished.

Aural discharge

This is most commonly seen in long-eared breeds such as the spaniel and is often accompanied by vigorous head shaking and frantic scratching of the ears. It may be caused by:

- Foreign bodies such as grass seeds.
- Ear mites.
- Infection.

The ears should be examined for evidence of any obvious foreign body. The use of an auroscope may be required.

Ocular discharge

This can cause considerable distress to a patient and signs such as pawing at the face and rubbing the head against the floor may be seen. This may be a symptom of:

- Distemper.
- Feline upper respiratory tract infection.
- Foreign body such as grass seed.
- Abnormal eyelid or eyelash structure.

The eyes should be examined carefully, taking care not to touch the surface of the cornea.

Vaginal discharge

This is associated with the reproductive cycle of the bitch or queen and may be normal or abnormal. Indications include:

- **Pro-oestrus**—blood-red discharge.
- **Oestrus**—straw-coloured discharge.
- **Imminent parturition**—dark green discharge.
- **Metritis**—brown/black discharge.
- **Abortion**—foul-smelling, black discharge.
- **Pyometra**—purulent discharge, often green or pale coffee colour.

An accurate history should be obtained to help to establish the cause of the discharge and to ensure that the correct course of action is taken.

Coughing

This may be heard in the hospitalised patient and may vary from a dry, harsh cough to one that is fluid and productive. Coughing may be caused by:

- Congestive heart failure.
- Roundworm infestation in young animals.
- Kennel cough.
- Bronchitis.
- Distemper.
- Inhalation of chemicals and irritant gases.

Any method of restraint that may aggravate the situation should be avoided.

Changes in colour of mucous membranes

The colour of mucous membranes is a good indication of the health of an animal and will sometimes indicate the need for emergency action:

- **Pale**—may indicate haemorrhage, anaemia or circulatory collapse.
- **Blue-tinged (cyanosis)**—may indicate respiratory obstruction.
- **Yellow (icterus)**—may indicate liver disease or leptospirosis.

Restlessness

Any animal that appears to be unduly restless should be examined to establish the cause and steps that should be taken if possible to alleviate its distress. Signs of restlessness include:

- Panting.
- Whining.
- Pacing.
- Scratching at bedding.
- Barking.
- Inability to settle.

These signs may be caused by:

- Pain or discomfort.
- Excess heat or cold.
- Need to urinate or defecate.
- Hunger or thirst.
- Loneliness or boredom.
- Dressings too tight.

Temperature, Pulse and Respiration

These vital signs should be monitored routinely in every hospitalised patient. The normal range of vital signs in the dog and cat are shown in Fig. 2.2.

Temperature

Thermometers

The most common type of clinical thermometer is the veterinary **mercury thermometer**. This consists of a graduated glass tube with a stubby bulb at one end containing mercury. When the temperature rises, the mercury expands so that it travels along the tube. The thermometer has a kink in the bulb end which prevents the backflow of mercury when it is removed from the animal. This allows an accurate reading of body temperature.

The thermometer may be calibrated in degrees Celsius or Fahrenheit. Although the veterinary nurse should be familiar with both readings, degrees Celsius is now the standard unit for measurement of temperature. A Fahrenheit reading may be converted to Celsius by use of the formula:

$$°C = (°F - 32) \times 5/9$$

The **electronic thermometer** is designed for rectal or oesophageal use and allows continual monitoring of body temperature. The temperature may be read from a digital readout. The **subclinical thermometer**

may be used to record subnormal temperatures in the critically ill patient.

Care and storage of the mercury thermometer

The mercury thermometer should be stored in a glass jar with a pad of cotton wool at the bottom. The jar should be filled with antiseptic solution. Both the cotton wool and the antiseptic should be changed daily. The thermometer should be cleaned with cool water and antiseptic. Hot water should not be used as it would cause the mercury to expand and the glass to break.

Thermometers should not be shared between infectious and non-infectious patients.

Procedure for taking the temperature using the mercury thermometer

It is usual to take the temperature of an animal via the rectal route.

(1) The patient should restrained by an assistant.
(2) Shake down the thermometer to ensure that the mercury returns to the bulb. (To avoid the possibility of breakage, this should never be done near hard surfaces.)
(3) Lubricate the stubby bulb end of the thermometer with vaseline, KY jelly, soap or oil.
(4) Gently insert the thermometer into the patient's rectum with a twisting motion. The anal sphincter of the dog will relax easily but slightly more pressure will be required to relax a cat's inner sphincter muscle. The thermometer should be directed against the upper surface of the rectum to avoid insertion into the faecal mass.
(5) Hold the thermometer in the rectum for the stated time (30 seconds to 1 minute).
(6) Then gently remove the thermometer and wipe it clean with cotton wool. Avoid touching the bulb.
(7) Hold the thermometer horizontally and rotate it until the mercury level is visible.
(8) Read and record the temperature.
(9) Report any abnormalities to the veterinary surgeon.

Pyrexia (high body temperature) may be caused by:

- Infection.
- Heat stroke.
- Convulsions.
- Pain.
- Excitement.

Low body temperature may be caused by:

- Shock.
- Circulatory collapse.
- Impending parturition.

NORMAL RANGE OF VITAL SIGNS IN THE CAT AND DOG		
	Dog	**Cat**
Temperature	38.3 – 38.7°C (100.9 – 101.7°F)	38.0 – 38.5°C (100.4 – 101.6°F)
Pulse	60 – 180 beats per minute (depending on size of dog)	110 – 180 beats per minute
Respiration	10 – 30 breaths per minute	20 – 30 breaths per minute

Fig. 2.2. Normal range of vital signs in the dog and cat.

Fluctuating temperature is known as diphasic and it may be one symptom of canine distemper.

Pulse

The pulse rate of an animal can be palpated at any point where an artery runs close to the body surface. Each pulsation corresponds with the contraction of the left ventricle of the heart. In the dog and cat, suitable sites include:

- The femoral artery, on the medial aspect of the femur (Fig. 2.3).
- The digital artery, on the palmar aspect of the carpus.
- The coccygeal artery, on the ventral aspect of the base of the tail.
- The lingual artery, on the underside of the tongue (in anaesthetised patients).

Procedure for pulse-taking

(1) The patient should be restrained by an assistant.
(2) Locate the artery with the fingers.
(3) Count the pulsations for exactly one minute. (With very rapid pulse rates, a shorter period may be all that is possible.)
(4) Record the rate.

Although the rate of pulse is important, the character of the pulse should also be assessed. In a normal patient, the pulse rate increases on inspiration and decreases on expiration, and this variation is known as **sinus arrhythmia**.

A pulse rate that is lower than a corresponding heart rate is known as a **pulse deficit** and is indicative of **dysrhythmia**.

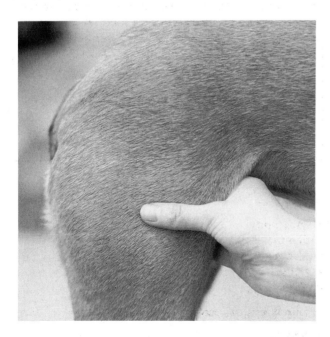

Fig. 2.3. Taking the pulse, using the femoral artery. Photograph courtesy of Roy Hancocks and Rachel Meredith.

Possible causes of abnormal pulse rates

Raised:
- Fever.
- Exercise.
- Hypoxia.
- Pain.
- Fear.

Lowered:
- Unconsciousness.
- Anaesthesia.
- Debilitating disease.
- Sleep.

Weak:
- Shock.
- Diminished cardiac output.

Strong and jerky ('water hammer' pulse):
- Valvular insufficiency.
- Congenital heart defects such as patent ductus arteriosis.

Respiration

The rhythm and rate of respiration can be assessed by careful observation of the patient or by gently resting the hands on either side of the chest cavity. The respiratory rate should be taken when the patient is at rest but not sleeping or panting. Count *either* inspirations *or* expirations, for exactly one minute. Also assess the depth of respiration, which indicates the volume of air inspired with each breath.

Possible causes of abnormal respiration

Tachypnoea (increased respiratory rate):
- Heat.
- Exercise.
- Pain.
- Poisons.

Bradypnoea (decreased respiratory rate):
- Poisons (narcotic or hypnotic).
- Metabolic alkalosis.
- Sleep.

Dyspnoea (difficult breathing):
(1) Inspiratory dyspnoea:
  - Obstruction or stenosis of the respiratory tract.
(2) Expiratory dyspnoea:
  - Bronchitis and emphysema of the lungs.
  - Pleural adhesions.
(3) Mixed dyspnoea:
  - Pneumonia.
  - Pneumothorax.
  - Hydrothorax.
  - Pyothorax.

Cheyne–Stokes respiration often occurs shortly before death and is characterised by alternating periods of deep, rapid and shallow breathing followed by **apnoea** (cessation of breathing).

General Care of the Patient

The specific needs of hospitalised patients obviously depend on their condition. However, all patients have a basic requirement for nutrition, warmth, comfort, hygiene and mental stimulation.

Nutrition

Correct nutrition is of vital importance to the hospitalised patient. A palatable, high-energy diet is required to support the animal during its recovery.

Easily digested foods such as scrambled eggs and chicken may be offered to the inappetent patient. Alternatively, a wide range of commercial diets is available. Strong-smelling foods such as pilchards or meat extract are useful in encouraging animals (especially cats) to eat.

All food should be warmed to blood temperature before feeding. Meals should be fed little and often and any food not eaten after 15 minutes should be removed.

There are various ways of ensuring that hospitalised patients receive sufficient nutrients. These include:

- Placing food on nose and paws of patient.
- Spoon-feeding.
- Syringe-feeding.
- Orogastric tubing.
- Nasogastric tubing.
- Pharyngostomy tubing.

Warmth

It is important that all patients are kept warm and free from draughts. The temperature of the hospital ward should be kept constant with adequate ventilation. Additional warmth may be provided by several means:

- **Blankets and towels** are readily available and often used in the veterinary hospital, but care should be taken that they do not become soaked with urine, which could lead to urine scalds in a recumbent or weakly patient.
- **Vetbeds** are ideal for use in the ward. They are comfortable, warm and easily washed. Their main advantage is that the base of the vetbed absorbs any fluid, thereby ensuring that the patient remains dry.
- **Heat lamps** should be used with great care. Animals that are unable to move can easily become overheated and possibly burnt if a lamp is used injudiciously. It should be no closer to the patient than 61cm (24in) from the patient and constant observation should be maintained.
- **Hot water-bottles** are a good source of heat for weakly patients, although there are certain disadvantages. The bottles require refilling at regular intervals and should always be covered with a towel or blanket. It is possible that the stopper may become loose or that patients may chew the rubber, and scalding may occur as a result. Boiling water should never be used.
- **Heated pads** are useful, but again must be used with care. They should be covered with a towel and the patient checked and turned at regular intervals. Animals with a tendency to chew should not be allowed heated pads, because chewing the flex could lead to electrocution.
- **Incubators** are ideal for smaller critical patients and for newborn puppies and kittens. The environment can be automatically maintained at the desired temperature. Newborn animals are **poikilothermic** (body temperature varies with ambient temperature) and therefore a constant temperature of 30–33°C should be maintained for these patients.

Comfort

The patient should be provided with adequate bedding materials. It should be allowed to assume a position that it finds comfortable. Fractured limbs, open wounds and dressings should be kept uppermost. Familiar bedding brought in by the owner may provide extra comfort and security.

Recumbent animals should be provided with extra padding, such as foam wedges, to prevent the occurrence of decubitus ulcers. Bony prominences such as the hock, elbow and sternum should be especially protected and the application of a bandage or vaseline to these areas may be beneficial. The recumbent patient should be turned regularly every 2–4 hours.

Hygiene

A high standard of hygiene must be maintained on the hospital ward. All faeces, urine, vomit and discharge should be removed from the kennel immediately and the patient cleaned thoroughly. Uneaten food should not be left in the kennel as it will be unpleasant for the patient and may attract flies in hot weather.

The patient's mouth, eyes and nose should be kept free from discharge by wiping with damp cotton wool.

Mental Stimulation

It is important to maintain the morale of the hospitalised patient. This can be achieved by talking, fussing and stroking with constant use of the animal's name. It should, however, be allowed periods when it can sleep and rest without distraction.

- Regular daily grooming should be carried out, especially in long-haired breeds. Clipping of hair and bathing may be necessary.

- Long-stay patients may benefit from visits by the owner, although this may not be advisable in all cases as patient and owner alike may become distressed when parting.
- Toys and chews from home maybe allowed at the veterinary surgeon's discretion.
- Whenever possible, the patient should be taken outside to enjoy fresh air and a change of environment.

Transport of the Patient

Animals should be suitably restrained when they are moved to and from the hospital ward. Dogs that are able to walk should be held on leads and cats confined to a secure basket or carrier.

Anaesthetised or unconscious patients should be supported by stretcher or trolley and observed constantly for struggling, vomiting or respiratory distress. A patent airway must be maintained by extending the head and neck and pulling the tongue forwards. Body temperature of the patient must be maintained during transport and subsequent recovery.

Emesis

Emetics are used to induce vomiting in order to empty the stomach contents. This may be necessary prior to surgery or more often as a means of eliminating poisonous substances following accidental ingestion. The veterinary nurse may be required to carry out the procedure of emesis or may need to advise clients on how to give an emetic in an emergency.

WARNING
Emesis is contraindicated in cases of corrosive poisoning or for unconscious or convulsing patients.

Methods for emesis
- **Apomorphine** may be administered under veterinary direction. It may be given via the oral, subcutaneous, intramuscular or intravenous routes. It is contraindicated in cats.
- **Sodium carbonate** (washing soda crystals) may be placed on the back of the patient's tongue. Two large crystals are effective and quick in most dogs.
- **Salt** or **mustard** may be dissolved in water and administered by spoon or syringe. This method tends to be less effective.

Bandaging

The veterinary nurse should be:

- competent in carrying out routine bandaging procedures;
- familiar with the more specialised techniques;
- capable of advising the client on care and protection of the bandage;
- able to recognise the need for attention or removal of bandaging.

Reasons for bandaging

Support:
- Fractures or dislocations.
- Sprains or strains.
- Healing wounds.

Protection:
- Self-mutilation.
- Infection.
- Environment.

Pressure:
- To arrest haemorrhage.
- To prevent or control swelling.

Immobilisation
- To restrict joint movement.
- To restrict movement at fracture site.
- To provide comfort and pain relief.

Dressing Materials

Various types of dressing are available. They are applied in direct contact with the surface of the skin:

- **Dry dressings** absorb pus or fluid from the wound.
- **Impregnated gauze dressings** may be applied to wounds that need to be kept moist, e.g. burns and scalds. These dressings are petroleum or vaseline based and may be impregnated with antibiotic, corticosteroid or chlorhexidine.

Padding Materials

These provide the intermediate layer of many dressings. They cushion and support the wound, and they also provide protection to bony prominences and prevent excoriation. They may be made from natural or manmade fibres, including:

- **Cotton wool**, a natural fibre which is cheap and has good absorptive properties.
- **Soffban**, a soft, natural padding material available on rolls of varying width and thickness.
- **Foam**, a useful padding material also available on rolls.

Bandaging Materials

These are applied to protect the wound and to hold dressings in place. They include:

- **White open-weave**, a natural bandage which is strong and firm, has the disadvantage of not conforming to the patient's body and a tendency for the cotton fibres to fray.
- **Conforming bandage**, the bandage of choice for most dressings, provides a strong, neat bandage that conforms to the shape of the patient's body.
- **Cohesive bandage** has self-adhering properties but does not stick to hair or skin. It is strong, flexible and conforming.
- **Tubular bandage**, an elasticated cotton or nylon bandage applied with the use of an applicator, is particularly useful for bandaging limbs or the tail.
- **Crepe bandage**, not commonly used in veterinary practice, has the advantage of being washable and therefore may be reused. It conforms to the larger parts of the animal's body and is useful for head and thorax bandaging.

Covering Materials

These form the outer layer of the dressing and provide support and protection:

- **Zinc oxide tape**, an adhesive, inelastic, relatively non-conforming material with a tendency to fray. More commonly used as a traction tape.
- **Elastoplast**, an adhesive, elastic material which provides a neat, conforming protective layer.
- **Non-adhesive tape**, material that will adhere to itself but not to the patient.

Casting Materials

- **Fibreglass cast**, a rigid, lightweight material that provides a strong, fast setting cast.
- **Plaster of paris**, a roll of gauze impregnated with calcium sulphate dihydrate. It is applied by immersing the roll in water and winding the material around the affected part in the manner of a bandage. Once dry, it sets to a hard, supportive, conforming cast.

Common Bandaging Techniques

Limb

Limbs are frequently bandaged in veterinary practice to provide protection and support for cuts, torn dew claws and surgical procedures. Various materials may be utilised, including narrow open-weave bandage, conforming bandage and elasticated tubular gauze.

(a)
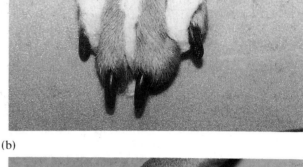

(b)
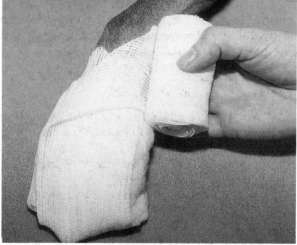

(c)
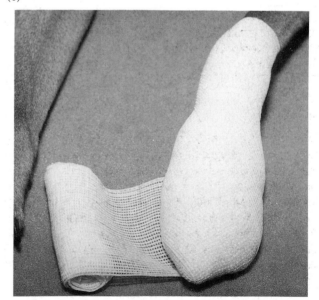

Fig. 2.4. Procedure for limb bandage: (a) padding between the toes; (b) applying the conforming bandage longitudinally; (c) winding the conforming bandage in a figure-of-eight. Photographs courtesy of Roy Hancocks and Rachel Meredith.

Standard procedure for limb bandage (Fig. 2.4)

(1) The patient is suitably restrained.
(2) In order to absorb sweat and prevent irritation, place cotton wool between the patient's toes, pads and dew claws.
(3) Apply a layer of cotton wool or soffban around the foot.
(4) Apply the conforming bandage longitudinally to the cranial and caudal surface of the limb and then turn it to wind around the limb in a figure-of-eight pattern. This ensures an even tension throughout the bandage. Anchor the bandage over the hock or carpus.
(5) Apply an external layer of adhesive tape in the same manner.

Ear

One or both ears are often bandaged following trauma, bleeding from ulcerated ear tips, or surgical procedures such as aural haematoma or resection.

Procedure for single ear (Fig. 2.5)

(1) Place a pad of cotton wool on the top of the patient's head. Fold the ear back on to the pad.
(2) Apply a dry dressing and place a further pad of cotton wool over the ear.
(3) Apply conforming bandage over the ear and then under the chin; anchor it on either side of the free ear.
(4) The bandage may be covered with adhesive tape.

It is important that the ear bandage is not applied too tightly. The patient should be able to open its mouth normally and its respiration must not be obstructed.

Abdomen

The abdomen is occasionally bandaged following trauma or surgery. Apply conforming bandage around the abdomen and secure it with adhesive tape or tubular gauze. The bandage may have to be extended forwards to the axilla to stop it 'bunching up' later. Care should be taken to prevent the bandage from rubbing on the exposed ventral surface of the abdomen—use cotton wool padding or apply vaseline.

Chest

The procedure for bandaging the abdomen also applies to the chest (Fig. 2.6). The bandage may be anchored between the front legs in figure-of-eight fashion.

(a)

(b)

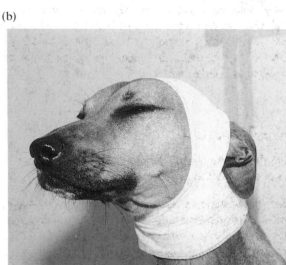

Fig. 2.5. Procedure for ear bandage: (a) padding the top of the head; (b) the conforming bandage in place. Photographs courtesy of Roy Hancocks and Rachel Meredith.

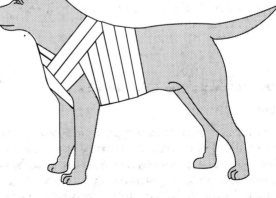

Fig. 2.6. Chest bandage.

Tail

A light bandage may be required following trauma to the tail or amputation of vertebrae. This can be one of the most difficult areas for keeping a bandage in place (Fig. 2.7).

Specialised Bandaging Techniques

The three most common special techniques are:

- **Ehmer sling**, to support the hindlimb following reduction of hip luxation.
- **Velpeau sling**, to support the shoulder joint following luxation or surgery.
- **Robert Jones bandage**, to provide support and immobilisation to fractured limbs in a first aid situation or following surgery.

Procedure for Ehmer sling (Fig. 2.8)

(1) Apply padding material to the metatarsus and stifle.
(2) Flex the leg and rotate the foot inwards. This will force the hip joint into the acetabulum.
(3) Apply conforming bandage to the metatarsus, bringing it medial to the stifle joint.
(4) Continue the bandage over the thigh and back to the metatarsus in a figure-of-eight pattern.
(5) Repeat until full support of the hip is achieved.
(6) The bandage is then held in place with adhesive tape.

This dressing is usually kept in place for 4–5 days.

Procedure for Velpeau sling (Fig. 2.9)

(1) Apply a layer of padding material to the foreleg.
(2) Apply conforming bandage to the paw.
(3) Hold the leg in flexion and apply the bandage over the elbow, then over the shoulder and round the chest.
(4) Repeat until full support of the shoulder is achieved.
(5) The dressing is then secured using adhesive tape.

Procedure for Robert Jones bandage (Fig. 2.10)

(1) Apply zinc oxide traction tapes to the dorsal and ventral surfaces of the foot.
(2) Take cotton wool from the roll and wrap it tightly around the leg and foot.
(3) Apply conforming bandage firmly to the padded leg.
(4) Incorporate the traction tapes into the bandage to prevent slipping.
(5) Cover the bandage with adhesive tape for protection and extra support.

On completion, the foot should be visible so that checks may be made for oedema and temperature. This bandage may be kept in place for up to 2 weeks. Occasionally the toes are included in the bandage.

Care of Bandages and Dressings

Once the bandage has been applied, constant checks should be maintained until it is removed. Any

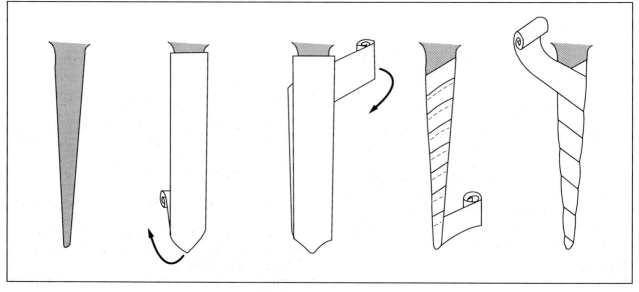

Fig. 2.7. Tail bandage.

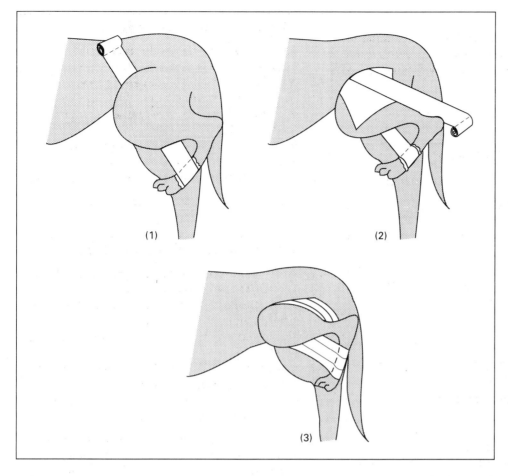

Fig. 2.8. Ehmer sling.

evidence of odour, oedema, discharge or skin irritation should be reported to the veterinary surgeon. The bandage should be checked to ensure that it is not too tight or uncomfortable.

It is important that the dressing does not become soiled or wet. This may be prevented by covering it with a plastic bag when the patient is taken outside.

Constant chewing or licking at the bandage by the patient should be discouraged. If this persists, try one of the following measures:

- Discipline.
- Elizabethan collar (Fig. 2.11).
- Muzzle.
- Application of foul-tasting substance to dressing.
- Sedation.

Local Applications of Heat and Cold

Heat may be provided by applying cotton wool soaked in hot water or by means of a poultice prepared with medicants such as kaolin. The hot application will cause vasodilation and therefore increased blood supply to the affected area. This will provide white blood cells for wound healing and assist in fluid removal from the area. The application of heat is indicated in cases of:

- Oedema.
- Infected wounds.
- Abscesses.

Cold may be provided by applying gauze soaked in cold water or an ice pack. Burns and scalds should be flushed with cold water from the tap. The cold application will cause vasoconstriction, therefore reducing heat and blood loss. The application of cold is indicated in cases of:

- Pain.
- Haemorrhage.
- Minor burns and scalds.
- Heatstroke.

Administration of Medicines

Drug classification, dosage and administration are considered in depth in Chapter 13. The following section is a short introduction to the subject.

Medicines may be administered via various routes:

- **Orally** in the form of tablets, capsules, liquids, pastes or powders.
- **Rectally** in the form of an enema or suppository.
- **Parenterally** by intravenous, subcutaneous or intramuscular injection.
- **Topically** to the skin, eyes, ears, nose or mucous membranes.

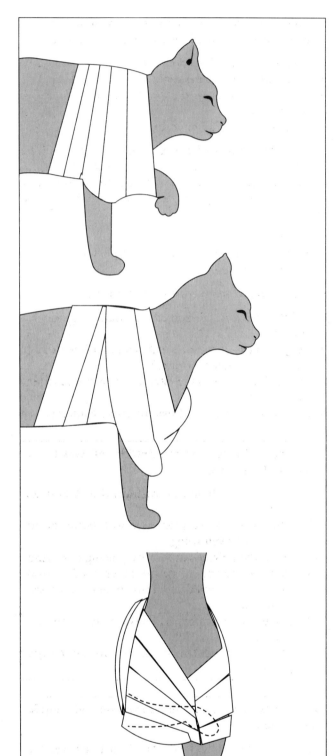

Fig. 2.9. Making a Velpeau sling.

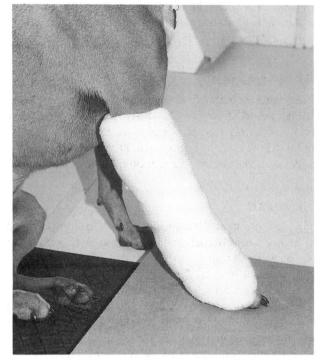

Fig. 2.10. Robert Jones bandage in place. Photograph courtesy of Roy Hancocks and Rachel Meredith.

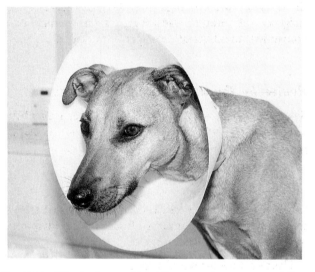

Fig. 2.11. Elizabethan collar. Photograph courtesy of Roy Hancocks and Rachel Meredith.

Choose the route that is the most appropriate for the patient and for the drug. The following factors should be considered before drugs are administered:

- Pharmacological properties.
- Rate of absorption.
- The patient.
- Convenience for the administrator.

Pharmacological properties

It is essential that the drug to be administered is compatible with the chosen route. Some drugs will not be adequately absorbed from the gastrointestinal tract if given orally, whereas others (e.g. pancreatic enzymes extract) must be given via this route as they act on the digestive system. Some drugs may be dangerous if not administered via the recommended route. If thiopentone sodium is injected subcutaneously, it causes irritation and sloughing of the skin.

Rate of absorption

The requirements for the onset of action of the administered drug should be considered. Generally an intravenous injection will have the fastest action, followed (in descending order) by intramuscular injection, subcutaneous injection and the oral route.

The patient

The condition and temperament of the patient will influence the route of drug administration. It may not be possible to administer drugs to an aggressive patient via the oral, topical or intravenous routes, and therefore an alternative route should be used. Administration of oral drugs to patients with respiratory embarrassment or mouth trauma such as a fractured jaw may cause pain or distress and should be avoided. Continued use of the same injection site may cause soreness and pain and should be minimised if possible.

Convenience for the administrator

Most clients will be able to give drugs orally to their animals and this will allow treatment to be given in the familiar surroundings of home. For the veterinary surgeon or nurse, however, it may be more convenient to administer drugs parenterally.

Routes for the Administration of Drugs

Systemic routes are those by which the drug affects the body as a whole. They include oral, rectal and parenteral routes.

Oral

Drugs are administered orally in the form of tablets, capsules, powder/granules or liquids. The advantages of oral medicines are:

- Usually the least painful route.
- Easily administered by client.
- Least risk of introduction of infection, as the skin is not penetrated.

  The disadvantages are:

- Possibility of aspiration of medication into respiratory tract, causing choking.
- Variable rate of absorption, depending on metabolic rate, age and condition of patient, motility and contents of digestive tract.
- May cause irritation or vomiting.
- Patients may not tolerate administration.
- May be difficult to ensure the correct dosage.

Tablets consist of a compressed, moulded mass of drug and may be coated for the following reasons:

- To protect them from moisture.
- To disguise an unpleasant taste.
- To protect the drug (e.g. from hydrochloric acid in the stomach).
- To give a recognisable colour.

Capsules consist of two sections, made of soluble gelatin, fitted together to enclose a powdered drug.

Powders/granules arc produced for addition to food or water. They are particularly suitable for the treatment of:

- Young animals.
- Small creatures, such as birds or hamsters.
- Digestive diseases.

Liquid medicines may be in the form of:

- **Solutions**—drugs dissolved in liquid (e.g. glucose solution).
- **Suspensions**—insoluble substance dispersed in liquid (e.g. kaolin and water).
- **Syrup/linctus**—drugs contained in a concentrated sugar solution.
- **Emulsion**—a mixture of two immiscible liquids.

Procedure for oral administration of tablets or capsules (Fig. 2.12)

(1) The patient should be restrained as gently as possible.
(2) The tablet may be lubricated with butter or oil for ease of swallowing.
(3) Open the animal's mouth by placing one hand over the muzzle, while the other hand is used to hold the tablet and also to pull down the lower jaw.
(4) Place the tablet on the base of the patient's tongue.
(5) Close the mouth and stroke the neck to ensure swallowing.

Procedure for oral administration of liquid medication

(1) The liquid should be placed in a syringe for ease of administration.
(2) The patient's head should be tilted back.
(3) Place the syringe into the side of the mouth behind the canine teeth.
(4) Slowly administer the liquid to the back of the throat.
(5) Stroke the neck to ensure swallowing.

Rectal

The rectal route is not commonly used in small animal practice, but drugs such as liquid paraffin or glycerine may be administered in the form of an enema or suppository. Details of enemata are given in Chapter 20 (General Nursing).

Parenteral

This term describes the administration of medicines via routes not involving the alimentary canal. This may be achieved using hypodermic injections given via the following routes:

- Subcutaneous.
- Intramuscular.
- Intravenous.
- Intracardiac.
- Intraperitoneal.
- Intrapleural.
- Intra-articular.
- Epidural.

The choice of route should be decided by considering the condition and temperament of the patient, the properties and volume of the drug to be administered, and the desired speed of effect. Hypodermic injections are most commonly administered via the subcutaneous, intramuscular and intravenous routes.

Subcutaneous injections. The loose skin from the back of the neck to the rump is the most common site for the administration of this injection (Fig. 2.13). This area is suitable because of its poor supply of nerves and large blood vessels. Only non-irritant drugs should be administered via this route as there may be irritation or necrosis of tissues. Action following subcutaneous injection will take effect after 30–45 minutes.

Procedure for subcutaneous injection

(1) Prepare the injection by selecting a sterile needle and syringe. Draw up the required volume of drugs.
(2) The patient should be suitably restrained.
(3) Raise a fold of skin from a suitable area.
(4) Moisten the skin with a spirit swab to flatten the hair and remove surface dirt. (Spirit should not be used when injecting a vaccine, as it may inactivate the drug.)
(5) Insert the needle under the skin and withdraw the syringe plunger slightly. If blood appears in the syringe, a blood vessel has been punctured and a new site must be selected.
(6) If no blood appears, the drug may be injected into the patient.
(7) Massage the injection site gently to disperse the drug.
(8) Make detailed records of the medication given.

Intramuscular injections. The most common site for intramuscular injections is the quadriceps group of muscles in front of the femur (Fig. 2.14). The lumbodorsal muscles and triceps muscles may also be used. The gluteal muscles of the buttocks and the hamstring muscle group should be avoided, as there is a danger of bone or sciatic nerve damage.

Because of the density of muscle tissue, large amounts of fluid may be very painful if injected via this route. The maximum administration should be 2ml in the cat and 5ml in the dog.

Action following intramuscular injection will take effect after 20–30 minutes.

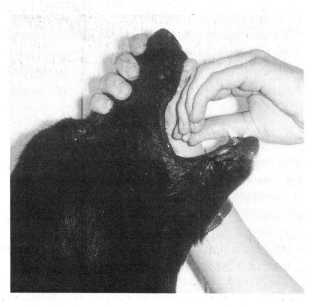

Fig. 2.12. Administration of a tablet via the oral route. Photograph courtesy of Roy Hancocks and Rachel Meredith.

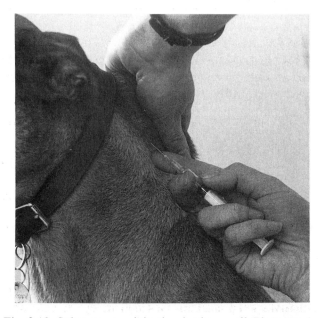

Fig. 2.13. Subcutaneous injection in the scruff. Photograph courtesy of Roy Hancocks and Rachel Meredith.

The technique is similar to that for the subcutaneous route except that the needle should be inserted at right angles into the muscle mass.

Intravenous injections. The common sites for intravenous injection are the cephalic vein in the forelimb, the lateral saphenous vein in the hindlimb and the jugular vein in the neck. The sublingual vein may be used in an anaesthetised or unconscious patient.

Action following intravenous injections will take effect in 0–2 minutes.

Procedure for a cephalic vein injection (Fig. 2.15)

(1) The patient, either sitting or in sternal recumbency, should be restrained by an assistant.
(2) The assistant should restrain the patient's head with one hand and use the other hand to extend the leg and 'raise' the vein by applying pressure around the elbow joint with the thumb.
(3) The operator should stabilise the vein and insert the needle through the skin into the vein. Blood should flow gently into the syringe.
(4) The assistant should then release the pressure on the vein and the operator may gently force the drug into the circulation. If large volumes of fluid are to be injected, regular checks should be made to ensure that the needle remains in the vein (by occasionally drawing back a little blood).
(5) Once the injection has been administered, the needle may be removed from the vein and pressure applied to the injection site for a minimum of 30 seconds, to prevent haemorrhage.

Topical

This refers to the application of medication to the external surfaces of the body, e.g. the skin, the eyes and the ears.

The skin. Skin treatment may be applied in the form of:

- **Shampoo**—a solution applied to the whole body by bathing.
- **Ointment**—drugs in a base of wax or jelly acting on the skin surface.
- **Cream**—a semi-solid emulsion which penetrates the skin surface.

The eyes. Eye medication may be applied in the form of drops or ointment. For either medium, the animal's head is tilted back and its eye is held open with the fingers. When applying any substance to the eye, the surface of the cornea should never be

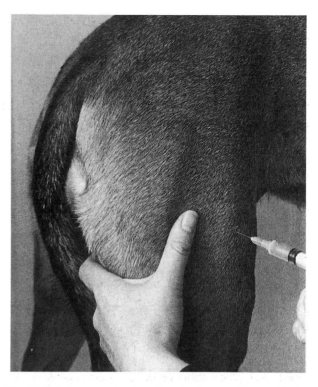

Fig. 2.14. Intramuscular injection in the quadriceps. Photograph courtesy of Roy Hancocks and Rachel Meredith.

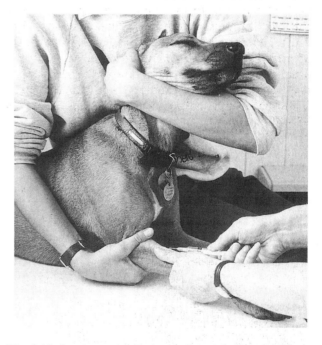

Fig. 2.15. Intravenous injection in the cephalic vein. Photograph courtesy of Roy Hancocks and Rachel Meredith.

touched by the fingers or the nozzle of the applicator.

Drops are applied by dropping liquid on to the centre of the eyeball (Fig. 2.16).

Ointment is applied by gently squeezing a line of the drug across the surface of the eye. It is often best to approach the patient from the side when using eye ointment, rather than a face-to-face confrontational approach.

After the medication has been applied, the patient should be allowed to blink to disperse the drug evenly over the eye.

The ears. Ear medication may be applied in the form of drops or ointment. The ear should be free from wax and discharge before application. The patient should be restrained and its pinna held firmly. Introduce the nozzle of the applicator into the ear canal and apply the contents gently (Fig. 2.17). Gently massage the external auditory meatus to ensure maximum coverage by the medication.

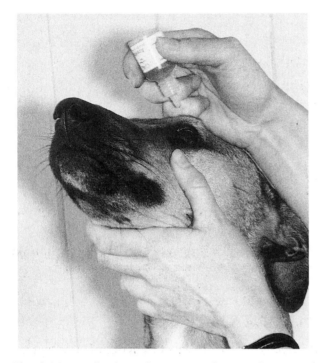

Fig. 2.16. Application of drops to the eye. Photograph courtesy of Roy Hancocks and Rachel Meredith.

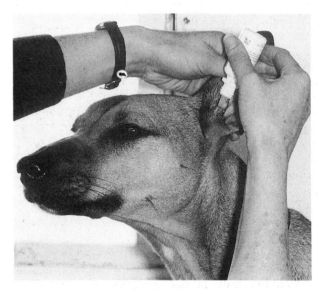

Fig. 2.17. Application of drops to the ear. Photograph courtesy of Roy Hancocks and Rachel Meredith.

3
First Aid

S. M. HISCOCK

First aid is the immediate treatment of injured animals or those suffering from sudden illness.

Limitations

Under the terms of the Veterinary Surgeons' Act of 1966, no person is allowed to practise veterinary surgery unless registered in the veterinary surgeons' register maintained by the Royal College of Veterinary Surgeons or in the supplementary register of veterinary practitioners. However, amendment to Schedule 3 of that Act in 1991 made special provisions for those whose names are entered in the College's list of veterinary nurses, and their rights and powers are described in more detail in Chapter 6 (Ethics and Legislation).

These changes in the law empower a listed veterinary nurse to do considerably more than a lay person, but only **at the direction of a veterinary surgeon**. In an emergency, when no veterinary surgeon is immediately available to give directions, the veterinary nurse is no different in law from any other lay person and, in common with lay persons, has the right to administer first aid treatment to an animal by whatever means are available, **but only as an interim measure, designed to preserve life and alleviate suffering until a veterinary surgeon is able to attend the animal**.

For example, the passing of a stomach tube in a case of gastric dilatation will instantly ease the pain and suffering of the patient and may well be life-saving, and therefore it is perfectly permissible. However, any attempts to give medical treatment or gastric lavage through that stomach tube (unless directed to do so by a veterinary surgeon) would exceed the powers given to a veterinary nurse under Schedule 3 as they would not constitute first aid treatments. They are long-term rather than interim measures and do not save the animal's life or lessen its suffering. Wherever possible the veterinary nurse should ask for directions from the veterinary surgeon once first aid has been given.

Although in theory veterinary nurses do not have greater powers in law than lay people, in practice they have greater knowledge and training and are obviously far better equipped to assess an emergency case and provide appropriate first aid treatment for the animal until a veterinary surgeon arrives.

Aims and Rules of First Aid

First aid treatment is based on three aims and four rules.

The three aims are:

(1) To preserve life.
(2) To prevent suffering.
(3) To prevent the situation deteriorating.

The four rules are:

(1) Don't panic!
(2) Maintain the airway.
(3) Control the haemorrhage.
(4) Contact the veterinary surgeon as soon as possible.

If you forget everything else when faced with an emergency case, don't forget these four rules!

Telephone Calls

An emergency can be classified as one of three types:

- Life-threatening emergencies, requiring immediate action by the owner at home and the nurse at the surgery.
- Emergencies requiring immediate attention at the surgery but where life is not immediately threatened.
- Minor emergencies where telephone advice enables the owner to alleviate suffering until a veterinary surgeon is able to attend the patient.

Examples of each type are given in Fig. 3.1.

Immediate classification of an emergency may not be easy over the telephone because owners are often in a panic when they ring the surgery for help. It must be remembered that animals are usually very precious to their owners—emotionally, financially or both. Therefore the owner is rarely able to judge the severity of the illness or injury and may consider that questioning by the veterinary nurse is a waste of valuable time. Bearing these points in mind, the nurse must remain calm but sympathetic and patient (which may not be easy!) and ask specific questions clearly and concisely.

When taking the history, it is always best to speak directly to the owner because 'second-hand' conversations are frustrating and time-consuming and lead to inaccuracies. There are seven basic questions to be asked:

(1) What is the nature of the injury (e.g. scalding due to a household accident, haemorrhage from a deep cut, insect sting)? If **poisoning** is suspected, does the owner know which poison is involved? (On this subject, further questions during

EXAMPLES OF TYPES OF EMERGENCIES		
Life-threatening	**Immediate attention**	**Minor**

Unconsciousness
Conscious collapse with
  dyspnoea or cyanosis
Severe haemorrhage
Severe burns
Prolapsed eye
Poisoning
Snake bites
	Conscious collapse
	Dyspnoea
	Fractures/dislocations
	Haemorrhage
	Gaping wounds
	Severe dysuria
	Dystocia
		Insect stings
		Minor wounds (where the
		  haemorrhage is easily
		  controlled by bandaging)
		Minor burns (where there is
		  only slight discomfort)
		Abscesses
		Slight lameness (where animal
		  is able to bear some weight
		  on the leg)
		Haematuria
		Aural haematomata

Fig. 3.1. Examples of types of emergencies.

history-taking are suggested in the Poisoning section of this chapter, p. 35.)

(2) What is the extent or degree of the injury? Is the animal conscious or unconscious? Is it able to breathe freely? How severe is any haemorrhage? What is the general appearance of the animal?

(3) When did the accident happen, or when was the illness first noticed? If the animal is collapsed, was it seen to fall or was it found in the collapsed state? Has the animal's condition improved or deteriorated and how rapidly has any such change occurred?

(4) What age, sex and breed is the patient?

(5) Is it receiving any current veterinary treatment (e.g. insulin injections if a diabetic, or NSAID if a gastric haemorrhage is reported)?

(6) If injured or taken ill away from home, where exactly is the animal?

(7) What is the owner's name, address and telephone number? (This is very important in case the veterinary surgeon needs more information before deciding on a course of action.)

It is often best to ask these questions in the order set out above because it immediately allows the owner to talk about the problem. It shows that the person receiving the phone call is experienced in dealing with emergencies and this in itself gives the owner confidence. There is nothing more frustrating and upsetting for an anguished owner than someone insisting on taking their name and address whilst refusing to listen to details of their pet's illness. Once they have talked to the veterinary nurse and received some reassurance, or been told to what to do, they very often calm down and can lucidly give their names, addresses and 'phone numbers. For safety, addresses and 'phone numbers should be repeated back to the caller.

History taking is very important because it enables the nurse to:

- decide on the type of emergency;
- give the owner relevant instructions on immediate first aid measures to be carried out in the home (e.g. how to maintain the airway of an unconscious pet); and

- make the necessary preparations to receive the patient at the surgery (e.g. prepare dressings for open wounds).

Handling and Transport of Injured Animals

Unless life is endangered by falling masonry, fire, poisonous atmosphere etc., no attempt should be made to move an accident victim until it has been given a brief examination. This will ensure that injuries can be adequately protected during handling.

General advice on handling and transport is given in Chapter 1 but emergency situations away from the surgery often call for different techniques and a degree of ingenuity.

Approaching the Injured Animal

An injured animal is usually frightened and shocked, which means that it is liable to bite and scratch viciously if cornered or approached too quickly. The gentle approach is usually best but it should not be hesitant. Slow, deliberate movements accompanied by the continuous gentle reassurance of the human voice can do much to calm the anxious patient.

Cats

Shocked and injured cats are not usually aggressive when approached. Observe the animal closely whilst extending the hand to stroke it under its chin. If this is permitted, slide the hand around the cat's face to stroke its neck and then gently grasp its scruff. The animal is now restrained and an examination can be made. If the animal reacts aggressively when approached, do not persist as this may only provoke an attack or an attempted escape. In these cases an inverted box or basket should be lowered gently over the cat to confine it, and a thin piece of hardboard or strong cardboard slid slowly under the inverted box so that the cat comes to lie on it. The whole may then be lifted and made secure for transport to the surgery.

Dogs

Frightened injured dogs are much more inclined to snap at an approaching human, especially a stranger. Even the dog's owner may be bitten if a normally placid pet is in pain from its injuries. If there is any indication of aggression, form a looped lead as a running 'noose' and try to drop it over the dog's head. Leather leads are better than chain or material ones because the noose tends to hang as an open loop and it is easier to position it around the dog's neck.

Some dogs react to the lead, biting and snapping at the noose as it is lowered towards the head. This makes restraint difficult and, unless there is a 'dog-catcher' available, it is often necessary to ask someone else to stand in front of the dog (at a safe distance), talking to it and **maintaining constant eye contact**. The veterinary nurse can then approach the dog from behind and lower the lead over its head.

Many dogs immediately feel more secure if they are on a lead with a human in control but they still might bite. A muzzle should therefore be tied in place before handling **unless the dog is dyspnoeic or the dog's face is injured**. Once the animal is under control, a brief but thorough examination should be carried out:

- The **airway** must be checked and cleared if necessary (see Asphyxia, p. 92).
- **Haemorrhage** must be controlled (see p. 42).
- **Fractures** should be immobilised with splints or dressings if possible (see Fractures, p. 58).
- **Wounds** should be dressed (see Wounds, p. 49).

The patient should then be restrained as gently as possible until it can be transported to the surgery or until a veterinary surgeon can attend the animal. The patient should be allowed to assume the position which it finds most comfortable and most injured animals will lie on the wounded side. This distresses owners but the patient should not be interfered with if it seems to be comfortable. The owner should be asked to stay with the animal to reassure and comfort it.

Transport to the Surgery

The aim is to remove the injured animal to the surgery with minimal discomfort to the patient and without disturbing any dressings that have been applied. There are two groups of animals: the ambulatory (able to walk) and the non-ambulatory.

Ambulatory

An ambulatory dog is one that can rise to its feet and is able to walk, even if only to limp slowly. Often these dogs are transported less painfully and with less stress if they are allowed to move themselves rather than submitting to the restrictions of being carried. Gentle encouragement should be used to guide the animal to the transport vehicle, but the patient may need assistance in climbing into it.

Non-ambulatory

Lifting in the owner's arms.

> WARNING
> None of the following methods should be used in cases of suspected spinal fracture, and the last method must not be used in cases of suspected abdominal or thoracic injury or if the patient is severely dyspnoeic.

Small dogs and cats may be held firmly round the neck with one hand (taking care not to obstruct the breathing), whilst the other hand and arm are slid around the hindquarters and under the sternum to scoop the body up, supporting the weight along the length of the forearm (Fig. 3.2). The foreleg furthest from the handler's body can then be held firmly in the left hand, to prevent the animal scrabbling to get free, whilst the handler's right hand continues to hold the neck gently in extension, like a wide collar, so that the animal is unable to turn its head round or down to bite the handler.

Medium-sized dogs may be lifted with one arm encircling the front of the sternum, the other around the back of the pelvis to support the hindquarters. The animal is then held against the handler's chest to support its trunk (Fig. 3.3). If possible, the injured side should be held next to the handler's chest. Always lift the dog with an almost straight back, using bent knees to provide most of the lifting effort, and always ask for help if the dog seems too heavy for one person.

Large heavy dogs should be lifted by two or more people. One person stands at the dog's shoulder with one arm curled round under the dog's neck, holding its head against the handler's shoulder to control it, with the other arm under and around its thorax, just behind its forelegs. The second person stands by the hindquarters and places one arm under the abdomen, just in front of the hindlegs, and the other around the pelvis (Fig. 3.4). Again, remember to keep your back straight and bend the knees when lifting, and ask for more help if the load is still too great.

Boxes and baskets. These are suitable for cats and small dogs. Types range from wire, wicker or wooden cages to cardboard boxes, laundry baskets, washing baskets and any other containers that might be to hand in an emergency. There are three important criteria:

- The basket should be **escape-proof**. Cardboard boxes, etc., should have a lid firmly secured across the open top.
- **Ventilation** must be adequate. Mesh sides are safer than solid-wall boxes.

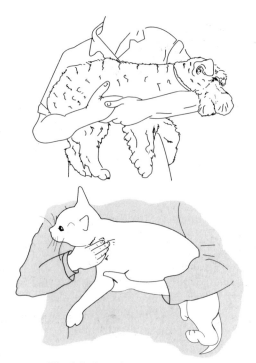

Fig. 3.2. Carrying a small patient.

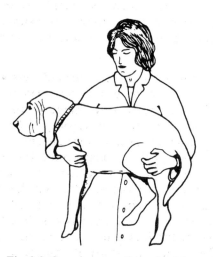

Fig. 3.3. Carrying a medium-sized dog.

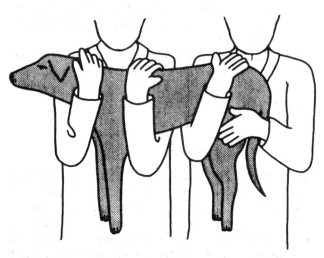

Fig. 3.4. Carrying a large dog.

- **Constant observation** of the patient must be possible. Wire baskets and plastic laundry baskets are best for this.

Lifting the patient into the basket is usually straightforward unless the animal is collapsed and severe injuries are suspected, when it should be lifted with great care to lessen the pain and distress and to prevent further injury. Find a sheet of hardboard or thick cardboard which is the same size as the basket or box (or slightly smaller) and slide this gently under the patient. The animal can then be picked up on the support and placed in the container with minimal disturbance.

If no such support is readily to hand, hold the animal's scruff with one hand (to control the head and stop the animal from biting). Slide the other hand, palm up, under the body trunk at the hindquarters and work the hand forwards until the patient's body is laid along the forearm. The animal can then be lifted, using the forearm as a rigid stretcher, and laid gently in the container by reversing the procedure (Fig. 3.5).

If the patient is too aggressive to allow either procedure, it may be less distressing and painful if it is lifted up bodily by the scruff in one hand, with minimal gentle support of the hindquarters by the other hand, and placed gently and carefully in the basket.

Stretchers. Stretchers should always be used to transport the following cases if the animals are too large to fit into boxes or baskets:

- Suspected spinal fractures.
- Collapse with dyspnoea.
- Collapse with thoracic or abdominal injuries.
- Collapse and unconsciousness (these dogs are very difficult to pick up without some support).
- Other severely injured animals, e.g. those with severe lacerations or multiple broken bones, where handling would be too painful for the patient.

The principle is to have a flat, rigid object which is big and strong enough to support the animal in lateral recumbency, yet small enough to fit into the transport vehicle. Stretchers can be improvised from:

- Wood or hardboard sheets (very good for small or medium-sized dogs).
- Wire mesh or plastic-coated fencing wire. (This can only be used if there are two handlers to stretch the wire taut when lifting the animal so that the wire provides a firm support.)
- Sacks or coats mounted on wooden poles. (These are described for human patients in *First Aid, Junior Manual*, British Red Cross Society.)
- Blankets. These offer little support for injured spines but may be slid underneath the patient easily (Fig. 3.6) and are usually readily available.

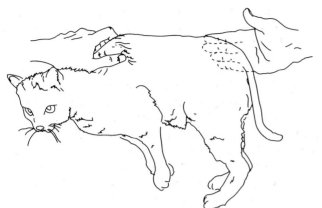

Fig. 3.5. Supporting the collapsed cat.

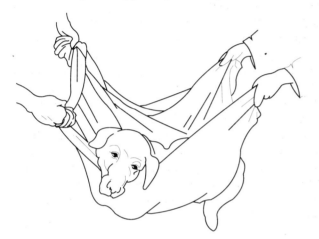

Fig. 3.6. Lifting a large dog with the help of a blanket.

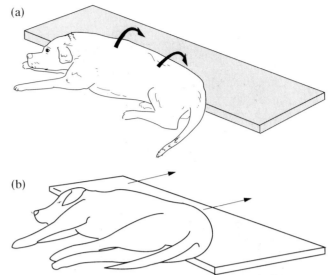

Fig. 3.7. (a) Rolling a dog on to a stretcher. (b) Pulling a dog on to a stretcher.

To transfer the patient to the stretcher:

(1) Place the stretcher close to the patient's back as it lies on the ground.
(2) Apply a tape muzzle to a conscious patient if possible, as these animals are often in pain and might bite when handled.
(3) Roll the patient half on to its chest and push the stretcher underneath the animal as far as possible. Then allow the animal to collapse on to its side again and thus on to the stretcher. Several people should help in the transfer and should try to move the animal as a unit, avoiding any twisting of the spine if a spinal injury is suspected (Fig. 3.7a).
(4) Alternatively, grasp the skin along the back at several points—above the scapula, midway along the back and above the pelvis. The patient may now be pulled the short distance on to the stretcher (Fig. 3.7b). This is particularly useful in cases of spinal damage and fractured limbs as it does not involve twisting the spine, body or limbs. A tape muzzle is strongly advised for this procedure.

Care in Transit

Within the vehicle, the patient needs to be observed constantly and restrained to ensure that:

- the condition does not deteriorate;
- any dressings are not disturbed;
- the animal does not escape from its container (or fall off the seat if it is too large to be contained);
- the animal cannot interfere with the driver of the vehicle.

It is important to have a second person in the vehicle—preferably the owner, who will be able to give a full case history at the surgery and who will want to be with the pet anyway. The owner's presence may also help to calm the patient.

If it is impossible or impractical for a second person to accompany the animal, the ambulatory patient must be restrained on a lead which is securely fastened inside the vehicle. Often the simplest way is to shut the lead in the car door as it is closed, leaving the handle of the lead protruding on the outside of the car. This method has three advantages:

- The dog is securely restrained.
- The animal cannot escape from the vehicle at the last minute as the door is being closed, because the lead is either held by the handler or is jammed in the closed door.
- On arrival at the surgery, the handler can take hold of the lead before opening the door, thus avoiding losing the dog if it makes a bolt for freedom.

Arrival at the Surgery

On admission, the animal should be examined, a provisional diagnosis made and treatment given. To avoid errors in treatment when several casualties arrive at the same time, it may be necessary to identify each accident victim individually. Labels can be attached to dogs' collars or identity bands fixed around the front or back leg of each animal.

WARNING
Unconscious animals should always take priority and must be examined and treated immediately, as follows:
(1) Check the throat for obstructions and clear the airway as quickly as possible.
(2) Check the heart to see if it is beating. If nothing is detected, start cardiac massage immediately.
(3) Check for respiratory movements. If the animal is not breathing, start artificial respiration.
(4) If the patient is trying to breathe, supply oxygen to prevent hypoxia.
(5) Once the heartbeat is steady and the respiration is maintained (either by the animal on its own or by artificial respiration), the veterinary nurse may proceed with the more detailed examination.

Examination of the Patient

It is necessary to take a full case history and to examine the animal thoroughly in order to make a tentative diagnosis and give the appropriate first aid treatment. Any diagnosis must always be provisional until confirmed by a veterinary surgeon and, if there is any doubt as to the severity of the injury, **the worst should always be assumed** and the patient treated accordingly.

History-taking

A complete and accurate case history can be vitally important in reaching a correct diagnosis. The veterinary nurse will already have a good case history if the owner was able to answer the first six of the seven questions outlined previously on p. 27, but further questioning may be needed in cases of suspected poisoning.

It is essential to ask questions about the previous health and treatment (if any) of the animal before the accident or illness because the answers may hold the key to a correct diagnosis. For example, an unconscious bitch may be in an hypoglycaemic coma if she is a known diabetic; or a bitch which has recently had pups may have collapsed because she is hypocalcaemic.

General Examination

The first step is to determine by observation that the animal is alive and that its heart and respiration are functioning adequately as described earlier. The patient should be observed closely before any attempt is made to touch it, because the general condition and bearing of the patient are important in evaluating the severity of its injuries. The experienced nurse can assess the following three points

very quickly whilst taking the case history or even as the patient is carried into the consulting room.

State of consciousness

The unconscious patient must always be treated as a serious case but, in conscious patients, the severity of the injury and risk to life can be more difficult to assess. The animal which follows the movement of human hands with its eyes and responds normally to human voice or touch is less likely to be suffering from potentially fatal injuries. However, the animal which is withdrawn, lies still and seems afraid to move, staring with blank unfocused eyes, is likely to be in serious trouble and severely shocked.

Behaviour

Behaviour is abnormal in some cases. The animal may be excitable, over-reacting to stimuli (**hyperaesthetic**) or, conversely, it may be very depressed and sluggish. Also note any sign of incoordination, muscle tremors or convulsions.

Respiration

The character and rate of respiration should be taken into account. Figure 3.8 illustrates the wide variety of causes which alter the respiratory pattern.

THE CAUSES OF ALTERATION OF RESPIRATORY PATTERN	

Laboured breathing	Obstructed upper airway –
	   nasal passages e.g. by blood, exudates
	   pharynx e.g. by large solid foreign bodies
	   larynx, trachea e.g. strangulation injuries
	 Alveolar damage –
	   haemorrhage into lung spaces, fluid in lung
	   spaces e.g. drowning accidents, house fires
	 Collapsed lungs –
	   pneumothorax, haemothorax, diaphragmatic hernia
	 Severe blood loss (leading to hypoxia)

Rapid, shallow breathing	Shock
	 Pain –
	   thoracic wall injuries
	   abdominal crises e.g. gastric torsions, severe
	   wounds, fractures, etc.

Fig. 3.8. Causes of alteration of respiratory pattern.

Detailed Examination

Ensure that:

- the heart is beating steadily;
- respiration is maintained; and
- severe haemorrhage is controlled.

Then examine the patient methodically from nose to tail tip, leaving no area of the body unchecked. Figure 3.9 sets out the steps for such an examination.

The first aider must be able to appreciate any possible complications which may underlie a seemingly simple wound, e.g. broken bones or penetration of thoracic or abdominal cavities. The mere suspicion that there may be a serious complication can help the nurse to alleviate suffering, preserve life and prevent the situation deteriorating.

DETAILED EXAMINATION IN FIRST AID

Nose	Note any haemorrhage (*epistaxis*) and whether it comes from one or both nostrils. Note any swellings which may suggest fracture of the nasal bones.
Mouth	• Odours. Carefully open the mouth and smell the breath. Note any unusual smell: e.g. ketones ('pear drops') in cases of untreated diabetics; creosote or phenol in cases of poisoning; urine odour in cases of kidney failure.
	• Haemorrhage. Check for signs of haemorrhage and locate its source, e.g. gums, tongue (dorsal and ventral surfaces), palate, etc. If no injuries are apparent, the blood may have been coughed up from the lungs or issued from wounds in the throat area.
	• Tongue. Check for signs of redness or ulceration, which often occur after licking corrosive poisons.
	• Fractures. Examine the bony structures for signs of fracture: splitting of the hard palate down its centre, jaw fractures.
	• Teeth. Look for any signs of food caked in the crevices. Pesticides are often highly coloured and some evidence may be seen on the teeth if the animal has eaten poisoned bait.
	• Mucosa. Note the colour of the mucosa, which may be: (i) normal (pale pink); (ii) congested: brick-red (in toxic or septicaemic animals and heatstroke patients, for example). (iii) pale: may appear white (e.g. in severely shocked patients and those suffering severe haemorrhage); (iv) cyanosed: purple (e.g. patients with severe dyspnoea); (v) jaundiced: orange or yellow (e.g. patients with acute liver damage). Note whether the mucosa is dry or normally moist, or if the animal is salivating so profusely that it drools. Certain poisons affect the rate of production of saliva. If the gums or lips are not darkly pigmented, test the capillary refill by pressing the mucosa to blanch it. In an animal with normal blood pressure, the pink colour returns rapidly within 1–2 seconds of the pressure being removed. In an animal with a low blood pressure, it may take up to 5 seconds before the capillaries refill with blood and the mucosa becomes pink again. This simple test is very helpful in assessing whether the animal has suffered a severe haemorrhage.
Eyes	The eye is a very delicate and sensitive organ and must be treated gently. It is best to examine the animal in a dimly lit or darkened room, where the patient is more likely to open its eye. For detailed examination, an auroscope head or torch may be used to illuminate the eye.
	• Discharges. Note any discharges of fluid and their appearance and quantity. Clear fluid may indicate that the eyeball has ruptured; purulent discharges could be evidence of a foreign body.
	• Eyelids. Eyelids can easily be examined for signs of injury and may be opened gently and everted slightly to allow examination of the conjunctiva and nictitating membrane (third eyelid). Check the palpebral reflex and examine the colour of the conjunctival mucosa for an indication of anaemia (pale pink or white), jaundice (yellow) or cyanosis (mauve).
	• Eyeball. Check for bruising to the sclera or conjunctiva and note any sign of jaundice. Note any injuries to the eyeball, haemorrhage into the anterior chamber, collapsed eyeball, corneal opacity. Note the position of the eyeball in the socket in cases of unconsciousness and any *nystagmus* (involuntary flicking movement of the eyeball from side to side).
	• Pupils. Note the size of the pupil in each eye and check for response to light. Brain-damaged patients often show a difference in the size of the two pupils; poisoned patients may have very constricted or very dilated pupils which do not respond normally to light.
Skull	Look for signs of depressed fractures, swelling, pain or crepitus. Be *very* gentle when checking for a suspected fracture of the cranium as heavy handling could depress the bone fragments into the brain cortex and cause enormous damage to the cerebral hemispheres.
Ears	Examine for signs of haemorrhage from the ear canal as this can occur with brain damage.
Limbs	Palpate all limbs, bones and joints, for signs of swelling or pain. In cases of suspected deformity, it is useful to compare the injured leg with its normal partner. If a fracture is suspected, treat it as such pending diagnosis by the veterinary surgeon. Record the way the limb is held and note any seeming *paralysis*: • Flaccid. When the muscles are totally relaxed; • Spastic. When the muscles are contracted to fix the limb rigidly in extension or flexion.

Fig. 3.9.—continued

DETAILED EXAMINATION IN FIRST AID	
	Note any loss of feeling, which may be tested by pinching the toes. If the animal is able to feel this stimulus, it will look round at the foot, try to move away or attempt to bite the cause of its discomfort as well as flexing the leg to draw it away from the painful stimulus. This is known as conscious proprioception and should not be confused with the simple withdrawal reflex when the limb is simply flexed to remove it from the pinching stimulus without the animal showing any signs that it is aware of the pain.
Rib cage	Gently palpate for signs of fractured ribs. Listen to any wounds to detect a 'hiss' sound on inspiration which indicates penetration of the pleural cavity.
Abdomen	Palpation of the abdomen is a skilled procedure and can cause considerable harm if attempted by the inexperienced: do not attempt it. Haemorrhage from the penis or bruising or swellings of the abdomen wall should be noted.
Spine	Note any obvious deformities in the spinal column and gently palpate to detect any gross abnormalities. The spinal column is covered by large muscle trunks and severe spinal fractures are not always obvious. Always assume a fracture is present if there is any doubt.
	Fractures or dislocations in the cervical region may cause paralysis of all four legs, *quadriplegia* or, more rarely, paralysis of one side of the body, *hemiplegia*. Fractures or dislocations of the thoracolumbar region may cause paralysis of the hindlegs, *paraplegia,* and many cases show rigid extension of the forelegs and flexion of the hindlegs, with the back arched at the fracture site. It is important to realise that the spinal cord may continue to function normally above and below the fracture site. Thus limb withdrawal reflexes are often unaffected as they are a local reflex arc and do not require input from the brain. However, conscious proprioception may be absent from areas caudal to the spinal injury if nerve impulses are unable to pass to the brain.
Pelvis	Gently palpate the pelvic bones for signs of instability, pain, crepitus and deformity.
Perineal region	The prepuce, vulva and anus should be examined for signs of haemorrhage because signs of blood at these orifices may indicate that internal organs (e.g. the bladder) have been damaged.
	In cases of paralysis, it is useful to note the presence or absence of the anal ring reflex by watching for anal sphincter contraction when a thermometer is inserted into the anus.
Tail	Observe the signs of voluntary movement, e.g. correct carriage of the tail, wagging, etc.
General body surface	Note any matting of the fur which may indicate an underlying wound. If in doubt as to the severity of the wound, assume the worst and treat accordingly. If foreign bodies are present, removal may be attempted unless they are embedded. Dislodging embedded foreign bodies may provoke more serious injury and must therefore be avoided.

Fig. 3.9. Stages of a detailed examination.

Recording the Information

Following the examination and first aid treatment of the animal, make notes of the findings and mark the time of the examination. Brain injuries in particular can rapidly deteriorate or improve over short periods, and it is vital to chart the course of events as accurately as possible.

General Nursing Care

Accident victims and very ill patients are likely to be severely shocked. Many of the actions taken in first aid nursing are aimed at countering the effects of the shock, a subject which is covered in depth in Chapter 21 (Shock and Fluid Therapy).

Signs of shock:

- Pallor of mucous membranes (gums, inside lips, conjunctiva).
- Slow capillary refill.
- Increased respiration rate, which may rise markedly if the animal tries to struggle in any way.
- Rapid, feeble pulse. The pulse may be so weak that it cannot be felt.
- Coldness of the inside of the mouth, limbs and tail.
- Dull and depressed attitude—the animal is withdrawn.
- Convulsions and collapse if the brain becomes short of oxygen (**hypoxic**) and ceases to be able to function normally. This is likely to happen in the patient which is haemorrhaging badly (**hypovolaemic shock**).

Treatment of the Shocked Patient

The exact treatment given depends on the cause of the shock but the following principles apply to all cases:

(1) **Prevent any further haemorrhage**.
(2) **Do not apply direct heat or give alcohol or other peripheral vasodilator drugs** (e.g. acepromazine). Both actions will cause dilation of the cutaneous blood vessels, which are a non-essential part of the circulatory system so far as the shocked

patient is concerned. The cutaneous blood vessels constrict in shock so that the circulating blood volume is directed towards maintaining sufficient blood supply to vital organs such as the brain, heart and lungs. This is why the extremities (paws and tail) feel cold to the touch and also why the mucosae are pale. If these non-essential blood vessels are encouraged to dilate, the blood pressure will fall as there is more circulatory 'pipework' to be filled by the circulating blood. Vasodilation in the skin is also more likely to restart haemorrhage from surface wounds.

(3) **Make the animal comfortable and prevent heat loss** by laying the patient on an insulated surface (such as thick blankets, vetbeds or polystyrene bean-bags) and covering the animal with further insulation (warmed blankets, towels etc.) to prevent heat loss from the body.

(4) **Set up an intravenous fluid drip**. The drip of choice is warmed Hartmann's solution but normal saline is adequate in an emergency. This measure not only helps to correct the metabolic acidosis of shock but also expands the circulating blood volume quickly and improves the supply of oxygen to all body tissues. It allows the kidneys to function more normally again.

  If there has been extensive blood loss, a blood transfusion may be required or a plasma expander used. In cases of brain damage, some veterinary surgeons use hypertonic solutions to decrease the oedema of the brain tissues (e.g. mannitol solutions). These fluids may be warmed, ready for administration if the veterinary surgeon needs them.

(5) **Give fluids by mouth** unless there are contra-indications e.g. vomiting, unconsciousness, severe mouth or throat injuries. Small volumes of fluid (25–100 ml, depending on the size of the animal) should be offered every 30 minutes. Oral Hartmann's solution (lactated Ringer's solution) will help to guard against the effects of shock, but plain water or a prepared solution of half a teaspoonful of salt and half a teaspoonful of bicarbonate of soda, dissolved in one litre of water, can be used if no Hartmann's Solution is available.

(6) **Check dressings** every 10–15 minutes to ensure that they are comfortable, that the animal is not interfering with them and that any haemorrhage is being controlled.

(7) **Maintain constant observation**. This is essential, especially in cases of brain injury, haemorrhage, dyspnoea and suspected poisoning. The condition of the patient can deteriorate rapidly and the veterinary nurse must always remain on the alert. The state of consciousness, pupillary and palpebral reflexes, mucosal colour, capillary refill, and character and rate of pulse and respiration should be monitored every 10 minutes, or more frequently if the animal seems very distressed. **Make notes of the findings and time of each inspection and record them on the kennel chart.**

(8) **TLC.** All the above measures are aimed at reversing the effects of shock and will therefore make the animal feel more comfortable. However, the emotional needs of the patient should not be overlooked. These animals are often in much pain; they are confused and disorientated because they are alone in a strange and hostile environment (few animals like the surgery!) and they need sensitive and sympathetic handling. It should also be remembered that brain-damaged patients may have lost some faculties (e.g. sight or hearing) in the accident and need even more careful handling.

The nurse can help patients greatly by keeping them in a quiet, warm, darkened room and moving quietly and calmly whilst talking in a soothing manner. It does not matter what you say, rather how you say it. When checks are made, the animal should not be rushed—a gentle approach is much less stressful. Contact with human hands is very important, especially to dogs, and a little fussing is a good idea if time permits, but attention should *never* be forced on the patient. If any apprehension is shown, the animal is best handled as little as possible and it may even be advisable to cover the front of the kennel or basket to allow the patient some privacy between the regular check-ups.

As soon as possible, veterinary assistance should be obtained, and comprehensive notes should be handed to the veterinary surgeon in charge of the case. Meanwhile, the veterinary nurse may prevent delays by preparing dressings, drips, transfusions, instruments, anaesthetic machines and the operating theatre in readiness for any further treatment which the veterinary surgeon deems necessary once the patient's condition is stabilised.

Poisoning

Definitions

- A **poison** or **toxin** or **toxic agent** is a substance which, when it enters the body in sufficient doses, causes harmful effects.
- **Poisoning** is said to have occurred when the poison produces clinical effects in the animal.
- An **antidote** is a substance which specifically counters the action of the poison.

The Role of the Veterinary Nurse

The veterinary nurse should know of the common poisons and their effects in order to be able to act as follows:

(1) **Take a comprehensive case history**. From this the veterinary nurse should be able to recognise that the animal may have been poisoned or be able to

reassure the client that the substance is harmless. One of the most common false alarms is when a puppy eats an owner's contraceptive tablets. The hormones contained in these are usually rapidly metabolised and excreted with no harmful effects to the patient.

(2) **Give appropriate first aid advice over the telephone** if the type of poison can be clearly identified from the case history given and the symptoms described by the owner (Fig. 3.10).

(3) **Thoroughly examine the patient and provide the correct supportive treatment** for the animal at the surgery until the veterinary surgeon can attend the case.

(4) **Reserve any vomit, faeces or urine and a sample of the suspected toxic agent** (if it is available) for examination and possible forensic analysis. Even if you are reasonably certain that the patient has not been poisoned, it is always wise to take such samples. Many domestic poisons (e.g. rat and slug baits) are brightly coloured, and the presence of these coloured pellets in the vomit will help the veterinary surgeon in his diagnosis and treatment of the case. The other reason for taking samples is that the owner may require them for analysis at a future date if legal action is taken.

(5) **Label the samples clearly** with:

- the name and address of the owner;
- the animal's name and description (e.g. breed, age, sex);
- the time and date of collection.

(6) **Maintain a diplomatic silence** as regards accusations of malicious poisonings. Unfortunately, there are some owners who are all too keen to assume that poison is the cause for any acute illness and accusations against unfriendly neighbours can flow thick and fast. **It is very important not to agree with any such accusations and it is essential not to make any such suggestion to the owners**. The reasons for this are threefold:

- Cases of malicious poisoning are mercifully rare.
- It is often very difficult to prove exactly which poison is responsible for the illness.
- It is usually impossible to prove in a court of law that the accused person deliberately placed the poison where the patient could reach it in order to harm the animal.

(7) **Ensure that access to a poison information unit is available**. In the U.K., the Veterinary Poisons Information Service (VPIS) provides a round-the-clock information service to veterinary surgeons and is able to:

- supply data on the clinical effects of a great number and range of poisonous compounds;
- advise on methods of treatment of specific poisons;
- advise on antidotal therapies (where available).

In order to enable the staff at VPIS to give a speedy and rapid response, an accurate case history

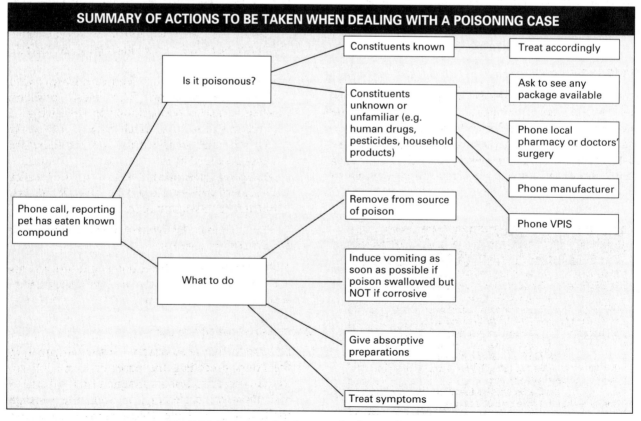

Fig. 3.10. Summary of actions to take for a poisoning case.

is needed. This should include as many precise details as possible about the suspected toxic agent (exact trade name, manufacturer, constituents etc.).

It is very important that the veterinary nurse should only contact the service with the consent of the veterinary surgeon. The VPIS is *not* a public access service and will only accept calls from veterinary practices. It will also make a charge for answering any enquiries, unless the veterinary practice in question already pays an annual subscription to the service, in which case the subscription number should be quoted when the 'phone call is made. To avoid delay, ensure that this number is available.

The VPIS can be contacted on 071 635 9195, 0532 430715 or 0532 316838.

Incidence of Poisoning Cases

Poisoning is not commonly seen in small animal practice but the veterinary nurse must always bear the possibility in mind when presented with an acutely ill patient. Sometimes the history offers a clue – for example, a cat which has been over-enthusiastically treated for fleas so that its coat is wet with flea spray. At other times, careful questioning is necessary to establish the cause of the problem. Many humans are incurable hoarders and ancient bottles and boxes may be found in many cupboards and garden sheds: strychnine has been banned from use in the U.K. for a long time but occasional poisonings still occur; some old houses still have linoleum, old lead pipes, lead paint etc. Figure 3.11 suggests possible sources of poisons around the house.

History-taking

Many poisons cause common symptoms. This means that, when asking routine questions over the telephone, it can be difficult to decide if an animal has actually been poisoned or has simply had severe gastroenteritis or an epileptic fit. The following points should be considered when trying to come to a conclusion:

CLASSIFICATION OF POISONS	
Type	**Possible sources**
Medicines	Sedatives, NSAID's, etc.
Pesticides	Herbicides e.g. weedkillers
	Insecticides e.g. flea sprays
	Molluscicides e.g. slug bait
Household chemicals	Rodenticides e.g. rat poison
	Garage – engine oils, antifreeze
	Garden shed – wood preservative
	Kitchen – disinfectants
Plants	Rare in small animal practice
Reptile bites	Adder bites
	Exotic species bite if snake etc. escaped
Insect stings	Wasp and bee stings

Fig. 3.11. Classification of poisons.

(1) **What species is the patient?**
   - **Pups** are indiscriminate chewers of everything from laburnum sticks to old lino, both of which are toxic, and many dogs will eat almost anything, including rat bait.
   - **Cats** are fastidious and cautious about what they consume, but they groom endlessly and are therefore more likely to ingest contact poisons on the coat. They also hunt more and may eat their poisoned prey. The cat also has a poorly developed enzyme system in the liver, which means it is far less able to metabolise and excrete certain poisons. These chemicals therefore build up to toxic levels in the body tissues and poison the animal. The classic example here is paracetamol.
   - **Birds** are more susceptible to inhalation poisoning because of the design of their respiratory system.

(2) **What could be the cause of any poisoning?** Most reported poisonings are due to:
   - **Accidents**, e.g. cats falling into containers of old sump oil, or dogs finding slug bait.
   - **Overdosing**, e.g. owners who do not read and follow directions correctly on cans of flea spray.
   - **Unusual reactions** to normally harmless substances, e.g. allergic (**anaphylactic**) reactions to wasp or bee stings, antibiotics or vaccines (some of these are not poisons but the reaction suggests it).
   - **Carelessness**, when an owner leaves medications where an inquisitive puppy can eat them. This is more of a hazard now that many human medicines are packaged in 'bubble packs'.
   - **Ignorance** of an owner who doses a pet with human preparations. The most common incident under this heading is the giving of paracetamol to cats, which have an extremely low tolerance of the drug and are therefore easily poisoned by it.
   - **Malicious poisoning**, which is in reality extremely rare—it should be considered, but not agreed to without proof.

   The questions the veterinary nurse should ask must therefore concern:
   - the species, age, whereabouts and movements of the patient prior to the onset of illness; and
   - the actions of the owner.

Questions about the patient

(1) Has the animal been observed eating anything in the hours preceding the onset of illness? If so, ask the owner to bring a sample of the substance with them or, preferably, to bring the package itself, if it is available. (Most poisons act within hours of ingestion.)

(2) Is there any contaminating substance on the coat, e.g. a smell of creosote, sticky engine oil, greasy paraffin?

(3) What were the patient's movements prior to the illness? For example, was the cat out overnight, or had the dog been shut into a garden shed where slug bait was stored, or is there evidence of chewed tablet packets? Has the animal been anywhere unusual in the last 24 hours—has the dog perhaps been walked in a different area where it may have found something?

(4) How old is the patient? The young are curious and may eat anything. The very young and the elderly are more susceptible to being poisoned since the liver and kidneys may not be functioning efficiently and therefore the poison cannot be detoxified and excreted so quickly. These animals need more rapid treatment and more intensive nursing care.

(5) Are other animals in the household affected (if there is more than one animal there)? Simultaneous illness is more likely to be caused by poisoning.

Questions about the home environment

(1) Any medication (human or veterinary) given in the last 24 hours?

(2) Any recent use of toxic products by owner in the house or garden, e.g. pesticides, wood preservatives, painting?

(3) Any recent upheavals in the house which may have exposed pesticides or toxic material previously inaccessible, e.g. moving to a renovated house, gutting a kitchen where rat bait has been laid, removing old (lead) pipework, stripping old paintwork where lead-based paints were originally used?

(4) Any recent accident in the home, e.g. over-heating of fat or non-stick cooking utensils, accidental spillage of substances onto the animal's coat?

Treatment

Successful first aid treatment of the poisoned animal depends on four important principles:

(1) Prevent further absorption of the poison.
(2) Identify the type of poison.
(3) Treat the symptoms.
(4) Give the antidote if a specific one is available.

Identifying the type of poison

Until the nature of the poison is known, correct treatment cannot be given. For example, an animal that has ingested corrosive poisons must *not* be made to vomit because the poison will cause further damage when it is regurgitated over the already damaged tissues of the oesophagus, pharynx and mouth. Animals poisoned by depressant compounds or those likely to cause fits should also not be made to vomit.

Prevention of further absorption

Some of the following first aid measures can be applied by the owner at home, and all may be continued at the surgery as appropriate:

- Remove the animal from the source of the poison.
- Induce vomiting.
- Give gastric lavage.
- Prevent absorption of the poison from the alimentary tract.

Removing the animal from the source of the poison. This includes any other animals in the household which may not yet be showing any symptoms.

If the poison was eaten or inhaled, the animals must be penned in a *known safe area*. Picking up one pile of rat bait may not be the answer as there could be other similar piles around the house.

If the coat is contaminated:

(1) Prevent the animal from washing, grooming or preening itself whilst preparing the bath to wash the patient or whilst transporting it to the surgery. Paws and tails may be lightly bandaged, Elizabethan collars can be used or, if the whole body is affected, the animal may be placed in an old pillowcase or bag (with only the head protruding) or wrapped in a towel. Birds should be confined in a darkened box as they are less likely to preen in the dark. The patient must also be kept under constant observation to ensure the dressings are not disturbed.

(2) Wash and rinse contaminated coats and plumage *thoroughly.*

Cleaning contaminated coats

Suitable cleaning solutions are described in Fig. 3.12. Cats pose the greatest problem: they not only groom themselves assiduously, regardless of any nasty taste, but also hate water and are armed with teeth and claws. Many compounds are extremely toxic to cats in very small doses and so it is very important that the toxic material is totally removed from the coat. This can be a lengthy procedure, requiring as many as three or four repeated washings.

Towelling the coat dry helps to remove any remaining contamination, but the patient will be extremely soggy so that it is also necessary to use a hair-dryer or heat lamp to complete the process and to ensure that the animal does not succumb to hypothermia.

If the animal is too fractious to allow thorough cleansing, a general anaesthetic or some form of sedation will be necessary. Whilst awaiting the

CLEANSING SOLUTIONS	
Non-oily compounds (e.g. disinfectant solutions)	Wash from the coat with copious amounts of water. The immediate use of detergents can actually *increase* the absorption of the toxic material: they make it fat-soluble, which means that it can be absorbed through the skin.
Liquid oily compounds (e.g. sump oil, creosote)	The most efficient way to remove these is to smear the coat liberally with 'Swarfega' (use liquid paraffin or cooking oil if 'Swarfega' is not available) and work it well into the hair. The coat must then be washed clean with 3–4 baths of detergent in warm water until the smell of the contaminant has completely disappeared.
Solid oily contamination (e.g. tar)	If possible the contaminated fur should be clipped away but often (especially when paws are affected) the tar has become so closely attached to the skin that this is impossible. In these cases, liquid paraffin, vegetable oil or butter can be applied and rubbed well into the area. Solvents such as a mixture of acetone and liquid paraffin are sometimes used.

WARNING – It is wise to wear gloves when using these solvents to clean oily contaminants from the coat since regular skin contact with many of these compounds carries a known risk of cancer in humans. If the tar fails to loosen, the area should then be bandaged for 15 minutes, when the heat of the body and the action of the solvent may allow easier removal. If this fails, sedation or anaesthesia may be necessary but the area should be kept bandaged to prevent the animal chewing it. Following successful removal, the area should be well washed with soap and water.

Fig. 3.12. Cleaning solutions for oiled animals.

veterinary surgeon's arrival to administer the anaesthetic, the owner and veterinary nurse may continue to remove as much of the contamination as possible by gentle cleansing or, if this is impossible, they must ensure that the animal does not lick itself and ingest more poison.

Following bathing, an anaesthetised animal must be carefully observed to ensure that it does not become overheated or burnt. It will be unable to move away from the heat source if it becomes too hot.

Oiled birds

Oiled birds present a real problem, especially wild birds unaccustomed to confinement and close association with human beings.

WARNING
To clean the plumage thoroughly and then maintain the patient whilst the bird's water-proofing oils are revived by natural grooming over a long period requires considerable experience, special facilities and weeks of attention, none of which can be easily provided by busy veterinary nurses in a routine small animal practice. There will also be the problem of returning a wild bird to its natural habitat, and this process of rehabilitation (which is vital to its survival) requires a great deal of knowledge and skill.

The role of the veterinary practice is to admit the bird and then take the following steps:

- Decide if it is well enough to survive. Many oiled birds are in too poor a condition or too badly poisoned, and euthanasia is often the kindest treatment.

- Prevent further ingestion of the poison—give superficial cleansing only.
- Correct hypothermia. Many oiled seabirds are hypothermic because the caked feathers become waterlogged.
- Rehydrate the patient.
- Refer it to the nearest RSPCA treatment centre as soon as possible for proper cleansing and rehabilitation.

Suggested first aid measures are therefore as follows:

(1) **Prevent ingestion of poison** by carefully wiping as much contamination off the feathers as possible with a clean towel or paper towelling. Take great care not to break the feather shafts and work methodically from the head of the bird to its tail, wiping both topside and underside of each oiled feather. Do not use solvents as this could increase the absorption of the poison.

(2) **Darkness, warmth and quiet** are the most important requirements. Darkness will calm the stressed bird; it will be less likely to preen and so the danger of absorbing more poison is reduced. Warmth and quiet will counter hypothermia and stress, improving the bird's chances of survival. The worst places for such patients are busy reception areas or noisy kennels.

   The bird should be placed in a cardboard box of suitable size (such as a cardboard cat carrier for a domestic duck) lined with thick newspaper. Put the box under a heat lamp or next to a radiator or on a hot water-bottle so that the bird is kept in an environment of 17–20°C.

(3) **Rehydrate by intubating the gullet**. The recommended equipment is a catheter mounted on a syringe. The catheter should be measured against

the bird and cut to a length which will pass into the bird's oesophagus and down its neck until well clear of the laryngeal opening (Fig. 3.13). Intubating the gullet is relatively simple: the larynx can be readily seen attached to the base of the tongue as the bird gapes and it is easy to slide the catheter around the larynx and down the gullet.

If the bird is bright and alert:

(a) Give warm water to flush the poison from the alimentary system and wait for 20–30 minutes to allow this to work. The volume given will vary according to the size of the patient.

(b) Give Lectade solution diluted in warm water to rehydrate the bird.

(c) Give a slurry mixture of BCK granules and water to prevent absorption of any remaining poison.

If the bird is collapsed, give the Lectade solution every 2 hours to attempt to stabilise the patient's condition.

(4) **Feeding**. Ideally, a wild bird should not be fed until it has been taken into the care of the RSPCA. In any event, do not feed for at least 30 minutes after giving fluids to ensure that any oil has been flushed out of the intestines. Toxins are more easily aborbed if there is food present. When food is offered, it should be suitable—a mixture of chick pellets, chopped greens and chopped hard boiled eggs is suitable for land

birds (a 1:1 mixture of hard-boiled egg and digestive biscuit is a useful substitute in an emergency). Sea birds may be fed small slivers of fresh fish or sprats. Cat food is *not* suitable for birds as it usually causes diarrhoea.

(5) **Refer to a RSPCA centre as soon as possible** for thorough professional cleaning and rehabilitation. If there is an unavoidable delay, but only with very great care and appropriate handling of the bird, give the feathers a preliminary clean to remove the worst of the oil, paying particular attention to the breast feathers and 'wing pits'. Mild detergents such as 'Co-op Green' or 'Fairy Xcel' washing-up liquid are recommended as these two are most readily washed out of the plumage. The bird must be thoroughly rinsed in at least 2–3 bowls of clean water warmed to 40–45°C.

Inducing vomiting

If the poison has been eaten, the patient should be made to vomit as soon as possible except in certain circumstances. Figure 3.14 suggests agents which can be used to induce vomiting.

WARNING

- Do *not* suggest that vomiting should be induced if the poison is known or suspected to be corrosive, i.e. petroleum products, disinfectant solutions, strong acids or alkalis.
- Do *not* suggest that vomiting should be induced if the patient is comatose, unconscious or in a fit, or if the poison is of a type likely to make the patient collapse in any way. Collapsed animals can easily inhale the vomit.
- Do *not* suggest that vomiting should be induced if the poison was eaten 4 hours or more previously. The stomach empties in about 4 hours and there is little point in inducing vomiting after this time, as the poison will already be in the small intestine.
- Do *not* suggest the use of salt as an emetic. It is not very effective and the salt swallowed is absorbed and will cause severe electrolyte inbalances, which could be more harmful to the patient than the ingested poison.
- Do *not* encourage the owner to persist in attempting to make the animal sick at home. Most owners find it very difficult to place foul-tasting concoctions on the back of their pets' tongues to make them vomit. If there is no success after 5 minutes, the animal should be brought straight to the surgery as valuable time is being lost.

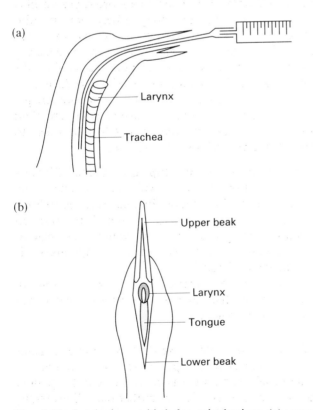

Fig. 3.13. Intubating a bird for rehydration: (a) cross-section; (b) open beak.

(a)

Larynx

Trachea

(b)

Upper beak

Larynx

Tongue

Lower beak

Gastric lavage

This procedure requires the patient to be unconscious or under a general anaesthetic and should

AGENTS USED TO INDUCE VOMITING

Washing soda	One or two pea-sized crystals on the back of the tongue.
Apomorphine	0.1mg/kg s/c (only available at the surgery and to be given only under the direction of the veterinary surgeon, but very effective).
Xylazine	3.0mg/kg i/m (subject to the same restrictions as apomorphine).
Mustard	2 teaspoonfuls in a cup of warm water if nothing else is available.

Fig. 3.14. Agents to induce vomiting.

AGENTS USED TO BIND POISONS

BCK granules:	1–3 tablespoonsful (depending upon the size of the patient) mixed to a slurry with water.
Charcoal:	Weigh the patient and allow 1g activated charcoal/kg bodyweight. Make up to a suspension by adding 5ml water for every gram of charcoal used.

Fig. 3.15. Agents to bind poisons.

only be performed under the direct supervision of the veterinary surgeon. Warm water or saline is given by stomach tube and then the stomach is drained to wash out the poison. After several flushings, the fluid coming out of the stomach should run clear and then absorbent material (e.g. charcoal, fuller's earth, universal antidote, BCK granules) can be pumped in to absorb any remaining poison. This is a time-consuming and messy procedure, but can be very rewarding.

Preventing absorption from the alimentary tract

If the poison is corrosive or was eaten more than 4 hours previously, there is nothing which can be done except the following:

- Hasten the passage of the ingesta as much as possible so that the poison passes through quickly (by using saline purges). This is not advisable in an already shocked patient or one with intestines already inflamed by the passage of a corrosive poison.
- Give inert, absorptive material by mouth so that the poison is bound to the ingesta in the gut lumen and is not available for absorption through the intestinal mucosa into the circulation (Fig. 3.15).

Treating the symptoms

In many cases, drugs are needed to control the symptoms of poisonings. These can only be administered by the veterinary surgeon but in the meantime the veterinary nurse can ensure that everything is prepared so that there is no delay caused by searching for the appropriate drugs. However, there are some vital nursing procedures which can be initiated immediately:

- Maintain oxygenation of the depressed patient.
- Give demulcents for gastrointestinal irritation.
- Administer fluids.
- Keep the patient comfortable.
- Prepare drugs to counter symptoms.

Maintaining oxygenation of the depressed patient. If the animal is **dyspnoeic** (struggling to breathe), cyanosed or unconscious, it should be treated as for asphyxiation. Doxapram may be given in the form of drops if breathing ceases.

Giving demulsants for gastrointestinal irritation. The principle is to coat the alimentary lining with a soothing substance. Mix a beaten raw egg with a little milk and one teaspoonful of sugar and give by mouth. The proteins of the egg and milk coagulate and are deposited on the mucosal surface; the sugar acts to soothe the tissues.

The owner can be advised to give this demulcent at home (especially in cases of corrosive poisoning) to attempt to lessen the damage to the tract and it can also be useful where vomiting and diarrhoea are already evident **but only if the patient is fully conscious and there are no other symptoms** such as excitability or depression. The owner *must* be told that, if other symptoms develop, the animal should be brought to the surgery.

Administration of fluids. As most poisons are metabolised or detoxified by the liver and excreted through the kidneys, it is important to give fluid therapy (Chapter 21) to enable a more rapid flushing of the poison from the body. Many poisons also actively damage the kidney tissue as they are excreted, but this effect can be decreased by ensuring that the urine is as dilute as possible so that the concentration of the poison in the urine is reduced.

Although a conscious animal may be encouraged to drink, it is impossible to ensure adequate fluid intake by mouth and the only effective ways to promote kidney dialysis are as follows:

- **Set up an intravenous drip.** Use lactated Ringer's solution because this will also correct any metabolic acidosis caused by toxic damage to body tissues. As usual, the drip should be warmed unless the poison is one which has caused hyperthermia and the rectal temperature is climbing off the scale.
- **Make ready a diuretic** to increase the rate of excretion by the kidneys to use on the veterinary surgeon's instructions.

Keeping the patient comfortable. Some poisons (e.g. alphachloralose) depress the body temperature. If the rectal temperature is below normal, the patient should be treated for hypothermia. Conversely, poisons such as dinitro herbicides (2,4-dinitrophenol and dinitro-orthocresol) raise the body temperature so that these patients may suffer from hyperthermia and need to be kept as cool as possible. Treatment for hypothermia and hyperthermia is described in the section on Unconsciousness (p. 85).

Giving drugs to counter symptoms. The veterinary nurse may not administer prescription-only medicines without the knowledge and consent of a veterinary surgeon but drugs may be prepared so that they are ready for administration as directed by the veterinarian in charge of the case:

- **Barbiturates** (e.g. thiopentone, pentobarbitone) or **diazepam** may be required for convulsing or over-reactive (**hyperaesthetic**) patients.
- **Doxapram** may be given where the depression of the central nervous system is so severe that breathing ceases.

Preparation of specific antidotes

Unfortunately, most poisons do not have specific antidotes or ones that are readily available in veterinary practice. There are a few exceptions, such as warfarin-type rat poisons, where the antidote is vitamin K, and organophosphorus compounds, where the antidote is atropine. Again, these are prescription-only medicines and the veterinary nurse may not administer them unless directed to do so by a veterinary surgeon.

Specific Poisons

This section is included only to give the veterinary nurse an indication of the relative toxic effects and treatments of the most common poisons encountered in veterinary practice (based on the *Veterinary Poisons Information Service Report*, 1992). When the owner makes the initial telephone call to report an incident involving a *known* substance, the veterinary nurse must be able to give accurate advice immediately or within minutes, but the notes in Fig. 3.16 are *not* designed to ensure that the veterinary nurse can diagnose which poison has been consumed or absorbed. There are so many toxic compounds encountered in everyday life that it requires a toxicology textbook to describe all the effects, signs and treatments of all toxic agents and the veterinary nurse should consult the publications listed at the end of this chapter for further information.

Haemorrhage

Haemorrhage is bleeding from any part of the body and is usually caused by injury, but may also occur when blood vessels are affected by disease.

Any haemorrhage must be regarded as serious, for a sudden or severe loss of blood may result in death. Even a slight haemorrhage which continues over a long period may result in loss of blood which jeopardises the life of the patient.

Classification

Haemorrhage classification (Fig. 3.17) depends on the answers to three questions:

- **What** type of blood vessel is damaged?
- **When** does the haemorrhage occur?
- **Where** did the blood escape to?

Type of blood vessel damaged

- **Arterial haemorrhage.** This is the most serious form of haemorrhage. Blood from an artery is bright red and spurts forcefully from the wound, the spurts synchronised with the heart beat. The blood may escape with such force that it sprays walls and floor 2m away or more, but this depends upon the size of the severed artery. If the wound is large, the blood will be seen to be coming from the side of the wound nearest the heart. Usually a definite bleeding point can be detected.
- **Venous haemorrhage.** This is slightly less serious than arterial haemorrhage but rapid blood loss will still occur if a large vein is damaged. Venous haemorrhage is usually easier to control, since the force of the blood loss is never as great as with arterial haemorrhage. Blood from a vein is darker in colour than arterial blood and issues from the wound in a steady stream. When a large vein is damaged, however, the blood loss may pulsate slightly in time with the heart beat but there is no forceful spurting as is seen in arterial haemorrhage. In large wounds, the blood will issue from the side furthest from the heart and a definite bleeding point is visible.
- **Capillary haemorrhage.** Bleeding from damaged capillaries occurs in all wounds, as the fragile capillary wall is easily damaged. The blood escapes from multiple, pinpoint sources in the tissues and oozes from the wound with very little force. No definite bleeding points are visible.
- **Mixed haemorrhage.** The arteries and veins of the body usually lie very close to one another, so that often all three types of blood vessel are injured simultaneously. When an artery and vein are severed at the same time, the haemorrhage may be so great that the characteristics of arterial haemorrhage are not detectable.

Time of blood loss

- **Primary haemorrhage.** This occurs as the immediate result of damage to the blood vessel wall.
- **Reactionary haemorrhage.** The primary haemorrhage will cause a drop in blood pressure, which may be sufficiently severe to slow the rate at which the blood escapes from the wound. As the blood flow lessens, a blood clot can form around the end of the damaged vessel and seal it. However, if the blood pressure rises again within the next 24 hours (e.g. as the animal recovers from shock or is given

COMMON POISONS – EFFECTS AND TREATMENTS

	Causes	Effects	Treatment
Medicines ACP misuse	Accidental overdosing with tablets in the house. Idiosyncratic reaction to the drug.	Depression or collapse. (Cats may become hyperaesthetic.) Vasodilation leads to decreased blood pressure and increased susceptibility to heatstroke on warm days. Brachiocephalic dogs are especially likely to suffer. Increased likelihood of fits in epileptic animals.	Induce vomiting if many tablets have been eaten (unlikely, since few surgeries prescribe more than a few tablets for specific occasions.) Treat symptoms of collapse/shock, heatstroke and epilepsy as described elsewhere in this chapter.
Abnormal response (Anaphylactic reaction)	Allergic-type response to medication, e.g. vaccination, antibiotics.	Depression, occasionally vomiting and diarrhoea, swelling of injection sites. Severe reactions result in.collapse, with signs of shock.	Swellings may have cold compresses applied. Treat for shock if collapsed and maintain if unconscious. Prepare corticosteroid injection.
Non-steroidal anti-inflammatory drugs (NSAIDs)	Owners using human preparations on their animals (dosing their pets with so called pain killers). Dogs 'stealing' owners' medications. *Aspirin* – particularly toxic in cats. *Ibuprofen, Flurbiprofen and Naproxen* – May be rapidly fatal in some dogs. *Phenylbutazone* – more toxic to cats than dogs.	*Aspirin* – Depression. Gastric irritation, leading to vomiting and anorexia. Cats may show some incoordination. *Ibuprofen and Flurbiprofen* – Gastric ulceration and perforation in dogs leads to vomiting and haematemesis, followed by diarrhoea with melaena. Kidney damage may cause acute and fatal renal failure. Dehydration due to fluid losses. *Naproxen* – Gastric inflammation and ulceration leading to vomiting and melaena. Anaemia due to low-grade blood loss. Dehydration.	Stop medication with the drugs. *Before symptoms show*, induce vomiting as soon as possible. *If showing symptoms*, give absorptive preparations and/or demulcents. Dosing with activated charcoal is vital in cases of aspirin poisoning and should be given immediately after vomiting ceases. Prepare intravenous fluids. Prepare **cimetidine** for intravenous injection in cases of naproxen poisoning.
Paracetamol	Owner administered dose or tablet packet chewed.	Dogs tolerate paracetamol well but cats are easily poisoned by as little as half a 500mg tablet. Poisoning with paracetamol results in haemoglobin being changed to methaemoglobin, which is incapable of transporting oxygen. *Signs* Cyanosis. Depression or excitement. Incoordination due to hypoxia. Facial swelling.	Induce vomiting if no symptoms shown. Give absorptive material by mouth but NOT before consulting veterinary surgeon – if **N-acetyl cysteine** is to be used, the absorptive material may also prevent the absorption of this antidote. Provide oxygen if any sign of cyanosis; ensure that the animal rests as much as possible. Prepare **methionine** or N-acetyl cysteine (human preparation 'Parvolex') for oral administration.
Salbutamol	Human preparations that are used to treat asthma and for premature labour.	Stimulation of the sympathetic nervous system, causing peripheral vasodilation and rapid heart rate (tachycardia). Panting respiration. Muscle weakness.	General first aid treatment but beta blockers may be needed if the heart rate becomes excessively high.
Herbicides Chlorates	Ingestion of weedkillers or drinking from contaminated puddles – this substance does not degrade readily after use.	Vomiting and diarrhoea with abdominal pain. Cyanosis of mucosa, turning to a muddy brown colour (blood becomes chocolate in colour because poison causes the formation of methaemoglobin – see Paracetamol).	General first aid treatment. Prepare **methylene blue** injection.
Dinitro compounds	Ingestion of 2,4, dinitrophenol (2,4,D) or dinitro-orthocresol (2,4,5,T).	Depression, listlessnes, muscle weakness. Rapid respiration and dyspnoea. Hyperthermia with sweating. Urine is almost fluorescent yellow/green.	General first aid treatment. Monitor rectal temperature to detect hyperthermia.
Paraquat	Ingesting weedkiller (though this product is rapidly absorbed onto the soil after application, which renders it harmless). Paraquat has been used in malicious poisonings, but most cases are due to accidents.	Inflammation of the mouth and tongue. Vomiting and diarrhoea, with abdominal pain. Depression and progressive respiratory distress and cyanosis over a period of days, resulting in death.	**Induce vomiting** as soon as ingestion of this chemical is suspected. Even though this is an irritant poison, the effects of the absorbed poison are so severe that treatment is usually hopeless and the only hope is to remove the poison from the alimentary tract as soon as possible. Administering fuller's earth is also helpful because the poison will bind to the fuller's earth and be rendered inactive.

Fig. 3.16.—continued

COMMON POISONS – EFFECTS AND TREATMENTS

	Causes	Effects	Treatment
Insecticides Borax	Ant killers (e.g. 'Nippon') which are based on honey and therefore very attractive to dogs.	Vomiting and diarrhoea. Collapse, convulsions and possible paralysis. Poisoning may be fatal.	General first aid treatment.
Organophosphates	Overdosing with insecticidal sprays, chewing insecticidal collars, etc.	Vomiting and diarrhoea. Salivation. Constricted pupils. Muscular twitching, excitement, followed by weakness, incoordination. Depression or convulsions.	General first aid treatment. Prepare **atropine sulphate** for injection.
Organochlorines	Woodworm treatments and other insecticides (aldrin, dieldrin, gamma BHC etc). Many products are now withdrawn from sale but old stocks still exist.	Involuntary twitching of muscles, especially facial, fore and hindlimbs and convulsions. Behavioural changes, e.g. aggression, pacing, apprehension, frenzy.	Wash off contamination. Administer absorptive material and/or liquid paraffin to decrease absorption. **Fatty foods and drinks** (including milk) **must not be given** as they may increase absorption of the poison. Prepare **barbiturate** injection to control convulsions.
Molluscicides Carbamate	See Organophosphates		
Metaldehyde	Ingestion of slug bait, which some dogs and cats seem to find very palatable.	Incoordination leading to hyperaesthesia and convulsions. Rapid pulse and respiration and possibly cyanosis.	General first aid treatment. Dosing with liquid paraffin may delay adsorption of poison as long as it is given before the patient shows any symptoms (do not dose the unconscious patient). Prepare **barbiturate** injection to control convulsions.
Rodenticides Alphachloralose	Rat baits and preparations to control pigeon and seabird populations.	Poison acts by lowering the body temperature. Progressive depression, incoordination and coma with hypothermia.	General first aid treatment but warmth is essential.
Anticoagulant preparations	Rat baits. Several different compounds come under this heading: Warfarin, Coumatetralyl, Chlorophacinone, Difenacoum, Brodifacoum, Bromadiolone.	Interference with clotting mechanism results in haemorrhages in the mucosae, bruising and haematomata, swollen joints, etc.	General first aid treatment. Prepare injections of vitamin K. Large and repeated dosing may be necessary.
Household chemicals Alcohol	Ingestion of alcoholic drink or fermenting grain (especially likely with pups).	Hyperaesthesia, incoordination, collapse and even death.	Induce vomiting and provide general first aid treatment.
Disinfectants	Household disinfectants, when diluted to correct strength, do not cause a problem but are often used undiluted or incorrectly diluted by over-zealous owners.		
	Phenols – **Cats are particularly susceptible to poisoning by phenols.** Licking paws after walking on wet surfaces recently cleaned with undiluted or incorrectly diluted solutions of disinfectant. Grooming coat after accidental spraying or splashing with strong disinfectant solutions.	**These are corrosive poisons with a strong, distinctive odour** e.g. pine disinfectants. Convulsions, coma and death in acute poisoning cases. Less acute cases may have inflamed mouths (stomatitis) and occasionally ulcers in the mouth. Animals may also vomit and have diarrhoea and abdominal pain.	**Do not induce vomiting**. General first aid treatment, including thorough washing of contaminated fur.

Fig. 3.16.—continued

COMMON POISONS – EFFECTS AND TREATMENTS

	Causes	Effects	Treatment
	Quaternary ammonium compounds – as for phenols.	These are also corrosive poisons but are odourless. Depression and anorexia. Occasionally vomiting. Salivation, stomatitis and mouth ulcers, especially on the tongue tip. Skin ulcerations if compound not washed off quickly.	As for phenols.
Ethylene glycol (antifreeze)	Ingestion of water drained from car radiators (dogs seem particularly prone to drink this).	Incoordination, depression and rapid breathing. Later animal may become uraemic.	General first aid treatment. **Ethanol** is the specific antidote and intravenous injections may be prepared if available at the surgery.
Petroleum products	Usually a problem in cats which have fallen into containers of sump oil, drained from cars. Accidental spillages of petrol, paraffin etc. Caking of tar in the paws.	These are very corrosive poisons with a distinctive odour. Depression, vomiting, collapse and death if enough ingested. If submersed in the liquid, may also suffer an aspiration pneumonia, which is very severe because of the extremely irritant nature of the inhaled liquid. Inflammation of the in-contact skin and mouth, especially the tongue if the animal has been allowed to groom.	**Do not induce vomiting.** General first aid treatment, including giving olive oil by mouth to decrease the absorption of the toxins.
Reptile Bites	The only indigenous venomous snake in Britain is the adder (*Vipera berus*) but other exotic reptiles are now being kept in greater and greater numbers by the public and should one of these animals escape, it is possible that it might bite the family pet. Although cats are rarely bitten, snake bites can be a problem in dogs because they are more likely to try to attack an escaping snake or to disturb one whilst out walking. The adder has a characteristic dark "V" or "X" marking on the head, and dark zig-zag markings along the length of its body. It is commonly found basking on warm sunny days on dry well-maintained heathland. When disturbed, it may strike and therefore bites are usually inflicted on the head, neck or legs of the sniffing dog.	Following a bite from an adder, the tissues swell rapidly and to such an extent that the two fang marks are rarely visible. The swelling is very painful and oedematous, and may be serious if it affects the mouth or throat area to cause narrowing or blockage of the airway. The patient is often dull and depressed, but may show signs of great distress, and may, on occasion, collapse. The effects of bites from other reptiles depends upon the species involved. Some reptiles are non-poisonous, when the only sign wil be a set of puncture wounds but other snakes can be so venomous that the patient dies very quickly.	If the reptile is a non-poisonous species, the bite should be treated as described. If the bite was poisoned, the normal principles must be applied: (a) Identify the poison involved. In the case of an exotic reptile, the owner will usually know the species responsible. (b) Prevent further absorption of the poison. The wounds should be thoroughly flushed with cold sterile saline if possible to wash out as much toxin as possible and to encourage vasoconstriction in the area so the absorption of toxins into the blood stream is kept to a minimum. Ice packs should be applied to maintain the vasoconstriction and alleviate the pain (packing a plastic bag with crushed ice or frozen peas etc. makes a useful ice pack!) and the animal should be made to rest so the general circulation is slowed as much as possible. (c) Treat the symptoms. The main symptoms will be shock, followed by collapse, unconsciousness and death and general first aid measures should be applied. Corticosteroids, antihistamines, diuretics, antibiotics, calcium and Vitamin D have all been used in the treatment of these wounds. (d) Antidotes. Antivenom for adder bites is called Zagreb and should be held at all major accident and emergency departments of local hospitals. It may well save valuable time if the veterinary nurse can telephone the local casualty department, explain the situation and ask if any antivenom is available. Antivenoms for rare and exotic species are kept at the VPIS in London and at the Liverpool School of Hygeine and Tropical Medicine. Therefore, the VPIS should be contacted for advice on antidote sources for these bites.

Fig. 3.16.—continued ⬥

intravenous fluid therapy), this clot may be displaced and the haemorrhage will recur.

- **Secondary haemorrhage.** This is haemorrhage that recurs from the damaged vessel because bacteria have invaded the wound and destroyed the blood clot and the new repair tissue. It may occur any time after the first 24 hours but is usually seen at 3–10 days following the injury.

COMMON POISONS – EFFECTS AND TREATMENTS			
	Causes	**Effects**	**Treatment**
Toad Poisoning	The Common Toad secretes toxic venom on to its body surface and, although very few animals will try to pick them up, it is not unknown for the unwary pup to do so and be poisoned.	Dogs mouthing toads may show signs of excessive salivation, and occasionally some distress. If part of the toad has been eaten, nervous signs may be shown.	Little treatment is usually necessary, since the dog usually drops the toad hurriedly and the salivation washes the venom out of the mouth. Nervous signs, if shown, may need symptomatic treatment and may require treatment with atropine or corticosteroids.
Insect Stings	Wasp and bee strings are very common in the summer and early autumn months and usually affect the young puppy or kitten as it chases and catches the insect. The areas most affected are therefore the mouth or around the lips, but occasionally the feet may be stung if the kitten "bats" the insect with its paws.	Stings in the mouth are rarely severe but may cause considerable swelling, excessive salivation and discomfort. This soon subsides rapidly after about an hour. Stings in the pharyngeal area could cause sufficient swelling to obstruct the airway. The dog will often paw at its mouth and, if the swelling is marked, the breathing may become laboured. Some animals develop a severe allergic reaction to the sting and may collapse, with pale, cold mucous membranes.	In event of collapse, the animal should be given first aid for shock and the assistance of a veterinary surgeon obtained as soon as possible. Intravenous corticosteroid injections may be prepared. If the owners report that the animal has been stung at the back of the mouth, they must be warned of the possibility of airway obstruction and advised to keep the patient under close observation for the next hour. In the event of airway restriction, the animal should be brought to the surgery immediately and treated as prescribed under "Asphyxia". Wasps rarely leave the sting behind, but bees invariably do. In all cases, the area should be examined to see if the poison sacs remain. The sting shaft is barbed and the barbs point backwards, so that once the stinger has penetrated the skin, it cannot be withdrawn and the posterior segment of the abdomen is torn away as the bee flies away. The muscles in the sting continue to work, forcing the sting deeper into the body tissues and emptying the poison sacs at the same time to cause greater and greater inflammation. Therefore, owners should be advised to scrape the sting away immediately before it has time to penetrate the tissues. A scraping action ensures that the entire sting is removed without disturbing the poison sacs, whereas grasping the sting with tweezers will empty the poison sacs and worsen the inflammation and pain. If the sting has been present for a few minutes, it is impossible to scrape off the sting because it is too embedded. Tweezers have to be used but it is best to try to grasp the top of the sting, not the poison sac portion. Removal can be difficult because of the barbs on the sting shaft. Bee stings inside the mouth can then be washed with an alkaline solution (one dessertspoon of bicarbonate of soda to half a litre of water or one tablespoon of household ammonia to quarter of a litre of water); wasp stings may be washed with a dilute solution of vinegar. A small sponge or pad of cotton wool can be used to apply the solutions to the area. Following gentle swabbing, ice packs should be used to alleviate the pain and reduce the swelling. These can be usefully fashioned at home by filling a small plastic bag with frozen peas or similar vegetables, if not, crushed ice is immediately available. If the swelling does not respond to any of these measures, the patient should be brought to the surgery. The veterinary nurse should prepare injections of corticosteriods and possibly calcium and vitamin D preparations, which some veterinary surgeons use because these compounds stabilize the cell membranes and prevent further swelling and oedema of the area.

Fig. 3.16. Toxic agents.

CLASSIFICATION OF HAEMORRHAGE TYPE		
Type of blood vessel damaged:		
Arterial	**Venous**	**Capillary**
Bright red blood Pumps forcefully	Dark red blood No or little spurting from wound	Bright red blood A small volume which oozes slowly from damaged tissues throughout the wound
Issues from side nearest heart Definite bleeding point	Issues from the side furthest from the heart Definite bleeding point	No definite bleeding point
Time at which bleeding occurs:		
Primary	**Reactionary**	**Secondary**
Immediately	Within 24–48 hours	3–10 days post trauma
Destination of blood loss		
Externally – to body surface and clearly visible	Internally – into body tissues/cavities. Hidden	

Fig. 3.17. Classification of haemorrhage.

Destination of blood loss

- **External haemorrhage**. When the blood escapes on to the body surface, it is termed external haemorrhage. It may come from obvious open wounds or escape from regions such as the nose, ear, mouth, stomach linings, bowels, urinary tract or uterus.
- **Internal haemorrhage**. If the blood is lost into the tissues or into a cavity such as the thoracic or abdominal cavity, it cannot be seen and is termed internal haemorrhage. Such haemorrhage occurs:
- if there is severe muscular bruising;
- when an internal organ is damaged (such as lungs, liver or spleen);
- if there is disease (e.g. tumours) which erodes blood-vessel walls.

It is very difficult to detect internal haemorrhage although it may cause swelling of the tissues or distension of a body cavity such as the abdomen or joint capsules. In most cases, the only way to detect severe internal haemorrhage is by recognising the general signs of shock which the haemorrhage produces.

Natural Arrest of Haemorrhage

Four factors tend to stop initial bleeding:

- Retraction of the cut ends of the blood vessels.
- Falling blood pressure.
- Back pressure.
- Blood clotting.

Retraction of cut ends

Retraction of cut ends of arteries, arterioles and large veins is due to the elastic nature of their walls. When the cut ends recoil, the elastic tissues contract and bunch up the end of the vessel. This closes or reduces the size of the aperture through which blood is flowing. Tearing of the vessel produces a better

recoil as the vessel is stretched before it breaks. Therefore a lacerated wound bleeds less than an incised wound. A lessening of blood flow allows a more rapid clot formation to seal the blood vessel completely.

Fall in blood pressure

Loss of blood will result in lowered blood pressure so that less blood reaches the affected vessel and there is less pressure to force it out of the cut end of the vessel.

Back pressure

Internal haemorrhage will eventually fill the cavity (e.g. abdomen) or distend the surrounding tissues (**bruising**) until the lowered blood pressure *in* the severed vessel is equal to the pressure of the fluid *surrounding* the severed end of the vessel. When the pressures are equal, no further blood can escape from the damaged blood vessel.

Blood clotting

Clotting takes place in the wound, both within and around the cut end of the vessel. This clot acts as a plug, sealing the severed vessel and preventing further blood loss. (This mechanism cannot work in cases of warfarin poisoning.)

Repair of Blood Vessels

When haemorrhage has been arrested, the body will repair the damaged vessel. If this is not possible (e.g. in complete severance of a vessel, where the two ends have recoiled away from each other) the vessel will become permanently sealed. The flow of blood will be redirected via other vessels, which enlarge to cope with the increased flow. New vessels will develop to re-establish the natural circulation. This bypass system works well unless all arteries

48   S. M. Hiscock

supplying a part of the body are severed. The circulation cannot then be re-established in time to prevent the tissues dying, as is often seen in crushing injuries to the tail and digits.

First Aid Treatments of Haemorrhage

A number of methods can be used to stop bleeding:

- Direct digital pressure.
- Use of artery forceps.
- Pad and pressure bandage.
- Pressure points.
- Tourniquet.

The risks, advantages and disadvantages of each method are described in Fig. 3.18.

Direct digital pressure

Haemorrhage is controlled by applying pressure to the wound with *clean* hands. It is best to apply the fingers to the *intact* skin on either side of the wound and to pinch the wound edges together gently to avoid further bacterial contamination of the wound itself. The finger pressure will collapse the walls of the severed blood vessels, so preventing blood loss from the cut ends (Fig. 3.19).

If the wound is too large to apply effective pressure along its entire margin, clean hands or a piece of clean, non-fluffy material (e.g. a tea towel) should be placed in the wound and direct pressure applied to the bleeding points in the wound itself.

METHODS FOR STOPPING BLEEDING: RISKS, ADVANTAGES AND DISADVANTAGES			
	Risks	Advantages	Disadvantages
Direct digital pressure	If a foreign body is suspected in the wound, care must be taken not to push it deeper. Similarly, in the case of underlying fractures, care must be taken not to displace fracture fragments.	(i) Direct pressure on a wound, particularly when applied to a bleeding point, is both quick and effective and stops blood loss immediately. (ii) It needs no equipment other than a clean finger and thumb – instruments which are always available. (iii) This method alone may be sufficient to control venous haemorrhage because constant digital pressure for five minutes stops the flow for a sufficient time to allow a clot to form and this clot may well seal the blood vessel. However, a constant pressure must be maintained for this time because lessening the pressure even for a few seconds allows the haemorrhage to start again, destroying any clot structure which may have begun to form in the blood vessel. It is a wise precaution to apply a pressure bandage to the wound in any case, even if the haemorrhage has completely stopped, because the blood vessels may also start to haemorrhage again as the animal moves and the blood pressure rises. (iv) If there is a protruding foreign body, direct digital pressure can be applied without disturbing the foreign body as pressure can be applied to the wound edges rather than into the wound itself.	This is a temporary emergency measure and is not suitable for the longer term control of haemorrhage.
Use of artery forceps	Arteries and nerves commonly lie close together and fishing blindly in a wound with artery forceps may crush these nerves to functionless pulp. The artery forceps should never be used as a clamp across a bleeding wound.	This method permanently controls haemorrhage.	(i) It can be difficult to identify the cut end of an artery when blood is pumping out of the wound. To clear the field, it is often necessary to apply direct digital pressure or a tourniquet to stop the haemorrhage temporarily so that the wound can be examined and the end of the cut vessel identified, clamped and ligated. If the vessel cannot be identified (and these vessels may be surprisingly small), the digital pressure or tourniquet should be released gradually whilst the wound is examined carefully to detect the first sign of bleeding which will mark the location of the offending blood vessel.

Fig. 3.18.—continued

METHODS FOR STOPPING BLEEDING: RISKS, ADVANTAGES AND DISADVANTAGES

	Risks	Advantages	Disadvantages
			(ii) This method requires specialised equipment (artery forceps and ligation material). In an emergency, household tweezers and cotton thread may have to be substituted to save the animal's life.
Pad and pressure bandage	Where there is an embedded protruding foreign body or shallow underlying fracture, a ring pad should be used so that the foreign body is not driven deeper into the tissues or the fracture is not complicated or displaced. The ring pad may be fashioned from material or several thick rolls of bandage can be arranged as a ring around the wound and bandaged in position to create the same effect. If the foreign body is large and protudes a long way, it may also be necessary to carefuylly cut off the protruding end so that the ring can be effective. The principle behind ring pads is that they should only prevent overlying pressure bandages from applying direct pressure to the protected area. However, since the pressure bandage will still apply pressure to the ring pad, it forces the pad down and, in so doing, effectively creates a ring of direct digital pressure around the wound. This will prevent haemorrhage from superficial blood vessels but does not affect the haemorrhage which wells up from the deep tissues around a fracture site. The deep haemorrhage is controlled by back pressure as the area in the centre of the ring fills with blood until the pressures equalise. (Penetrating foreign bodies usually act as a plug in the wound they have created and so deep external haemorrhage is rarely a problem in these cases).	(i) Pressure bandages are easy to apply and comfortable for the animal. (ii) The bandage can be left in place until the veterinary surgeon attends the case, and needs little attention from the veterinary nurse except continued observation to ensure that the dressing is not disturbed and that blood is not seeping through the bandage. (iii) Most forms of haemorrhage respond well to this method of control and this is the commonest form of first aid for haemorrhage used in practice.	(i) This method requires first aid equpment and a certain degree of co-operation from the patient. (ii) Some areas of the body can be difficult to bandage effectively, e.g. the shoulder and upper thigh regions.
Pressure points	Only major arterial haemorrhage is controlled using this method so blood loss will continue from other vessels. As the tissues of the lower limb which are supplied by the artery will also be deprived of an arterial blood supply, this method can only be used for a limited period (see Tourniquet).	(i) Equipment (i.e. fingers) is always available. (ii) Arterial haemorrhage is quickly controlled, allowing identification of bleeding points and ligation of severed vessels. (iii) In cases where the damaged tissues are macerated beyond recognition (e.g. loss of limbs or severe injuries following road accidents), these pressure points allow haemorrhage control at a site far removed from the injured area, which lessens the pain for the animal.	(i) Pressure points can be difficult to find. Plenty of practice in detecting the pulse of normal animals in these sites is essential in order to be confident of finding the correct location in an emergency case, where the blood pressure may be very low. (ii) This procedure does not immediately cause all bleeding to cease, because venous bleeding is unaffected and will continue. (iii) As with direct digital pressure, this is only a temporary measure and some other form of control such as ligating the artery must be applied to contain the haemorrhage if veterinary help is delayed for any length of time.
Tourniquet	A tourniquet should be used for as short a time as possible because it cuts the circulation to all the tissues of the limb or tail so that they will start to die from the moment the tourniquet is applied. Therefore, a tourniquet should never be left in place for more than 15 minutes before being released for at least 1 minute to allow blood to circulate and revive these tissues.	(i) Tourniquets are quick and easy to apply. (ii) No special equipment is necessary. If nothing is available, the limb or tail may be held as tightly as possible by hand. This usually controls the haemorrhage sufficiently until a tourniquet can be found or the haemorrhage is controlled by some other means.	(i) All the blood supply to the limb or tail is cut off. (ii) Tissues are damaged at the point of application because of the pressure exerted by the tourniquet. (iii) Constant observation of the patient is essential.

Fig. 3.18. Methods of stopping bleeding: risks, advantages and disadvantages.

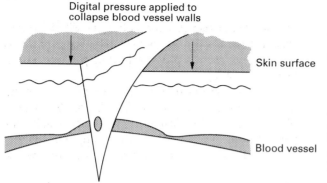

Digital pressure applied to
collapse blood vessel walls

Skin surface

Blood vessel

Fig. 3.19. Cross-section of a wound showing direct digital
pressure to stop bleeding.

Use of artery forceps

In cases of severe arterial haemorrhage, it is acceptable for a skilled nurse to attempt to use a pair of artery forceps to occlude the offending vessel and then ligate it with catgut. **This procedure must only be considered when the cut end of the artery can be clearly seen.**

Pad and pressure bandage

A pad of gauze swabs or gauze overlaid by a thick pad of cotton wool is applied to the wound and bandaged very firmly into position. If the wound is high up on a limb, the whole leg may need to be bandaged because otherwise the tissues below the bandaged area will swell.

If the bleeding continues, a second pad may be bandaged over the first; it is best not to remove the first dressing or the blood clots will be disturbed to restart the haemorrhage. Deep wounds may need to be packed with sterile gauze before the pressure pad is applied.

If internal bleeding is suspected, a crepe bandage may be firmly applied to the area, effectively

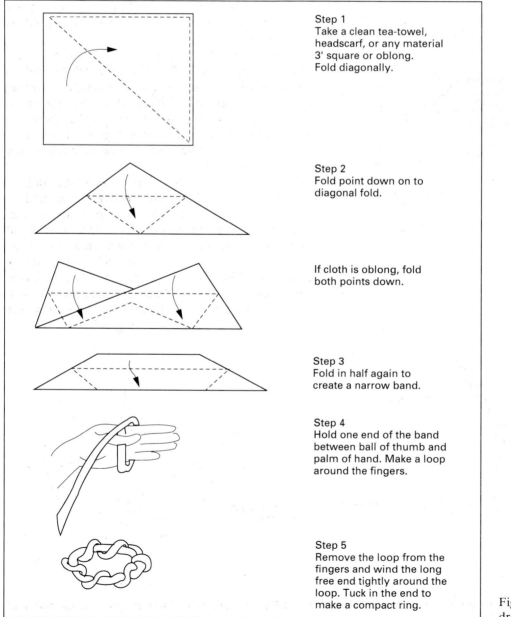

Step 1
Take a clean tea-towel, headscarf, or any material 3' square or oblong.
Fold diagonally.

Step 2
Fold point down on to diagonal fold.

If cloth is oblong, fold both points down.

Step 3
Fold in half again to create a narrow band.

Step 4
Hold one end of the band between ball of thumb and palm of hand. Make a loop around the fingers.

Step 5
Remove the loop from the fingers and wind the long free end tightly around the loop. Tuck in the end to make a compact ring.

Fig. 3.20. Ring-pad dressing.

increasing the back pressure in the affected tissues. Blood loss is quickly controlled and there should be minimal swelling and bruising of the tissues.

Pressure points

A pressure point is a site in the body where it is possible to press an artery against a bone. The pressure of the artery against the bone prevents the flow of blood along the vessel and its escaping from the wound further down the leg or tail. The method is limited to three points in the dog and cat:

- **The brachial artery** as it runs down the medial shaft of the humerus and swings cranially behind the fleshy biceps muscle (Fig. 3.22). The pulse can clearly be felt in the distal third of the humerus. Pressure applied to this vessel will arrest serious arterial haemorrhage from below the elbow. (Note that this pressure point is not easily found and so it is a good idea to practise finding the pulse on a healthy animal.)
- **The femoral artery** as it passes obliquely over the proximal third of the femur on the medial aspect of the thigh. It lies just in front of the small taut pectineus muscle, and pressure applied to this vessel will arrest arterial haemorrhage from below the stifle.
- **The coccygeal artery** as it passes backwards along the underside of the tail (Fig. 3.23). Pressure at the root of the tail where the pulse can easily be felt, ventral to the coccygeal vertebrae, will arrest arterial haemorrhage from the rest of the tail.

Tourniquet

A tourniquet stops bleeding by constricting all the arteries supplying blood to a wound on a limb or a tail. Correct application is essential, and the tourniquet should only be used in cases where there is severe haemorrhage that cannot be controlled by other methods.

Many forms of tourniquet are available, the usual one consisting of a flat elastic bandage with a fastening clip. In an emergency, a length of strong bandage or material, a piece of rubber tubing or thick elastic band or a narrow belt can be effectively applied. String and rope are not good materials as they dig in and cause severe tissue damage at the point of application.

The tourniquet is fixed firmly round the limb or tail, at a point a few inches above the wound. It should be adjusted so that the pressure is just sufficient to stop the haemorrhage. This is achieved by adjusting the clip of the conventional tourniquet. With other tourniquets, a half-hitch is tied firmly against the skin and then a stick or rod (e.g. ballpoint pen) is tied over the half-hitch. Twisting this stick will twist and gradually tighten the tourniquet until the haemorrhage is just controlled (Fig. 3.24).

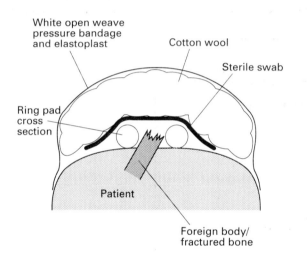

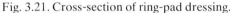

Fig. 3.21. Cross-section of ring-pad dressing.

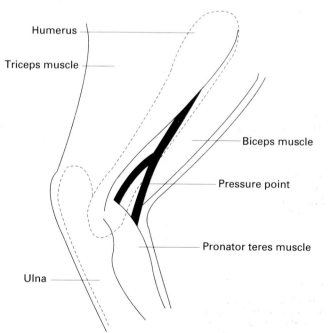

Fig. 3.22. Brachial artery pressure point, medial aspect of elbow.

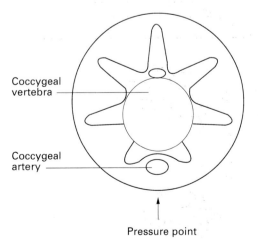

Fig. 3.23. Coccygeal artery pressure point, cross-section of tail base.

Some other method of control should be attempted as soon as the tourniquet has controlled the bleeding, e.g. ligating the large blood vessels or applying a pressure bandage. Then the tourniquet should be slackened off slowly and the wound or dressings observed for signs of further haemorrhage. If bleeding starts again and it is necessary to replace the tourniquet, it should be applied a little closer to the wound to allow the tissues at the original site to recover from the effects of the constriction. **At no time should a tourniquet be covered with a dressing and no animal should be returned to a kennel with a tourniquet in place.**

Wounds

The classification of wounds is set out in Fig. 3.25.

Definitions

A **wound** is an injury in which there is a forcible break in the continuity of the soft tissues.

An **open** wound is one where the injury causes a break in the covering of the body surface, i.e. skin or mucous membranes. These wounds can be seen and blood loss evaluated.

A **closed** wound is one where the injury does *not* cause a break in the body covering. This category includes anything from minor bruising to serious damage to internal organs, e.g. rupture of the spleen. The wounds cannot be seen and blood loss is difficult to evaluate.

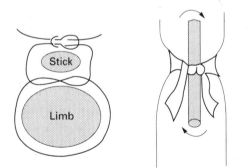

Fig. 3.24. Tourniquet.

CLASSIFICATION OF WOUNDS	
Open	Closed
Incised	Contusion
Lacerated	Haematoma
Puncture	Haemorrhage into body cavity
Abrasion	e.g. cranial cavity
	epidural space
	chambers of the eye
	thorax
	pericardium
	abdomen
	joint spaces

Fig. 3.25. Classification of wounds.

An **abrasion** is a wound where the epidermis has been eroded to expose the underlying dermis, i.e. the injury does not penetrate the entire skin thickness.

An **avulsed** wound is any wound in which a flap of skin has been forcibly plucked off or torn away from the underlying tissues and yet still remains attached at some point (Fig. 3.26(b) and (d)).

A **contused** wound is any wound in which there is bruising.

Open Wounds

Figures 3.26(a)–(f) and 3.27 illustrate and describe the characteristics of open wounds.

Incised wounds

Incised wounds may be caused by sharp cutting instruments such as knives or broken glass. Barbed-wire tears and claw injuries from cats may cause similar skin injury.

The edges are clean cut and clearly defined and usually gape, especially on movement. Avulsed incised wounds are often V-shaped and are commonly seen on the legs and feet where the pad has almost been sliced away when the animal stood on a piece of broken glass. Simple small incised wounds (say 1cm in length) may seal together very rapidly and remain closed, which can make them difficult to find. Incised wounds usually bleed freely as there is little elastic recoil from the cut ends of the blood vessels to allow natural arrest of haemorrhage. Such wounds often penetrate deeply to damage underlying structures such as nerves and tendons.

Incised wounds tend to heal quickly if the edges are held together, leaving little scar formation.

Lacerated wounds

These are the most common type of wound encountered in small animals, and are usually caused by road accidents, dog fights, tearing by barbed-wire etc. The wounds are irregular in shape, with jagged, uneven edges. Areas of skin may literally be worn away, especially following road accidents when the animal has been dragged along the road. The edges of any lacerated wound always gape because the skin has been torn apart.

The severity of these wounds depends on how deeply the wound penetrates, but often underlying muscle, tendons, ligaments and even bones may be affected. Haemorrhage, even from large wounds, is often surprisingly little as the ragged tearing of the blood vessels causes good elastic recoil and natural control of haemorrhage. There is, however, considerable risk of infection from ingrained dirt, saliva and bacterial contamination.

Healing is slow and there is usually considerable risk of extensive scar formation.

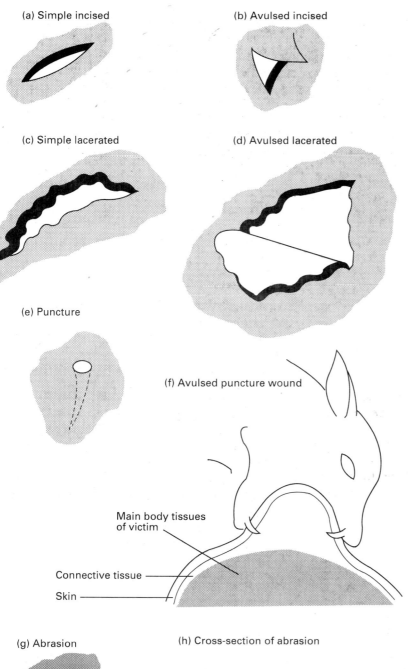

(a) Simple incised

(b) Avulsed incised

(c) Simple lacerated

(d) Avulsed lacerated

(e) Puncture

(f) Avulsed puncture wound

Main body tissues of victim

Connective tissue

Skin

(g) Abrasion

(h) Cross-section of abrasion

Epidermis

Dermis

Subcutis

Fig. 3.26. Open wounds and abrasions.

CHARACTERISTICS OF OPEN WOUNDS AND ABRASIONS			
Incised	**Lacerated**	**Puncture**	**Abrasion**
Any size	Any size	Small	Any size
Usually deep	May be deep	Deep wound	Superficial
Haemorrhage freely	Little haemorrhage	Little haemorrhage	Little haemorrhage
Gapes unless small	Gapes	Closes very quickly	No gaping skin edges
Rarely grossly contaminated	Often grossly contaminated	Often contaminated	Often contaminated
Heals rapidly by first intention	Heals slowly by granulation	Rapid healing if infection controlled	Rapid healing
May be avulsed	May be avulsed	Rarely avulsed	Cannot be convulsed
Rarely contused	Often contused	Often contused	May be contused
Little pain	Painful	Little pain unless infected	Painful

Fig. 3.27. Characteristics of open wounds and abrasions.

Puncture wounds

These are produced by blows from sharp pointed instruments such as nails, stakes, thorns or fish hooks, and also from the canine teeth in bite wounds. Airgun pellets and bullets also cause puncture wounds.

The actual skin wound may be quite small but this will often lead to a long narrow track which penetrates deeply into the underlying tissues. Puncture wounds commonly become infected because bacteria may be carried deep into the tissues at the time of injury. The small skin wound usually heals rapidly, trapping infection in the tissues, and an abscess will form. Bleeding from puncture wounds is often small and **such wounds are liable to be overlooked**. The only sign of such a wound may be a small tuft of matted, bloodstained fur over the site of the swollen wound.

In some staking injuries, the cause of the wound may be seen projecting from the surface. In other cases, the damaging foreign body may be hidden below the surface. Airgun slugs and shotgun pellets usually remain in the depths of the puncture wound but bullets can penetrate right through the body, leaving wounds at the points of both entrance and exit.

Occasionally avulsion wounds can occur (Fig. 3.26(f)) and are most often seen in the scruff following dog-fight injuries if the injured dog has been picked up or shaken by its opponent. The area of skin grasped by the teeth is pulled away from the patient's body, creating a cavern underneath the skin where the connective tissue holding the skin to the underlying body is torn apart. Little is seen on the outside except two or four puncture wounds at either side of the cavern, which were created by the canine teeth of the attacker, but the space will readily fill with pus if the wound becomes infected.

Successful healing of a puncture wound can only occur if the wound granulates from the bottom up, i.e. the skin wound remains open until the underlying tissues have healed so that any infection can drain out as the wound heals. Once the infection is controlled, healing is rapid because the wound edges do not gape as the wound is so small.

Abrasion

This is the name given to a graze or scrub wound. Such wounds do not penetrate the entire skin thickness (Fig. 3.26(g)) and therefore are not true open wounds, but they do affect the body surface and have been included here for completeness. They are usually caused by a glancing blow or road accident where the animal is dragged along the ground.

The wound is superficial and the haemorrhage consists of capillary bleeding, so that these wounds, though often contaminated, are rarely serious. They are, however, very painful, often more so than any of the other wounds because the epidermis may be worn away to expose large areas of the sensitive dermis with its multiple nerve endings. In open wounds, which penetrate through the total skin thickness, the dermal nerve endings are only exposed along the line of the wound, which is a relatively small area when compared with an extensive graze.

Healing of the abrasion takes place under the scab formed by coagulation and drying of the serum exuded from the damaged area after the bleeding has ceased.

Healing of open wounds

Wounds heal by one of two methods: **first intention** healing or **granulation** (Fig. 3.28).

First intention healing. The edges of the wound are not widely separated, and are held together by blood clots. New blood vessels grow into these clots from the sides of the wound, carrying with them the healing components that will produce the fibrous scar tissue to tie the wound edges together permanently. Epithelial cells quickly spread across the narrow scar and start producing a new skin layer over the scar tissue (Fig. 3.29). Provided that there is no sepsis to interfere with the process, healing will be complete in 5–10 days.

| HEALING OF OPEN WOUNDS ||
First intention	Granulation
Usual for incised wounds	Usual for lacerated and infected puncture wounds
Edges of wounds remain close together	Wound edges are widely separated
Healing complete in 7–10 days	Healing can take weeks or months
No infection present	Wound often contaminated and may become infected
Minimal scarring	Scarring is extensive

Fig. 3.28. Healing of open wounds.

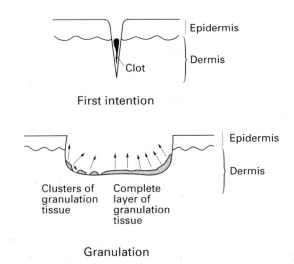

First intention

Granulation

Fig. 3.29. Healing of wounds.

norse with cut leg

First intention healing can only take place in incised wounds where the edges remain closely together. This may be achieved by stitching or bandaging whilst the healing takes place.

Granulation. Granulation tissue usually heals lacerated, avulsed and infected wounds and the repair process may take several weeks, as the wound edges are widely separated (Fig. 3.29). Clusters of cells are produced on the exposed tissue of the wound and they multiply rapidly to form areas of granulation tissue which gradually expand to cover the entire wound area. The tissue is moist and bright red, with a bubbly, uneven surface. It is easily damaged and bleeds if disturbed, as it has a very rich blood supply. It grows up towards the skin surface level, filling the gap between the wound edges. When it is level with the surface, new epithelial cells spread across the top to complete the healing process.

Factors delaying wound healing

Movement. If the wound edges move against each other, the delicate healing tissues are continually destroyed and need to reform. Injuries over joints will take longer to heal than injuries where skin movement is minimal.

Infection. Most wounds are contaminated because they have been inflicted by unsterile objects which leave bacteria in the body tissues. For example, lacerated wounds caused by road accidents are usually grossly contaminated by dirt, grit and hair, all of which are covered with bacteria that may be harmful to living tissues. If the wound is not treated correctly or the body defence mechanisms are poor, the bacteria will multiply and invade the body tissues, killing them. The healing tissues are destroyed and wound healing is seriously delayed. Infected wounds show all the signs of inflammation and may discharge pus.

Disturbance in circulation. Heavily contused wounds may take longer to heal as the local circulation to the wound edges is impaired. The skin at the edge of the wound dies and the wound edges cannot heal until this dead tissue has been removed.

Avulsed wounds also may result in areas of skin which lose their blood supply and die. The dead skin becomes hard and dry and will eventually separate from the healthy tissues. The wound created by this loss of skin then has to heal by granulation.

Self-trauma. Continual licking will cause movement of the wound, introduce infection and damage the healing tissues.

Treatment of open wounds and abrasions

The aims of treatment are:

- to arrest haemorrhage;
- to treat shock; and
- to prevent sepsis.

The first two are the most important, and it is sometimes preferable to delay the treatment against infection until the general condition of the patient has improved.

There are certain pitfalls to be avoided when presented with the patient and it is best to follow a set course of action:

(1) Treat for shock.
(2) Remove any dressings applied by the owner.
(3) Control any severe haemorrhage.
(4) Remove the cause of the injury.
(5) Clip the hair around the wound.
(6) Remove any contaminating foreign bodies.
(7) Cleanse the wound.
(8) Dress the wound.

Treating for shock. If the animal is collapsed, fluid therapy should be commenced at an early stage.

Removing dressings applied by the owner. This allows the veterinary nurse to inspect the injuries sustained.

Controlling haemorrhage. Immediate steps must be taken to control any severe haemorrhage. All instruments used in treating the wound should be sterilised if possible, and hands should always be washed (preferably in surgical scrub) to prevent further contamination of the wound. Blood that has clotted should never be removed by the person applying first aid as this will invariably restart the haemorrhage.

Removing the cause of the injury. The cause should be removed where this is possible, particularly if it is likely to cause further damage. Items such as traps or fish hooks may be removed, but deeply penetrating foreign bodies should be left alone. Glass fragments can be triangular, with only the tip showing above the skin: attempts to remove them will cause the animal pain, and may only serve to drive the glass deeper into the tissues. Stakes penetrating the chest wall or abdomen may have entered the thoracic cavity or ruptured a large blood vessel, and the attempted removal of these foreign bodies may cause a pneumothorax or may disturb clots formed around the blood vessel, restarting a serious haemorrhage.

Large penetrating foreign bodies which protrude from the body should be cut off so that they only just protrude above the skin surface. A ring-pad dressing can then be applied over the whole wound.

Clipping the hair. The hair around the wound should be clipped carefully. If the hair is matted with blood, it can be clipped away quite cleanly; but normal fur should be smeared with cream, or at least dampened with saline, so that it sticks together in clumps when cut and therefore falls from the body as a piece, thus avoiding contaminating the wound with multiple individual hairs.

Contaminating foreign bodies. Grit and dirt usually contaminate road accident wounds. Hair is commonly found deeply buried in gunshot wounds and bite injuries. Such foreign bodies should be removed if possible by the careful use of dressing forceps or similar instruments.

Cleansing the wound. The aim at this stage is to flush the wound mechanically, irrigating the damaged tissues with a soothing, non-toxic solution which will wash away the superficial contaminating dirt and bacteria. Isotonic sterile saline, syringed with gentle force into the wound, will achieve all these objectives (this is a good use for half-used sterile intravenous drips). If no sterile saline is available, a saline solution may be made up from half a teaspoonful of salt to one litre of cooled, boiled water. Failing all else, warm tap water may be used. In general, antiseptic solutions should not be used to cleanse wounds: although they hinder the growth of micro-organisms, they can also have harmful effects on the raw body tissues, especially if not made up to the precise strength recommended by the manufacturer.

Puncture wounds caused by canine, feline or reptile bites are the exception to this rule and should be gently but thoroughly flushed with a solution of hydrogen peroxide, diluted 1:4 with warm water, or a *correctly diluted* solution of povidone iodide could be used. These bites are usually heavily contaminated with pathogenic bacteria, many of which are anaerobes.

The cleansing procedure should be gentle but thorough. Make sure that the irrigating fluid penetrates into the depths of the wound, but **take care that clots in the wound are not disturbed** and that the wound is not further contaminated by dirt derived from the skin.

Dressing the wound

A suitable dressing should now be applied, preferably a non-adhesive wound dressing or sterile gauze covered with cotton wool and bandage. Cotton wool must never be applied directly as it will stick to the wound and the wisps will be hard to remove. (Bandaging techniques are described in Chapter 2.)

An antiseptic cream may be used if the wound is heavily contaminated, particularly where application of a dressing is not possible. Oily ointments should be avoided as they are difficult to remove at subsequent surgery.

Closed Wounds

There are three types of closed wound: contusions, haematomas, and injuries to internal organs.

Contusions

A contusion (bruise) is produced by a blow with a blunt instrument which causes rupture of blood vessels in the skin and in the soft tissues beneath. The escaping blood seeps into the surrounding damaged tissues and will eventually clot. As the damaged tissues heal, the red blood cells in the clot are broken down and the breakdown products of the haemoglobin pigment account for the yellow/green discoloration of the skin.

The signs of a contusion are heat, pain and swelling. White-skinned animals show discoloration of the skin, which is first red (immediately after the blow), then purple (within a few hours) and finally yellow/green (after several days). Deep bruising of muscles will cause a swelling which often increases in size as it heals. This severe bruising remains painful for a period of weeks until healing is complete.

Treatment of contusions.

- **Cold compresses** should be applied immediately to cause vasoconstriction in the damaged area. Constriction of the blood vessel walls will decrease the amount of blood entering the area and thus limit the volume of blood lost and help to prevent swelling of the tissues. The cold will also help to alleviate pain.
- **Firm bandaging** will increase the back pressure, control haemorrhage and limit swelling.
- If several hours have elapsed since the injury and the area is already swollen, **hot formentations** should be used: they will speed recovery by causing vasodilation to *increase* the blood supply to the damaged tissue so that the injury can be repaired more rapidly.

Haematomas

These injuries most commonly affect the earflaps of dogs and cats. If the flap is scratched or shaken violently, small veins may be ruptured and the escaping blood fills a pocket of connective tissue under the skin, ballooning it out until back pressure results in a natural arrest of haemorrhage.

Haematomas may also be seen following intravenous injections or blood sampling if pressure is not applied to the vein as the needle is withdrawn. Accidental puncture wounds which damage large blood vessels may also create haematomas.

Unlike a contusion or an abscess, the swelling of a haematoma is soft, usually painless and cool to the touch. In time, the blood will clot, and the clots contract over a period of weeks to become hard and knobbly.

Treatment of haematomas. The only first aid treatment of value is to bandage the affected area firmly, as soon as possible, or apply firm pressure with a cold compress if bandaging is impractical. Once the area is swollen, surgical intervention may be necessary to drain the haematoma of the earflap.

Damage to internal organs

Crushing injuries of the body may result in damage to internal organs. Details of first aid are given later in this chapter, in sections relevant to various body systems.

Burns and Scalds

Definitions

A **burn** is an injury to the body caused by:

- dry heat (house fires, contact with hot surfaces etc);
- excessive cold (frostbite, cryosurgery);
- corrosive chemicals (strong acids, petroleum products);
- electric currents or radiation (after a major disaster, e.g. a nuclear disaster).

A **scald** is an injury caused by the effect of moist heat (such as boiling water, tar or oil).

The distinction between burns and scalds is not of practical interest, for the signs and principles of treatment are the same in each case. It is far more important to identify the cause of the injury so that the correct first aid is given. For example:

- **Heat burns** must be cooled immediately.
- **Chemical burns** must be cleaned with a suitable solvent.

Classification

Classification depends upon the depth of the injury and the size of the area affected.

Depth of injury

This classification used to be divided into six degrees but the modern classification recognises only two types of burns or scalds:

- **Superficial**, penetrating no deeper than the skin surface (1st and 2nd degree burns).
- **Deep**, penetrating through the skin thickness into the tissues beneath (3rd, 4th, 5th and 6th degree burns).

Percentage of the total body surface affected

This is simply an estimation based on examining the patient. A burn which affects the whole of one side of an animal, for example, could be estimated to be a 40% burn. Evaluation of the skin area affected is of value because it gives some idea of the degree of pain suffered by the animal and the rate of loss of body fluids. Extensive burns can cause dehydration as appreciable volumes of body fluids evaporate from a large area of exposed flesh.

Clinical Signs

The clinical signs of all burns and scalds are very similar but appear at different times depending on the cause of the injury. Heat and electrical burns produce symptoms immediately but with chemical, cold and radiation burns it may take several hours or even days before the signs appear. The signs are also more severe in young animals, which have more delicate skin.

The signs may be summarised as follows:

- **Redness and heat**. The blood vessels of the skin dilate as the area becomes inflamed. Redness is most easily seen in white unpigmented skin.
- **Swelling**. The tissues swell and the surface becomes *moist* as the inflammatory changes allow tissue fluid to escape from the capillaries into the damaged tissues and on to the surface of the wound. Blisters are rarely seen in animals.
- **Pain**. Pain is variable but, as a rule, deep burns are less painful than large superficial ones. This is because the deep burn destroys the sensitive nerve endings, which the superficial burn leaves intact.
- **Loss of fur**. The fur will fall out after a few days (if it was not burnt away by dry heat at the time of the accident) with all but the most superficial of wounds. This is because the hair follicles in the dermis are damaged, so that the hair shaft is shed.
- **Skin surface becomes leathery**. Surface tissues are destroyed in deep burns and dry out to become leathery and totally insensitive in the days following the injury. The dead tissues will peel away from the surrounding healthy, healing tissues and the open wound created will heal by granulation.

Specific Injuries: Treatment and Complications

Figure 3.30 sets out the likely causes and clinical signs of heat burns, scalds, electrical burns and chemical burns.

Extensive heat burns and scalds

Burns and scalds from, for example, domestic fires can be extremely painful and animals resent interference. All cases of extensive burns or scalds should be treated by a veterinary surgeon as soon as possible. First aid measures involve:

(1) Cooling the damaged areas as quickly as possible.
(2) Keeping the patient warm once the initial cooling treatment is complete.
(3) Dressing the wound.

BURNS AND SCALDS		
	Causes	**Clinical signs**
Heat burns and scalds	House fires Kitchen accidents Burns to the feet as the result of walking on hot surfaces (e.g. unwary cats walking on hot ceramic hobs)	Any area of the body may be damaged but scalds usually affect the head, neck and dorsum of the back as the scalding liquid pours down over the animal. The wound shape is often like an inverted pear because the bulk of the fluid splashes onto the body and then drains down the skin in an increasingly narrow stream. The hair may be matted together by the liquid which then evaporates or solidifies, leaving an area covered by a thick crust of hair and dried fluids. In a burn, the singed or burnt fur clearly indicates the injured area.
Electrical burns	Burns are seen in pups that chew through electrical cables and also in cases of electrocuted animals.	Burns are seen at the points where the current flows into and out of the body. The pup which chews a wire may have red inflamed areas on the lips, gums or tongue. The electrocuted animal can show burns to very different parts of the body because the current will flow out of the body where it contacts the ground. The nose of a curious animal may be burnt because this was the part of the body which touched a live wire, but the paws will also show burn marks since this is where the current flowed out of the body. If the animal was lying down, the skin of the chest might be affected, rather than the paws. The burns resemble heat burns and the cause of the injury is often all to apparent.
Chemical burns	Splashing by strong acids or alkalis (e.g. quicklime) or accidental immersion in containers of corrosive or irritant substances (e.g. battery acid, sump oil).	These burns also resemble a heat burn, but may take several hours to develop.

Fig. 3.30. Burns and scalds: causes and signs.

(4) Splinting to limit movement if necessary.
(5) Preparing intravenous drips.

Cooling the damaged areas. Cold water should be gently hosed on to the burnt areas as soon as the animal is removed from the fire. This will rapidly decrease the heat in the tissues so that fewer cells die and tissue damage and pain are kept to a minimum. It will also guard against the risk of hyperthermia.

A gentle, continuous stream of water is better than an ice pack because larger areas can be treated and it avoids putting any pressure on the extremely painful, damaged tissues. This treatment must be discontinued if it causes the animal pain or the animal shows signs of becoming chilled, which can happen within a few minutes if large areas of the body are affected.

Keeping the patient warm. This is difficult because, although the body needs to be kept warm,

any heating of the burnt areas will cause considerable pain. **Heat lamps and other forms of direct heat must never be used in these cases.** It is best to conserve the body heat by wrapping the unaffected parts of the body in warm, dry blankets and shielding the animal from draughts. The injuries may be kept cool by covering the wound dressing (see below) with a cold, wet towel. Ice packs may also be used to control the pain, but only for short periods so that the patient does not become chilled.

Dressing the wound. Burns and scalds are sterile wounds as the initial heat destroys the bacteria on the skin surface. The wound should be gently cleaned with sterile saline to remove any loose or charred remnants of hair before a dressing is applied. However, it must be remembered that these wounds are extremely painful and thorough cleansing will probably be possible only under a general anaesthetic, when strict aseptic precautions can be observed.

As a temporary measure, the wound should be covered with a waterproof dressing to prevent loss of body fluids—further damage will be done to the exposed tissues if they are allowed to dry out and the patient will suffer a greater degree of shock if body fluids are allowed to evaporate through the damaged area. Sterile non-stick dressings or paraffin tulle covered by a minimal amount of sterile absorbent dressing, should be applied and bandaged in place. Polythene bags wrapped around the completed dressing will prevent evaporation of moisture.

If no dressings are available at the site of the accident or if the wound is too large or painful to be dressed using bandages, a *clean* sheet of polythene may be laid directly over the injured area and a cold, wet towel laid on top to keep it in place and cool the burnt area.

Splinting. Splinting can be used to limit movement if there are severe burns to the limbs, but must be applied in such a way that there is no pressure on the damaged area.

Preparing intravenous drips. These will be needed to replace the fluid lost by evaporation in extensive burns. Dextrose saline or normal saline are both suitable.

Less extensive heat burns and scalds

The treatment of minor scalds from kitchen accidents is similar:

(1) Cool the affected area as soon as possible to limit tissue damage and alleviate the pain.
(2) Clean the area, as for extensive burns. (In long-haired animals, the fur covering a scalded area should be clipped away if possible to allow the skin to cool before it is dressed.)
(3) Apply dressings, as for extensive burns.

Cooling the affected area. Scalds caused by fat or oil must be cleaned quickly before the fat congeals in the coat and seals in the heat. Detergent solution should be poured on to the area to loosen the fat, followed by cold-water washes to remove the detergent and cool the tissues. Scalds caused by water-soluble fluid (e.g. milk, boiling water) and burn injuries can be flushed *immediately* with cold, running water.

Ice packs are very useful to continue cooling the injured area and can be made from polythene bags filled with crushed ice. As only a relatively small area of the body is to be treated, there is no risk of causing hypothermia and the ice pack may be gently bandaged over the wound and left in place for 10 minutes, after which it can be renewed if necessary.

Complications of heat burns and scalds

Shock. The degree of shock is very severe in cases of extensive burning and is caused by:

- Pain.
- Tissue damage and inflammation.
- Loss of body fluids from the damaged areas.
- Infection in the days following the injury.

Tissue death and wound infection release toxins which, when absorbed into the bloodstream, may cause a toxaemia or septicaemia. This, in combination with the shock of fluid loss, may be severe enough to cause the death of the patient.

Dyspnoea or asphyxia. Animals rescued from house fires may suffer from pulmonary oedema (fluid on the lungs) as the irritant smoke inhaled in the fire can cause severe inflammation of the respiratory tract. These patients often develop bronchitis or pneumonia 2–3 days after the accident.

Infection. The moist tissues on the surface of the burn easily become infected and this will delay wound healing.

Scar formation. These wounds heal by granulation and scar formation may be extensive in a large wound. This will cause problems if the wound overlies a joint because the healthy, elastic skin is replaced by inelastic scar tissue which is unable to stretch freely as the joint is flexed and extended. Thus the range of movement of the joint is restricted.

Electrical burns

WARNING
Do not touch an electrocuted animal until the electricity supply has been disconnected.

Wounds should be treated and dressed in the manner described for heat burns.

The most serious complication associated with electrical burns is that of electrocution. Longer term problems could include the complications mentioned for heat burns and scalds. However, electrical burns are rarely extensive and so local infection of the wound is the most likely problem—if the animal survives the initial accident.

Chemical burns

Copious volumes of water should be used to wash the chemical off the skin. Addition of a mild detergent will ensure complete removal of the chemical. If the chemical is a known alkali (e.g. caustic soda or quicklime), prepare an acid solution by mixing equal quantities of household vinegar and water, and use it to wash away the chemical. If the burn is caused by a known acid, use a concentrated solution of bicarbonate of soda or washing soda.

Chemical burns are rarely deep but may be very extensive. The major complication in these cases is that of poisoning as the patient tries to clean the noxious chemical from its coat.

Fractures

Definitions

A **fracture** is a forcible break in the continuity of bony tissue, i.e. the bone is broken.

Fragments are the pieces of bone that are formed as the result of a fracture.

There are varying degrees of injury, but any damage to the bony cortex which is caused by force is still technically a fracture. Some fractures are as slight as a hairline crack but others may involve a severe break where the bone is shattered into two or more fragments.

The fragments are usually sharp and jagged and are thus likely to cause further damage, especially when they are displaced by muscular spasms and spear into surrounding tissues.

Fractures are also described according to the damage done:

- A **simple** fracture is one where the bone is broken cleanly into two pieces.
- A **compound** fracture is one where there is a wound communicating between the skin or mucous membranes and the fracture site. There is a real risk that infection can occur in these fractures.
- A **complicated** fracture is one where important structures or organs around the fracture site are damaged, e.g. blood vessels, nerves, the spinal cord, the lungs or the heart.
- A **multiple** fracture is one where the bone is fractured in two or more places, but where there is an appreciable distance between the sites of the fractures.

Signs of Fracture

- Pain at or near the site of the fracture.
- Swelling.
- Loss of function.
- Deformity.
- Unnatural mobility.
- Crepitus.

The last two signs will not be detected in incomplete fractures, and it must not be expected that all the above signs will be found in every case. If there is any reason to suspect a fracture, the injury should be treated as such pending diagnosis by a veterinary surgeon.

Pain at or near the site of the fracture

It must be remembered that pain increases shock and gentle handling is essential to avoid increasing the pain. The severity of the pain depends upon:

- **The amount of movement** which can occur between the bone fragments, and how much the fragments rub against each other. Incomplete fractures are less painful than complete fractures, as the fragments scarcely move. Overriding and distracted fractures tend to be less painful because the broken ends do not grate on each other.
- **The damage to other soft tissues**. In cases of vertebral fractures, the pain is usually intense because of the pressure exerted on the spinal cord by the displaced bones and fragments.

Swelling

Swelling occurs soon after the accident due to haemorrhage from the bruised muscles and inflammation of the soft tissues surrounding the fracture site. This haemorrhage will be worsened if the sharp fracture fragments are allowed to move freely following the accident and cause more soft tissue damage.

Loss of function

This may be partial or complete. There is always some limitation of use after a bone has been fractured and the animal is usually 90–100% lame.

Deformity

Fractures of limb long bones are often obvious because the fracture fragments can be severely displaced and the limb is markedly deformed. Fracture deformities of other bones may be more difficult to detect if the bones are buried deep in muscle tissue, e.g. the pelvic bones or the vertebrae.

Unnatural mobility

This is usually noted in fractures of the limb long bones. Movement may be noticed at the fracture site.

Crepitus

A grating sound may be heard or felt when the broken ends move against one another. This, and unnatural mobility, should not be tested for by the person giving first aid, but gives positive evidence of the presence of a fracture if noticed during the course of an examination.

First Aid Treatment

The principle of first aid treatment for a fracture is to minimise the movement of the fracture fragments. This alleviates pain and stops the situation deteriorating because the sharp fracture fragments are not allowed to jar against each other, nor can they cut into the surrounding soft tissues every time the animal moves. The following treatment routine is recommended:

- Handle the broken bone as little as possible.
- Control haemorrhage in a compound fracture.
- Support the fracture.

Handling

> **WARNING**
> **Under no circumstances should resetting of the limb or reduction of the fracture be attempted.** If a vertebral fracture is suspected, the patient must be moved with extreme care, keeping the whole of the spinal column supported *at all times* and avoiding any twisting movements of the spine. This means that the animal should not be turned over unless absolutely necessary (e.g. to examine wounds on its underside). If the patient does have to be moved, seek the assistance of several people to turn the animal.

Haemorrhage

Haemorrhage in a compound fracture should be controlled by applying a dressing if possible. Digital pressure must only be used with care as this could displace the fragments and cause complications. A ring pad dressing is very useful here. The wound may be cleansed as described earlier.

Support

Support for the fracture should be applied as soon as possible to limit movement and prevent further damage. However, splinting should be abandoned if it is impossible without a struggle—provoking the animal to thrash around will do it more harm than the splint will do good. Such animals are best kept still, warm and comfortable until professional help is available, or until the animal has calmed down and will allow a splint to be applied without a struggle.

Support Dressings for Fractured Bones

Robert Jones dressing

This is one of the most useful limb dressings which may be applied in veterinary practice. It consists of layers of cotton wool, which are then bound tightly with a roller bandage until the cotton wool is compressed and becomes almost rigid. It is thus a soft dressing, which conforms perfectly to the contours of the limb and is difficult to apply too tightly. It also controls soft tissue swelling superbly and, most important of all, is very well tolerated by the patient.

Application of a Robert Jones dressing.

- Cut two strips of 1 inch adhesive plaster, long enough to cover the length of the metacarpal/metatarsal region of the foot, plus a couple of inches. Apply these strips longitudinally to the anterior and posterior aspects of the metacarpals/metatarsals (Fig. 3.31).
- Using a roll of cotton wool as a roller bandage, cover the entire length of the leg with 4–5 layers of cotton wool (a 500 g roll should be sufficient for an Irish wolfhound). If orthopaedic bandaging is used (e.g. 'Softban'), as many as 12–15 rolls will be needed.
- Bandage the cotton wool firmly in place using white open-weave bandage. This is better than conforming bandage because it will not contract once applied. Conforming bandages can increase the pressure in the dressing to such an extent that the blood supply to the limb is cut off. White open-weave bandage relaxes slightly after application and so it is difficult to apply it too tightly and the blood circulation can function normally (for signs of an overtight bandage, see Application of splints).
- To test if sufficient tension has been used to compact the cotton wool, 'flick' the completed dressing with a finger. It should make a resonant sound similar to that heard when testing a ripe melon.
- Reflect the longitudinal strips of adhesive bandage upwards over the bandage and stretch them as tight as possible. These prevent the dressing slipping down the leg.
- Bandage these strips in place, using 2–3 in wide adhesive roller bandage wrapped around the layer of white open-weave bandage. The bandage now consists of the layers shown in Fig. 3.31. The toes are left exposed.

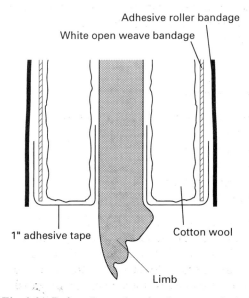

Fig. 3.31. Robert Jones dressing (cross-section).

Bandaging

The affected part of the body is bandaged firmly to unaffected parts of the body, so that the healthy body is used as a splint. This technique is used for the *scapula*, which can be bound against the rib cage, or for single fractured *metacarpals, metatarsals or digits* which may be bound to adjoining unaffected bones of the same foot by bandaging the foot. Such support will also decrease the amount of swelling following the fracture and thus minimise the pain.

Splinting

A splint is an appliance which restricts the movement of an injured part. Splints are of limited value:

- They can only be applied successfully to the bones and joints below the elbow and stifle joints. Above these joints, the bones are surrounded by large muscle masses and it is impossible to immobilise the fracture fragments by applying an simple external splint.
- They are time-consuming to apply and can cause the patient pain as they are fitted.

Therefore, the use of splints is restricted to those cases where professional help may be delayed for some time (e.g. the patient has to travel a long way to the surgery) or where the animal must be man-handled (e.g. the large, collapsed dog with a fractured tibia which has to be lifted into a car).

Criteria for a successful splint. The splint used should be:

- long enough to immobilise the joints above and below the fractured bone;
- rigid, so that it will not bend and allow movement of the injured part;
- smooth, so that there are no projections which can dig into the patient's underlying tissues;
- conforming, so that it holds the injured part firmly in position, does not allow movement and is comfortable for the patient.

Materials used for splints. Many materials can be used, depending on the initiative of the person at the scene of the accident and the size of the patient. Broom handles, rolled-up newspapers and magazines, ice-lolly sticks and wire coat-hangers have all played a part. More conventional splinting materials are as follows:

- **Wooden splints**—straight pieces of wood of appropriate length.
- **Preformed metal splints** made of tin or aluminium. Zimmer splints (malleable aluminium splinting of different widths, backed by foam) are very useful and can easily be bent to conform to the shape of the leg.
- **Plastic gutter splints** of varying diameters, lined with foam, may be snapped off at the desired length.

- **Plaster or resin**. Roller bandages made of coarse material and impregnated with plaster of paris or resin are commonly used in fracture treatment. The bandage should *not* encase the limb—this is beyond the scope of first aid—but may be used as a slab to form a gutter splint on one side of the leg only.

Plaster of paris splinting should not be used on a compound fracture because any wound dressings will become saturated with water and the wound may become contaminated by the plaster of paris. Resin materials hold hardly any water and will not contaminate the injury, and so these splints may be used over a dressed wound.

- **Inflatable airbags** could be used around a limb if of a suitable size to immobilise a broken leg. (There is a range of such appliances for human first aid.) There may be a risk of obstructing the circulation if the bags are too tightly inflated.

Application of splints. If the splint is not padded, the limb should first be covered with two layers of orthopaedic wool or a thin layer of cotton wool which is thick enough to prevent the hard splint from pressing on the skin and causing damage or discomfort, but thin enough not to prevent the splint from being placed as close to the fractured bone as possible. The splint is then applied to the leg and strapped in place to immobilise the limb.

Wooden, metal and plastic splints may be attached by strips of 1 in adhesive tape, bound firmly but not tightly around the leg (Fig. 3.32). Where possible, these strips should not encircle the limb at the actual fracture site for fear of causing complications. The whole leg is then bandaged with a support dressing such as a thick layer of cotton wool firmly bandaged in place with white open weave or conforming

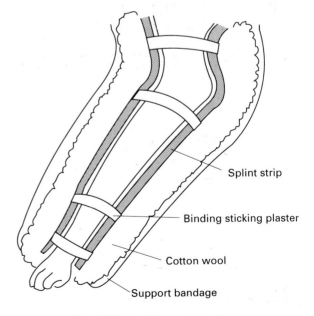

Splint strip

Binding sticking plaster

Cotton wool

Support bandage

Fig. 3.32. Applying metal splints.

bandage. This support dressing will also prevent swelling in tissues *not* bound by the adhesive strips.

Resin or plaster splints should fashioned as follows:

• Cut a suitable length of **resin cast** material from a roll and soften as appropriate before applying to the limb. Note that only *one* layer of resin casting material is needed, except when very large dogs are being treated (when it may be necessary to use two layers). This material is very strong, so that if several layers are used it may be impossible for the veterinary surgeon to remove the splint easily and give further treatment.

• A **plaster-of-Paris** bandage (Fig. 3.33) needs to be soaked in water, wrung out, unrolled on a smooth surface and folded on itself 3–4 times to form a slab of the desired length. It is then moulded upon the affected limb and secured in position by an ordinary roller bandage, used wet. (It may be easier to unroll the bandage and make a slab of the desired length *before* wetting the bandage – it is very difficult to wet an entire roll and also difficult to find the end of the bandage when it is wet. The

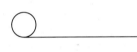

Step 1
Measure desired length against leg.

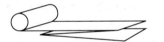

Step 2
Create a slab of wet and dry bandage (plaster of Paris only).

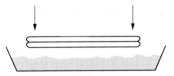

Step 3
Soak bandage and squeeze if necessary. (Hold in both hands for plaster of Paris. Use scissors etc. to immerse resin bandage in hot water).

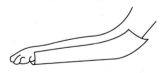

Step 4
Mould on to limb to form a gutter.

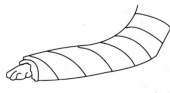

Step 5
Bandage in place and allow to set.

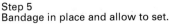

Fig. 3.33. Making a plaster splint.

ends of the dry slab should be held in either hand whilst immersing the bandage in the water so that the slab can easily be straightened out and applied to the limb after the excess water has been squeezed out of the dressing.)

The splint should be strapped firmly in place using crepe bandages and movement restricted until the casting material hardens.

Support dressing. If possible, the toes should not be completely covered by the final dressing, so that they can be examined frequently to ensure that the circulation is not hindered by too tight a splint. Overtight bandaging may obstruct the venous return up the leg and the toes will swell.

> **WARNING**
> If both arterial and venous flows are obstructed, the toes may become swollen and cold. If any swelling should occur, **the dressings must be removed immediately** and replaced by looser bandaging.

Observation. Finally, once any dressings are in place, patients should be observed constantly for signs of discomfort—usually indicated by biting at the splint. If this occurs, the dressings should be checked and, if the animal persists, the dressings should be removed and replaced.

The state of consciousness (in cases of trauma to the head and spine), the breathing (in cases of rib fractures) and the passage of urine and faeces (in cases of pelvic fractures) must also be continually assessed.

Dislocations, Sprains, Strains and Ruptured Tendons

Definitions

A **dislocation** or **luxation** is a persistent displacement of the articular surfaces of the bones which form a joint (Fig. 3.34).

A **sprain** is an injury which occurs when a synovial joint has been violently forced to move too far in one direction, stretching and damaging the synovial membrane, ligaments and other soft tissues in the process but where the anatomy of the joint remains normal (unlike dislocations).

A **strain** is the stretching or tearing of a muscle or tendon.

A **ruptured tendon** is a form of severe strain or injury in which the tendon is either partially or completely torn as a result of sudden violence. Wounds to the distal limbs should always be checked to find out if the tendons are damaged. The tendons may also rupture due to indirect violence, e.g. twisting the leg awkwardly can rupture the Achilles tendon.

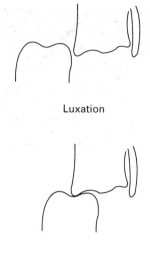

Luxation

Subluxation

Fig. 3.34. Luxation and subluxation of a joint.

Common sites, clinical signs and treatment of these conditions are given in Fig. 3.35.

Injuries to the Respiratory Tract

> **WARNING**
> Injuries to any part of the respiratory tract may be fatal because the respiratory tract is the only source of the body's oxygen supply. Therefore, all patients showing dyspnoea should be very carefully and continuously observed.

The most important criteria for treating any patient with **dyspnoea** are:

- **Rest**, so that the animal's demand for oxygen is kept to an absolute minimum (in practice, this involves confining the patient to a small basket or kennel in which it can lie down comfortably but has little space to move around).
- **Oxygen**, which should be given if the animal shows any signs of cyanosis or air hunger.
- **Close observation**, because the patient's condition may deteriorate very rapidly.

Nose

Epistaxis

Epistaxis, or bleeding from the nose, usually arises from the vascular turbinate mucosa and is not, in itself, a serious haemorrhage.

Causes

- **Trauma**—most cases occur following a direct blow to the nasal bones, which rarely causes any problems, but occasionally epistaxis is associated with severe skull fractures or bites from larger animals.
- **Tumours** of the nasal cavity may haemorrhage from time to time.
- **Persistent sneezing**, as might be seen with a nasal foreign body.

Signs

- **Haemorrhage**—the blood lost varies in each case:
  - Blows to the head usually result in haemorrhage from both nostrils, which is free-flowing immediately after the accident, but congeals within minutes, blocking both nostrils. In the following days, the patient usually sneezes a watery blood-stained discharge as the clots in the nose organise and contract. The haemorrhage rarely restarts.
  - Tumours bleed from time to time. The bouts of haemorrhage are therefore recurrent and are usually associated with sneezing (as in the case of foreign bodies) and often only one nostril is affected.
- **Sneezing** occurs because the lining of the nasal passages are irritated by a foreign body, blood clots or the presence of a tumour.
- **Mouth-breathing or noisy nasal breathing** occurs as the nostrils and airways are completely or partially blocked.
- **Swelling of the nasal or frontal sinus area** can be caused by trauma or tumours.
- **Crepitus**, **deformity** or evidence of **depressed fractures** at the point of impact of a blow.

Complications

- **Concussion**. If the blow to the head was sufficiently serious, the cranium may be fractured and the fracture fragments displaced into the cranial cavity. The pressure this produces on the brain can cause collapse, unconsciousness and possibly death.
- **Dyspnoea**. The patient will find it difficult to breathe because of the blocked nasal passages, but occasionally the nasal bones are fractured and collapse inwards, distorting and narrowing the nasal airways.
- **Vomiting**. The blood lost is usually swallowed. If much blood is ingested, it may cause the animal to vomit.

Treatment. The muzzle must *not* be taped to restrain the animal because of the risk of displacing any fractured nasal bones. It is also important for the patient to be able to mouth-breathe, as breathing through the nose may be impossible. The animal should be rested as much as possible.

Cold compresses applied externally to the nose will help to control the haemorrhage, reduce soft tissue swelling and alleviate pain, but in some cases adrenalin swabs inserted into the nostril opening may be needed to treat the condition. This should not be attempted without the consent of the veterinary surgeon: it is usually impossible to position the swabs effectively in a conscious animal and incorrect insertion will do more harm than good.

Constant observation is needed so that delayed concussion, if it occurs, can be detected at the

DISLOCATIONS, SPRAINS, STRAINS AND RUPTURED TENDONS

	Common sites	Clinical signs	Treatment
Dislocations	The carpus and tarsus (especially in conjunction with deep, lacerated wounds following road accidents, where the ligaments supporting these joints may be literally worn away by the abrasive road surface). The hip joint. The patella (but these are usually long-standing injuries).	Loss of function of the limb, resulting in 90–100 % lameness. Deformity. This is usually obvious in cases of complete dislocations of limb joints as the leg may be abnormally angled or shorter than its partner. Occasionally the dislocation is only a partial displacement of the joint surfaces (a subluxation -- Figure 3.34) which is more difficult to detect as the degree of deformity may be very slight. Limited movement of the joint. Pain on manipulation of the joint (much less in the chronic case). Swelling of the joint. Crepitus may be noticed, but it is much less obvious than between the ragged ends of broken bones because it is due to the smooth cartilaginous surface rubbing on intact bone.	No attempt should be made to reduce the dislocation. Limb joints may be dressed with a support bandage (e.g. Robert Jones dressing) or cold compresses may be applied to limit the swelling and alleviate pain. Analgesics may be given.
Sprains	The shoulder. The stifle, usually resulting in rupture of one or both cruciate ligaments. The carpus and tarsus.	Swelling of the joint capsule, which develops shortly after the injury and is due to bleeding from damaged tissues and inflammation of the synovial membrane. Tenderness on palpation of the actual joint and pain which is more severe when the joint is moved in the direction which stretches the damaged tissues. However, the pain is much less intense than in fracture or dislocation injuries. Loss of use, which is not so severe as in a fracture or dislocation injury but can result in 50--90% lameness. No gross deformity of the leg.	These injuries are minor emergencies (Figure 3.1). The affected joint should be rested as much as possible and the swelling minimised or prevented by applying a pressure bandage (crepe bandages are most useful and are usually to be found in most home first aid boxes). Robert Jones dressings may also be used but are more difficult for an owner to apply. Cold compresses alone do not prevent the swelling to the same degree as a firm bandage but may be incorporated under the crepe bandage to help alleviate the pain.
Strains	Muscles of the legs	Strains are commonly seen in the limbs and usually occur as the result of a sudden wrench. Racing dogs are particularly prone to these injuries. The signs of strain are 30--70% lameness on the affected leg. Locally, there is tenderness and swelling of the affected muscle but no gross deformity of the limb. Further exercise is impossible.	Rest must be enforced. If necessary, the limb may be splinted. Cold compresses and support bandages may be of value if applied immediately, because they will limit the swelling. Hot fomentations or electric heating pads should be used in the longer term, because the heat will help to alleviate pain and speed recovery (as for Contusions).
Ruptured tendons	Distal tendons of the legs Gestrocnemius tendon of the hind leg	Metacarpal and metatarsal tendons. These are often damaged in lacerated wounds to these areas, e.g. road accident injuries. The tendons may also rupture in racing dogs, causing the so called 'knocked-up toe'. If the flexor tendons are damaged (on the palmar and plantar aspects of the metacarpals, metatarsals and digits), the claws affected will stick upwards rather than curve neatly down to the ground (Figure 3.36). Gastrocnemius tendon (Achilles tendon). If this tendon, is severely damaged, the patient shows a peculiar lameness because it is unable to keep the hock extended when bearing weight. Therefore, as it places its foot on the ground, the tarsus sinks to the floor and the animal walks with the metatarsus on the ground like a kangaroo (Figure 3.37). The tendon may appear slack and the ruptured ends are usually palpable through the skin.	Tendons are normally held taut, and so when they are damaged the cut ends recoil and can be difficult to find at subsequent surgery. If possible, the limb should be splinted and kept as still as possible to prevent partially ruptured tendons from parting completely. Any wound should be dressed in the usual manner.

Fig. 3.35. Dislocation, strains, sprains and ruptured tendons.

earliest opportunity. If the patient already shows signs of concussion, it should be monitored.

Foreign bodies

Causes. Grass seeds, grass blades and occasionally splinters can gain access to the nose of the dog and cat. It is not uncommon to find that a blade of grass works its way forwards down the cat's nose from the pharynx (Fig. 3.38).

Signs. Nasal foreign bodies give rise to violent sneezing, head shaking and rubbing of the side of the

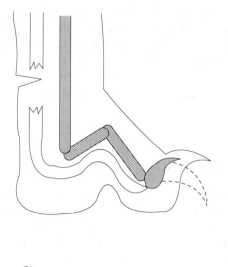

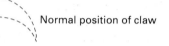
Normal position of claw

Fig. 3.36. Ruptured tendons: severed palmar/plantar flexor tendons ('knocked-up' toe injury).

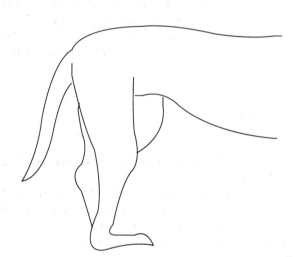

Fig. 3.37. Ruptured Achilles tendon, 'kangaroo' stance.

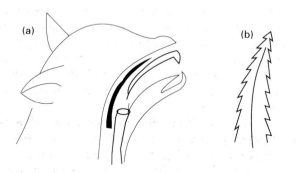

Fig. 3.38. (a) Grass in the nasopharynx. (b) A magnification of a grass blade showing barbed edges which prevent grass being swallowed and enable it to work forwards into the nasal passages.

nose with forepaws. Epistaxis may be induced by sneezing and there is often a purulent nasal discharge.

Complications. Infection is the greatest problem in these cases, as it cannot be controlled until the foreign body is removed from the nasal passages.

Treatment. The foreign body will sometimes be visible at the nostrils, and may be carefully removed. On other occasions, nothing is visible and the advice of the veterinary surgeon must be sought.

Pharynx

This area is considered in the section concerning the alimentary tract.

Larynx

Causes

- **Bite wounds**. Dog bite injuries occasionally result in severe wounds to the ventral neck area as the dog attacks its victim's most vulnerable part.
- **Lacerated wounds to the neck**, such as when a dog runs into a strand of barbed wire, hidden in the grass. These wounds are also occasionally seen following road accidents. Incised wounds may also occur if the animal falls through glass.
- **Strangulation injuries** usually occur because the animal's collar is caught on some projection as it falls or jumps from a height.

Signs

- **Swelling and pain**. The tissues of the neck may be swollen and painful because of extensive bruising and inflammation. **Subcutaneous emphysema** may develop around the injuries if the larynx has been punctured. The air in the larynx escapes into the tissues around the injury, creating a unique type of swelling: the swollen tissues 'crackle' under the fingertips when palpated as the tiny pockets of air in the tissues are popped.
- **Harsh, noisy breathing and dyspnoea**. The laryngeal cartilages may be distorted or collapsed and the lining of the larynx is inflamed and swollen, narrowing the air passageway.
- **Hissing and ballooning**. Any wound penetrating the larynx allows air to be sucked in and blown out of the wound during respiration, so that a 'hissing' sound may be heard on each inspiration as the air is sucked in through the tissues. On expiration, the tissues frequently balloon out as the air is forced into them.
- **Frothy haemorrhage**. Haemorrhage from these wounds is likely to be frothy as the blood is mixed with air.

Complications

- **Asphyxia**. If the trauma is severe and the lining of the larynx is very swollen or the laryngeal cartilages collapse, the patient will asphyxiate.
  If the wound penetrates the larynx, blood may be sucked into the respiratory tract as the patient inhales. Large volumes of blood will severely compromise the breathing as the clotting blood blocks the airways and fills the alveolar spaces.
- **Contamination of the airways**. Hair, dirt and bacteria may be sucked into the respiratory airways if an open wound penetrates the larynx.

Treatment

- **Asphyxia** should be treated as described on p. 92 (Unconsciousness). If the patient is having difficulty breathing, the veterinary nurse should have a suitable endotracheal tube prepared in case the animal loses consciousness. Prepare the site for a tracheostomy by clipping up the midline ventral neck and giving it a preliminary scrub.
- **Haemorrhage** should be controlled quickly to prevent any inhalation of blood and to save the patient's life. The haemorrhage may be fatal if branches of the jugular vein and carotid artery are also damaged in the accident.
- **Wounds** should be treated as described elsewhere but great care must be taken when cleansing the wound that no fluid is allowed to enter the air passages. Dressings may be applied, but only with great care because any pressure may further collapse the airway and make the situation worse.

Trachea

Causes, signs, complications and treatment are as described above for the larynx.

Lungs

Causes

- **Trauma**. Indirect violence such as a blow to the chest causes multiple minor haemorrhages into the lung tissues. Direct violence such as a displaced fractured rib, penetrating gunshot wounds or staking injuries can tear the delicate tissue.
- **Paraquat poisoning** causes irreversible changes to the lung tissue (see Poisoning section for signs and treatment).
- **Fluid in the alveolar spaces** as a result of drowning accidents, congestive heart failure etc.
- **Lung collapse** following damage to the chest wall.

Signs

- **Trauma**. External wounds and haemorrhage may or may not be present in both cases, but animals are usually shocked and breathing is often rapid and shallow because of the painful chest wall.

Bleeding from the lungs (**haemoptysis**) may be present, in which case bright red, frothy blood is coughed up. The haemorrhage is not severe and usually clears within a few hours.
- **Fluid in the alveolar spaces** causes the patient to cough continuously in an attempt to clear the lungs.

Complications

- **Infection of the pleural cavity** in cases of open wounds.
- **Haemothorax and/or pneumothorax** may be present in trauma cases. If the injury also damaged a major blood vessel in the chest cavity or tore the lungs so badly that a large volume of air escaped from the bronchioles, the lungs would collapse (see Chest Wall injuries, below).
- **Cyanosis, air hunger and death** if oxygenation of the blood is prevented, e.g. by fluid in the alveolar spaces.

Treatment. Lung injuries must always be regarded as serious because the complications may be so serious. **Rest is essential** and the animal should be allowed to assume the position which it finds most comfortable. Wounds, haemorrhage and shock should be treated as discussed elsewhere and additional oxygen supplied (see Resuscitation procedures, p. 86).

Chest Wall

Causes

- **Road accidents**, when the chest has been crushed by the vehicle.
- **Severe bites**, especially those inflicted to the chest walls of toy dogs which have been grabbed from above by larger dogs, picked up and shaken.
- **Staking accidents, gunshot wounds** etc.

Signs

- **Abnormal breathing patterns**. Breathing is painful for the patient and so animals with these injuries tend to have rapid, shallow respiratory patterns which cause minimal movement of the chest wall. However, if the lungs are collapsed, the need for oxygen overcomes the pain and the animal starts to gasp, trying to draw the air into the lungs. If the situation deteriorates, the patient will show increasing signs of 'air hunger' (see Asphyxiation—Unconsciousness).
- **Thoracic wounds causing an open pneumothorax**, often 'hiss' on inspiration as the air is drawn in through the wound (Fig. 3.39(a),(b)), but there are few external signs in cases of closed pneumothorax. Fractured ribs tend to stay in position because they are effectively splinted to those ribs on either side which are not damaged.

- **Subcutaneous emphysema** may be present in any case of pneumothorax (Fig. 3.39(b)) but it is usually more marked in a closed pneumothorax.

Complications. **Infection and contamination** of the pleural cavity may occur in cases of penetrating open wounds.

There are several possible reasons for lung **collapse** following injury to the chest wall:

- **Open pneumothorax** occurs when a wound penetrates into the pleural cavity. Air is sucked into the pleural cavity each time the animal inhales and the negative pressure in the pleural cavity is therefore destroyed so that the lungs will gradually collapse (Fig. 3.39(a),(b)).
- **Closed pneumothorax** occurs when there is no wound leading from the body surface to the pleural cavity. This can happen if the lung is torn during a crushing injury to the thorax or if the lung is pierced by a sharp fragment of fractured rib. In these cases, the air escapes from the damaged lung tissue and fills the pleural cavity (Fig. 3.39(a),(b)).
- **Haemothorax** occurs if a blood vessel is damaged in the thorax and a large volume of blood collects in the pleural cavity. The lungs float up to the top of the thoracic cavity but are unable to expand properly because of the fluid beneath them (Fig. 3.39(c)).
- **Diaphragmatic rupture** may occur if the chest wall is distorted (see Rupture of the diaphragm, below).

Anaemia and shock will follow extensive haemorrhage into the thoracic cavity.

Treatment

> WARNING
> **Any wound of the thoracic wall should be treated with caution since it may not be obvious how deeply it penetrates.** These animals should be handled with care because these injuries are very painful and fractured ribs may be displaced, causing further damage. The nose should *not* be muzzled unless absolutely necessary as these patients may need to mouth-breathe in order to satisfy their demand for oxygen.

The wounds should be cleaned carefully, taking care that no fluid is drawn into the pleural cavity. **Do not remove penetrating foreign bodies**, as this may lead to sudden lung collapse and death. Instead, the protruding portion should be cut off close to the skin and a ring pad dressing used to protect the remaining portion from being pushed deeper into the wound. The torn tissues may be folded back over the injury to seal the hole and a moist lint or gauze pad placed over the wound and bound to the thorax to keep the tissues in position. If the 'hissing' noise can still be heard after the tissues are folded down, an airtight dressing such as polythene or cling film should be

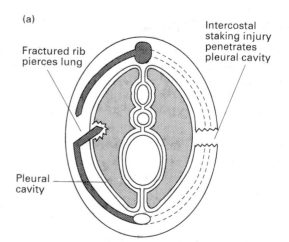

(a)

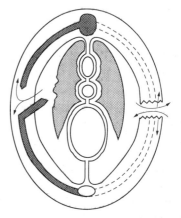

(b) Lungs collapse as pneumothorax develops

⟶ Direction of air flow during respiration movements.
Note subcutaneous emphysema developing under the skin of both injuries.

(c) Haemothorax

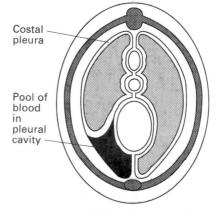

Fig. 3.39. Chest wall injuries.

placed over the wound before the lint and bandage are applied.

After the dressing is in place, the animal should be rested and oxygen given if necessary. Radiographs will probably be needed to assess the extent of the damage and chest drains required when the injury is surgically repaired. These can be prepared whilst awaiting the veterinary surgeon's arrival.

Rupture of the Diaphragm

Causes. This injury is seen more commonly in cats than dogs and is usually the result of a road accident or falling from a considerable height. The thin muscular diaphragm tears when the abdomen is crushed or the rib cage is distorted in the accident.

Signs. Diaphragmatic rupture alone causes no problem. It is only when the abdominal organs migrate through the diaphragm and cause lung collapse that any symptoms are seen. Very small tears may cause no problems immediately after the accident because the hole in the diaphragm is initially too small to allow large abdominal organs to enter the chest. Signs may occur later on as the omentum finds its way through and the hole gradually enlarges.

Complications. The complications of this condition are **cardiac compression** and **lung collapse**. Animals with large diaphragmatic tears, where the omentum and a liver lobe or two have entered the pleural cavity, may only show slightly laboured breathing at rest. The lungs are collapsed to some degree but still able to expand sufficiently to cope with the low oxygen demands of the resting animal. However, the animal may become quite distressed and dyspnoeic on exercise (e.g. if it struggles whilst being examined) because the lungs cannot expand sufficiently to cope with an increased oxygen demand.

Patients with extensive diaphragmatic tears may suffer severe dyspnoea or even partial asphyxia at rest because the omentum, liver, intestines and even the stomach and spleen have entered the pleural cavity and caused severe lung collapse. The abdomen of these animals often appears thin and sunken because many of the bulky abdominal viscera are in the chest cavity.

Treatment. There is no specific first aid treatment for these patients except to encourage the animal to lie on a slope, with the head higher than the hindquarters. This should allow the abdominal viscera to fall back into the abdomen, or at least to the back of the pleural cavity so that pressure is taken off the apical lung lobes, enabling them to inflate more efficiently.

As with any case of dyspnoea, the patient should be kept under constant observation, encouraged to rest as much as possible and given oxygen if necessary. No food should be given.

Injuries to the Alimentary Tract

The Mouth

Causes

- Curious cats and dogs may get their **heads or noses wedged** into plastic containers, discarded food tins etc.

- Lips—**Insect stings** commonly affect the lips. **Fishhooks** can also become embedded.
- Bony structures—**Compound fractures** of the hard palate and mandible are commonly seen following road accidents or in animals which have fallen from a great height (so-called 'tenement disease' after cats which fall from high up in blocks of flats).
- Teeth—**Foreign bodies** such as pieces of stick or bone sometimes become wedged transversely across the roof of the mouth between the molar teeth (Fig. 3.40) or portions of soft bone may become wedged on or between the teeth. In older animals, **teeth may become so loosened** in their sockets that they suddenly dislodge and remain hanging from the gum, which can be acutely painful for the animal.
- Tongue—**Foreign bodies** such as needles and fishhooks are occasionally found embedded in the tongue. Corrosive and irritant substances contaminating the coat will cause **tongue-tip ulceration**, especially in cats, as the corrosive chemical comes into contact with the tongue when the animal grooms itself. **Open wounds** are seen after an animal has licked out a sharp-edged can or bitten through its tongue after major trauma (e.g. a road accident). Dogs playing with sticks occasionally 'run on to' the stick, which can cause extensive lacerations, especially to the underside of the tongue and pharynx. Fragments of wood may break off and lodge in the wound.

Signs of oral pain. No matter what the cause, the signs of pain in the mouth are common to all:

- Profuse salivation and drooling.
- Pawing at the face or rubbing the face on the ground.

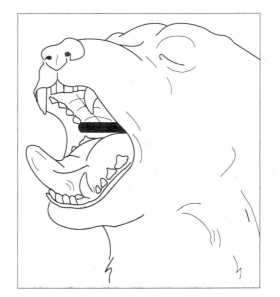

Fig. 3.40. Foreign body in roof of mouth: stick lodged between carnassial teeth.

• Dysphagia (difficulty in eating)—the animal is interested in food and may go to the bowl and sniff the food, but then turns away because it is too painful to feed.

Signs of specific injuries. **Inflammatory conditions** (e.g. stings, ulcerations) induce signs of acute pain. The swollen tissues around the area of the sting or the denuded, red raw tongue ulcers are usually easily spotted when the mouth is opened.

The pain associated with **foreign bodies** is usually less severe but the patient is more likely to paw at its face and may also continuously 'mouth' with its tongue and jaw as it tries to dislodge the problem. However, the animal with a penetrating foreign body (e.g. a needle) may remain very quiet and apprehensive, reluctant to move its tongue or swallow because of the pain that this induces.

Fractures in the mouth are usually easily recognised, if not easily seen:

• **Hard-palate fracture** presents as a thin reddened fissure running longitudinally in the midline of the roof of the mouth.
• **Mandibular fracture** results in one or both sides of the jaw being totally unstable. The most common site of such fractures is at the mandibular symphysis, when the two halves of the mandible can be freely moved against one another.

Wounds are also easily seen, except those affecting the underside of the tongue. Dogs which have 'run on' to sticks may show few signs at the time of the accident. The owner often reports that the dog yelped as it reached the stick, rushed back to the owner for reassurance and has been subdued ever since. There is usually surprisingly little haemorrhage from even quite deep and extensive cuts. If the injury is relatively long-standing (e.g. a foreign body that has been embedded for 2–3 days), there may well be halitosis because these wounds soon become infected.

Complications

• **Inability to eat or drink**. Some patients have such severe damage to the structures of the mouth that it is impossible for them to eat or drink. Such animals need to be supported with intravenous therapy and may need to have a pharyngostomy or nasopharyngeal tube implanted.
• **Unconsciousness**. Fracture of the hard palate may occasionally be associated with other cranial fractures which cause brain damage and unconsciousness.
• **Infection** following any injury, because the mouth is not a sterile environment.
• **Damage to pharyngeal tissues** and **deeply embedded foreign bodies** following the 'running on to a stick' injury. Many of these lacerations are very deep, often extending 15cm from the root of

the tongue into the pharyngeal tissue. It is not uncommon for a small fragment of stick to break off and remain buried deep in the wound, where it festers and may abscessate on to the skin of the neck weeks after the initial injury.

Treatment. For **insect stings** and **tongue ulceration**, refer to the Poisons section.

There is no specific first aid treatment for **fractures** unless the mandibular injuries are so severe that the lower jaw hangs down because both rami are fractured. In these cases, the fracture can be stabilised by gently bandaging the jaws together so that the upper jaw acts as a splint for the lower jaw.

Removal of **foreign bodies** (including loose teeth) should be attempted cautiously, as the animal will often resent handling of the mouth, and general anaesthesia may be required.

Sticks and bones lodged across the roof of the mouth are often easily levered out if a pair of closed artery forceps or dental forceps is gently slipped between the foreign body and the roof of the mouth. A small pair of forceps must be used as these objects are usually jammed tightly against the soft tissues. If the foreign body does not dislodge easily, do not apply excessive force: the object might have penetrated the tissues more deeply than it appears.

WARNING
No attempt should be made to pull out a fish-hook. Because of its barbed end, the shaft should be pushed still further into the tissues until the barb comes out through the skin (Fig. 3.41). This is not easy to do as fish-hooks are often rusty and blunt. Spraying the buccal mucosa with local anaesthetic can help to deaden the pain whilst this procedure is carried out, but it may be impossible to do with the animal conscious. Once the barb is pushed free of the mucosa, the shaft of the hook is cut through and the two halves are removed independently.

It is usually impossible to wash **wounds** in the mouth (as described earlier) but the theatre and instruments may be prepared for the suturing of extensive wounds.

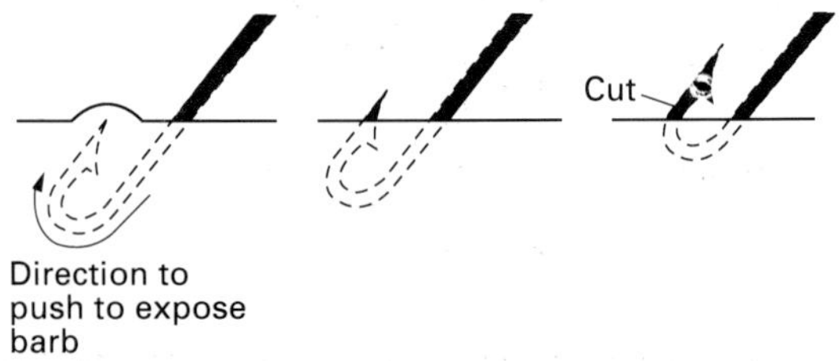

Direction to
push to expose
barb

Fig. 3.41. Removing a fish-hook.

Pharynx and oesophagus

Causes. **Foreign bodies** may lodge in the pharynx:

- The partly swallowed ball which lodges just behind the tongue on top of the larynx, being just too large to pass down the oesophagus, can be fatal (Fig. 3.42).
- Cats eating grass may get a blade of grass stuck in the pharynx as they try to swallow it (Fig. 3.38).
- Sewing needles and fish-hooks are occasionally found embedded in the walls of the pharynx or come to lie across the pharynx of young animals.
- Bones may also become lodged. The worst culprits are either fish bones (which usually lodge across the pharynx as a needle might) or rough irregular bones such as chop bones or chicken bones, where the projections prevent them from passing easily down into the oesophagus.

Inflammation of the pharynx as a result of trauma, stings etc. can cause severe problems if the walls of the pharynx become swollen.

Signs

- **Altered behaviour.** Cats are usually subdued and are reluctant to groom normally because the actions of the tongue move the foreign body in the pharynx and may cause severe discomfort. Dogs are often restless and may paw at the mouth or try to vomit to remove the foreign body.
- **Gagging, retching and gulping** when swallowing or when the pharynx is gently palpated externally. If the foreign body is sharp, handling this area will cause intense pain and may drive the object deeper into the pharyngeal tissues. Great care is needed when handling these animals.
- **Salivation.** If swallowing is too painful, the patient may drool; this is usually seen when sharp objects are lodged.
- **Dysphagia.**

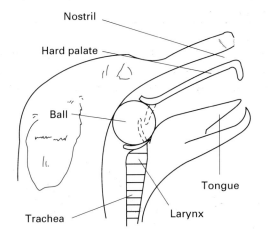

------ Normal positions of soft palate and epiglottis

Fig. 3.42. Pharyngeal foreign body: ball lodged in pharynx.

- **Dyspnoea** varying from heavy breathing to asphyxia, depending upon the degree of pharyngeal obstruction. If the walls of the pharynx are simply inflamed and slightly swollen, the breathing may be slightly harsher than normal. If the pharynx is completely blocked by a foreign body, the patient will very soon suffocate (Fig. 3.42).

Complications. **Asphyxia** has already been discussed. Another complication might be **nasal discharge** in cats with grass pharyngeal foreign bodies. If the grass is not or cannot be removed, it will usually start to track forwards into the nasopharynx and thence into the nasal passages over a period of days or weeks. It acts as a focus for infection so that a purulent unilateral nasal discharge commonly develops.

Treatment. **Remove the foreign body.** With the animal held firmly, the mouth should be opened as far as possible to inspect the throat. Pharyngeal foreign bodies are rarely removable without an anaesthetic, as they are usually lodged beyond reach, but it may be possible to attempt careful removal of a foreign body with fingers or forceps if it can be seen clearly. The Heimlich manoeuvre (see later section on Asphyxia) may be attempted to remove smooth foreign bodies.

A **thread** should not be pulled, but traced to determine if it is attached to a needle or fish-hook. If a **needle** cannot be dislodged, the two ends of the thread should be tied together to prevent it becoming unthreaded. The veterinary surgeon will then be able to trace the thread and easily locate the needle at surgery. If a **fish-hook** is involved, the line should not be tampered with for fear of worsening the injury.

Dyspnoeic patients should be kept under constant observation. Intubation may be necessary in cases of obstructing foreign bodies or if the swelling of the pharyngeal tissues gets steadily worse, as may happen in cases of allergic reactions to insect stings (see Asphyxia). Prepare a suitable endotracheal tube in case the animal loses consciousness. Also prepare the site for a tracheostomy by clipping up the midline ventral neck and giving it a preliminary scrub.

Oesophagus

Causes. The oesophagus is very distensible, with strong muscular walls, so that most smooth foreign bodies (e.g. balls) pass through uneventfully and enter the stomach. **Rough, irregular objects** such as chop bones might lodge in the oesophagus when the projections stick into the oesphageal wall. There are three sites where a bone or any other obstructing foreign body might lodge in the oesophagus:

- The thoracic inlet at the base of the neck.
- Over the base of the heart.
- At the cardia of the stomach.

Wounds to the oesophagus may occur in severe neck injuries (e.g. dog bite lacerations) but this is uncommon as it is a tough, elastic structure, buried under layers of muscle, and it tends to stretch rather than rupture.

Signs. Signs of foreign bodies include:

- **Vague discomfort**—the patient is usually slightly subdued and withdrawn.
- **Regurgitation**—food, if taken, is regurgitated almost immediately and is unchanged, i.e. there is no stomach acid present and no acidic smell to the vomit. Fluids often pass through unhindered because the obstruction is usually incomplete.

Traumatic damage to the oesophagus is usually only detected at surgery, when the wound is being sutured. Occasionally, swallowed saliva may be detected leaking from the wound.

Complications. Obstructing irregular or sharp foreign bodies may penetrate through the walls of the oesophagus, especially if they have been lodged there for some days because the owner does not realise the severity of the situation. If this occurs in the chest, the infected material surrounding the foreign body can leak out of the oesophagus and enter the pleural cavity, causing pleurisy or even a pyothorax if the condition is left untreated.

Treatment. There is no specific first aid treatment. In cases of suspected foreign bodies, the patient should be prepared for endoscopy and/or radiography and a barium swallow. Surgery will probably be necessary in long-standing cases.

Stomach

Causes:

- **Foreign bodies**. Many objects may be swallowed and lodge in the stomach—e.g. stones, bones and assorted household objects. Young, inexperienced and curious animals are the most at risk. Dogs tend to suffer more than cats because they do not mind what they eat and the greedy dog is the worst of all.
- **Infections or disease** causing persistent vomiting, e.g. parvovirus, renal failure.
- **Poisoning** by corrosive substances.
- **External trauma**, e.g. a blow to the abdomen sustained during a road accident.
- **Gastric dilation and torsion** (described later).

Foreign bodies

Signs

- **Vomiting**. Patients harbouring a foreign body are bright, alert and normally healthy for most of the time, but suffer bouts of acute vomiting if the foreign body jams in the pylorus and obstructs the emptying of the stomach. If the object then falls back into the stomach, the symptoms disappear again.
- **Pain**. The stomach is a roomy organ and it is rare that any foreign body causes much discomfort unless it lodges in the entrance or exit of the stomach.

Complications. Occasionally, a large foreign body may irritate the gastric lining, which leads to **haematemesis** (vomiting blood), but this is rare.

If the foreign body should squeeze through the pylorus into the small intestine, it may well obstruct and cause problems (see Intestines).

Treatment. Food and water should be withheld until the veterinary surgeon has been consulted. Radiographs and barium meals may be necessary to diagnose the problem and a laparotomy may have to be performed if a foreign body is present.

Inflammation

Signs

- **Vomiting**. Inflammatory conditions of the stomach result in more consistent, prolonged periods of vomiting, especially after food or water is ingested.
- **Haematemesis**. The vomit may contain blood, which haemorrhages from the sore and possibly ulcerated stomach lining. (Note that animals will vomit back ingested blood which they have swallowed, e.g. after licking wounds, and so haematemesis is not always a sign of gastric irritation/ulceration.) Fresh blood appears bright red or gives a pinkish tinge to the vomit. Blood which has remained in the stomach for any length of time is brown in colour and resembles coffee grounds as it is partially digested.
- **Pain**. The stomach lining is sore and becomes rapidly more inflamed as the vomiting persists. The animal is often depressed and obviously ill and may show abdominal guarding, a tucked-up abdomen or it may assume a 'praying position'. (Fig. 3.46)

Complications. Dehydration and electrolyte imbalance (loss of chloride ions) occur due to prolonged vomiting. Other complications arise because of the underlying conditions (see sections on poisoning, infectious diseases, renal failure etc.).

Treatment

- **Withold all fluids and food**. In some cases, great thirst may be exhibited, but no food or fluid should be given by mouth. A piece of ice placed on a flannel in a dish so that the water formed as the ice melts is absorbed and cannot be taken, may be given to the animal to lick.

- **Prepare intravenous fluids**. Normal saline will replace the chloride ions lost. In cases of kidney failure, Hartmann's solution should be used.
- **Treat for shock**.

Gastric dilation and torsion

Cause. The cause of this syndrome is not known, but it is an extremely serious condition. The stomach fills with gas and swells to enormous proportions (gastric dilation). Very often, the gas is unable to escape because the whole stomach has twisted around in the abdomen, effectively knotting the cardia and pylorus together and occluding both entrance and exit (gastric torsion). As the gas pressure continues to build, the condition becomes more and more serious and will be fatal within hours unless the first aider is prepared to take certain emergency measures.

The condition is almost always seen in large, deep-chested dogs, usually 2–3 hours after they have eaten a large meal. Dilations also occasionally occur in elderly small dogs.

Signs

- **Restlessness** and signs of discomfort are the first signs as the stomach begins to swell. Nothing else is usually noticed at this stage. The dog is unable to settle and may eat grass and try to vomit without success. In some cases, gas may be belched up.
- **Swelling** of the anterior abdomen follows as the pressure builds, distending the stomach so much that the posterior rib cage is pushed out. Gentle tapping on the abdominal wall with finger-tips produces a hollow, drum-like sound.
- **Breathing becomes laboured** as the swelling enlarges and the condition becomes more painful. The diaphragm is also pushed forwards by the hugely distended stomach, which makes breathing more difficult and painful. The stomach of a weimeraner-sized dog may be as big as a large washing-up bowl at this stage.
- **Collapse**. The dog collapses gradually into lateral recumbency, when the gas-filled, bloated stomach can be clearly seen to bulge on the left side, just behind the rib cage. The blood circulation has also been upset by this stage as the enormous stomach presses on the posterior vena cava and portal veins, slowing the return of blood to the heart from the posterior abdomen. The patient is now severely shocked and close to death.

Complications. Gastric rupture and death. If untreated, the dog will become unconscious, the stomach will rupture and the animal will soon die.

Treatment

(1) **Veterinary assistance must be sought immediately**.
(2) **Relieve the pressure in the stomach**. If the dog is collapsed and unconscious and veterinary help is delayed, the pressure must be eased or the dog will die. There are two possible courses of action: passing a stomach tube or, if that is unsuccessful, piercing the abdominal wall.
(3) **Treat for shock**.
(4) In all cases, **emergency surgery** will be necessary and the nurse should prepare the patient and the theatre accordingly.

Stomach tube. Attempts may be made to pass a stomach tube if the arrival is already unconcious once the airway has been maintained by intubating with a cuffed endotracheal tube. Some cooperative animals will swallow a stomach tube when fully conscious and a roll of bandage can be used as an improvised gag if placed between the molar teeth.

(1) The stomach tube is first measured against the outside of the patient: lay the tube on the dog so that it follows the course of the oesophagus down the neck, through the thorax to the posterior edge of the thorax. Make a mark on the tube where it lies level with the canine tooth (Fig. 3.43). This precaution ensures that the operator knows how far to pass the tube in order to position one end inside the stomach.
(2) Lubricate the blunted end of the stomach tube and pass it down the oesophagus.
(3) When the cardiac sphincter of the stomach is reached, there will be some resistance, but gentle pressure may overcome this. If not, **do not persist** in the attempt to enter the stomach. The stomach may have twisted on itself and force will only rupture the oesophagus.

Emergency deflation by piercing the abdominal wall

> WARNING
> **This procedure must only be performed with the knowledge and consent of the veterinary surgeon.** It must only be attempted if the patient has become unconscious, appears cyanosed and as an emergency measure to save the dog's life.

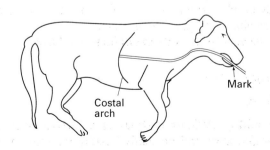

Fig. 3.43. Measuring stomach tube (gastric torsion).

If stomach tubing is unsuccessful, the gas may be allowed to escape by using a wide-bore (16 G) intravenous needle to pierce the **left** abdominal wall at the point of maximum distension.

(1) The skin is quickly clipped and prepared for surgery.
(2) The large bore needle is **inserted at right angles to the skin at the point of maximum distension**.
(3) As soon as the stomach is entered, a gust of gas will escape, and the pressure will reduce. The needle hub must be held in position, pressed against the skin at right angles as the abdomen slowly deflates.
(4) The release of gas may be slowed by a finger tip over the needle hub—this reduces the shock of too rapid deflation.

Intestine

Causes

* **Obstruction**. The small intestine can become blocked by
  (a) Foreign bodies similar to those found in the stomach. Various examples have been quoted, but often an object can be in the stomach for months before it finally moves into the small intestine and causes a problem.
  (b) Portions of intestine which 'telescope' into one another (**intussusception**).
  (c) Strangulation of hernias/ruptures of the abdominal wall.
* **Infection**. Organisms such as *Clostridium perfringens*, canine parvovirus, *Giardia* and feline enteritis can cause sudden and acute sickness and diarrhoea, involving severe inflammation of the intestine.
* **Poisonings**. Several poisons damage the intestines.

Foreign bodies

Signs

* **Vomiting** which, if the obstruction is complete, is often brown, foul-smelling faecal vomit. The patient may be sick every hour, day and night, as the normal bowel secretions are unable to pass down the intestine and have to be vomited back.
* **Pain** varies, depending on how much the intestinal wall is damaged. If the object is large or rough, with irregular, sharp projections (e.g. bones), the animal may suffer acute abdominal pain, shown by restlessness, adopting the 'praying position' and tucking up the abdomen (see Fig. 3.46). Some animals may suffer conscious collapse. Smooth objects do not cause the same discomfort and the animal may remain quite bright, despite regular bouts of vomiting.

* **Lack of faeces**. As nothing is passing through the intestine, faecal production gradually ceases or very few faeces are passed. When the temperature is taken, the rectum feels sticky and dry as the thermometer is inserted.

Complications. Rupture of the intestines and subsequent peritonitis—a sharp projection from a foreign body may erode the intestinal wall and rupture the intestine. In cases of intussusception, the wall may rupture as the telescoped tissues loose their blood supply and die.

Dehydration occurs due to the fluids lost by the continual vomiting.

Treatment

* Keep the patient comfortable and give nothing by mouth.
* Radiographs and barium meals may be needed to help diagnose the problem.
* Intravenous fluids will be required to correct the electrolyte loss (chloride ions) and dehydration.

Infections and poisonings

Signs

* **Vomiting**. Acute intestinal infections and certain poisons may cause bouts of prolonged vomiting. The vomit may be clear, bile stained or tinged with blood, which may be fresh or partially digested. It is rarely faecal vomit.
* **Diarrhoea** is often observed in these cases as the whole of the intestines are irritated and inflamed. In these acute cases, it is usually bloody and foul-smelling.
* **Collapse and shock**. These patients are acutely ill and rapidly dehyrate. The mucosa is pale and the pulse is thin and rapid.

Complications. Other animals may be infected by these patients. They should be isolated as soon as possible.

Dehydration is a real problem and needs to be corrected rapidly. In cases of poisonings, other body systems may also be affected, e.g. kidneys, central nervous system.

Treatment. Drugs may be needed to control the vomiting (e.g. metoclopramide) and the patient should be treated for shock. Intravenous Hartmann's solution is the drip of choice as the diarrhoea leads to loss of bicarbonate ions.

Rectum and Anus

Prolapse of the rectum

Cause. This condition involves a protrusion of the rectum through the anal opening. The rectum is literally pushed out of the anus and, not surprisingly, these prolapses are usually associated with conditions producing diarrhoea and/or **tenesmus** (straining to pass faeces).

Signs. Rectal prolapses are usually seen in young puppies or kittens but can also occur in hamsters of any age. They range in severity from partial prolapses (where only the mucosal rectal lining is prolapsed, Fig. 3.44(a)) to total prolapses (where the entire thickness of the rectal wall prolapses, Fig. 3.44(b)).

A **partial prolapse** appears as a pinky-red rosette centred on the anal opening. As the prolapse is small, it frequently disappears (i.e. reduces spontaneously) between bouts of straining and thus the mucosa usually remains moist and may escape ulceration.

Total prolapses present as red, oedematous, tubular structures protruding from the anus. The prolapsed mucosa is often coated with thick mucus and is frequently congested; it may dry out and ulcerate if not replaced promptly. The length of the prolapse varies, depending on how much rectal wall is involved, but can be surprisingly large – particularly in hamsters, where 2cm prolapses are not unknown. In the female it is sometimes difficult to distinguish this mass from a prolapse of the vagina.

Complications

- **Swelling.** The venous return and lymphatic drainage are often partially blocked by the pressure on the tissues at the anal ring. Thus the prolapse swells and becomes congested, which makes the patient strain even harder and makes it more difficult to replace the prolapse.

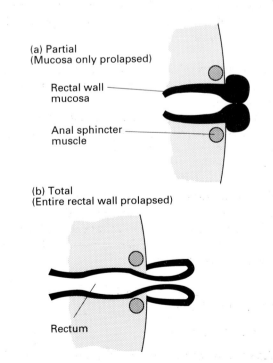

(a) Partial
(Mucosa only prolapsed)

Rectal wall mucosa

Anal sphincter muscle

(b) Total
(Entire rectal wall prolapsed)

Rectum

Fig. 3.44. Rectal prolapses.

- **Drying of mucosa.** Dry mucosa is very fragile and easily damaged and so ulcers and haemorrhage are common. The tacky mucosa is also easily contaminated by cat litter, bedding etc. and it can be very difficult to bathe these foreign bodies away without further damaging the mucosa.
- **Self trauma.** As the animal automatically tries to clean the area, its rough tongue inflicts much damage. It is not unknown for patients (particularly hamsters) to groom so obsessively that they severely mutilate or even chew off the prolapsed tissues.

Treatment

- **Moisten and lubricate** the prolapsed tissue. Warm saline (0.9% solution) should first be used to rehydrate the mucosa, followed by liquid paraffin to lubricate the tissues and prevent them from drying out again. Several applications of liquid paraffin may be required if the prolapse cannot be reduced to ensure that the surface stays moist.
- **Attempt to replace the prolapse.** Gentle pressure should be used—a finger-and-thumb 'pinching' movement on the end of the protrusion is usually the most successful, encouraging the tip of the prolapse to turn back in on itself. Once the exposed tip has been persuaded to invert again, the rest of the tissues usually follow—but not invariably. If the prolapsed mucosa starts to bleed, the attempt should be abandoned. Many cases require surgical treatment to reduce them successfully.
- **Prevent further straining.** An analgesic suppository may be inserted to prevent further straining or, if this is unavailable or impractical to use (e.g. the patient is too small or the tissues are too fragile to handle), the prolapse can be sprayed with local anaesthetic.
- **Prevent self-trauma.** The patient should be fitted with an Elizabethan collar and kept under constant observation.
- **Prepare the patient for surgery.** Even if the prolapse can be reduced, most cases readily recur and it is usually necessary to place a purse-string suture around the anal ring to keep the prolapsed tissues in place.

Anal foreign bodies

Cause. Sharp pieces of bone or small pieces of bone impacted into a mass may become lodged in the posterior rectum and anus. This is a particular problem of the middle-aged or elderly dog which has been given cooked bones to eat. As dogs age, they become less able to digest such 'treats' and the bone passes through the system virtually unchanged, gathering together in the colon to form a concreted mass of bony spicules. Pins, safety pins, needles, sharp bits of plastic etc. may lodge transversely across the rectum or anus, or penetrate their walls. This condition is seen more frequently in the young animal, which is more inclined to chew things up and swallow foreign bodies.

Signs

- The animal is restless and unable to sit comfortably; it may show persistent irritation by continually licking the anus.
- Constant straining which either produces only a mucoid discharge from the anus or may result in small, hard, blood-stained faecal pellets being passed.
- Pain when straining—non-penetrating foreign bodies cause some discomfort but the foreign body lodged across the rectum causes the animal to cry out as it strains to pass faeces.
- Haemorrhage may be seen if the obstruction penetrates the rectal wall.
- Vomiting is not uncommon in cases of constipation, possibly related to the continual strong abdominal straining.

Complications. Rectal prolapse due to the excessive straining (see above); wounding and inflammation of the rectal mucosa.

Treatment

- **Attempt to remove the foreign body**. The area should be lubricated with liquid paraffin and the bone may then be removed very carefully with fingers or forceps if it is not too firmly lodged. If a thread is found hanging from the anus, a search should be made to discover the other free end, and the two ends tied together. Gentle pulling may remove the needle, but no force must be applied. If the foreign body cannot be removed easily, the animal should be referred to a veterinary surgeon.
- **Attempt to remove the impacted mass**. A gentle 'milking' action, as used when emptying anal glands, may cause the impacted mass to pop out of the anus. Liquid paraffin should again be used to lubricate the area before this is attempted.

Impacted anal sacs

Cause. Blockage of the ducts of the anal sacs and subsequent impaction may lead to abscess formation. Such an abscess will usually break to the outside of the rim of the anus.

Signs. The animal shows initial irritation of the area but, as the abscess forms, the area is swollen and the skin becomes reddened, shiny and very painful. The patient becomes depressed and febrile, with a full, bounding pulse. The abscess soon bursts and the patient then recovers.

Treatment. Hot fomentations may speed the 'pointing' of the abscess and alleviate the pain in the earlier stages. A pad of cotton wool moistened with hot water can be held against the perineum.

When the abscess has burst, the matted hair should be clipped away from the area and the wound washed as described earlier. Antibiotics are usually needed to control the infection.

Injuries to the Abdominal Wall

Definitions

A **rupture** is said to have occurred when abdominal viscera escape through a traumatic tear in the muscles bounding the abdominal cavity, i.e. the muscular abdominal wall and diaphragm.

A **hernia** is said to have occurred when abdominal viscera escape through a natural body opening in the muscular abdominal wall, i.e. the inguinal canals and umbilicus.

Causes. Injuries to the abdominal wall may be caused by:

- road accidents, when the wheels of vehicles may pass over the abdomen causing severe crushing injuries;
- staking injuries, when the animal becomes impaled on a sharp object;
- severe bites;
- gunshot wounds;
- surgical procedures.

In the case of hernias, the natural openings in the body wall (i.e. the umbilicus and the inguinal canals) are larger than normal in affected animals but it may be years before any abdominal contents find their way through the enlarged openings and come to lie just under the skin. If these organs then become trapped and strangulate, the animal will become acutely ill and may present as an emergency.

Signs of injury. As with the thoracic injury, abdominal wounds must be treated cautiously as it can be difficult to appreciate the depth of the wound.

Open wounds. If the muscles making up the body wall have been ruptured, part of the abdominal contents (particularly the lacy fat of the omentum) can escape and protrude through the rupture (Fig. 3.45a). Fatty tags on the surface of the wound may indicate that the wound penetrates deeply into the abdominal cavity and is much more serious than a superficial wound.

Closed wounds. Occasionally, no external wound is apparent and yet the muscles of the abdominal wall have still been ruptured, allowing abdominal organs to escape from the peritoneal cavity. In these cases, there is little to see except the skin discolouration produced by the bruising, and an abnormal swelling under the skin. This swelling may not be obvious

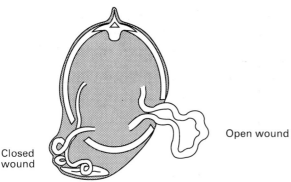

(a) Reducible hernias and ruptures

Closed wound

Open wound

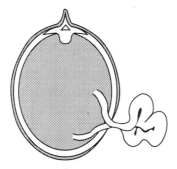

(b) Irreducible hernias and ruptures

Fig. 3.45. Abdominal wall injuries.

because the surrounding tissues are bruised and swollen themselves so that the edges of the swelling are not clearly defined.

The most serious of this type of injury is the **diaphragmatic rupture** (see injuries to the respiratory tract.) Other serious injuries commonly occur in the inguinal region.

Signs of strangulated hernia. The owner may report a sudden swelling in the umbilical or inguinal region which is soft and painless at first but, after a variable period, the swelling suddenly becomes hard and painful as the hernia strangulates. The skin over the swelling becomes inflamed and the animal shows considerable discomfort and may vomit because loops of intestine are obstructed.

Complications

Evisceration. Evisceration occurs when an organ or organs escape from a body cavity. The most common organs to escape from the abdominal cavity are the omentum and loops of small intestine.

Omentum tissue looks like small fatty tags in the depths of the open wound and can be difficult to distinguish from torn subcutaneous fatty tissue.

Loops of intestine are unmistakable. Usually several loops of intestine protrude from the wound and will dry out when exposed to the air. The surface

becomes tacky and is therefore often heavily contaminated by dirt, grit etc. The intestine appears bright red in colour but the walls remain soft and pliable (c.f. irreducible hernias and ruptures, below).

Irreducible ruptures and hernias. Any organs trapped outside the peritoneal cavity may gradually swell if the venous blood return from the organs is cut off or reduced. The organs then become very painful, swollen and inflamed and cannot be replaced into the abdomen.

Loops of intestine involved in irreducible ruptures appear dark red in colour, with turgid, stiffened walls. Small tears are often seen in the serosa. If the loops are parted, it is usually possible to see the bounding arterial pulse in the mesentery.

Irreducible ruptures and hernias also occur when a distensible organ such as the bladder is involved. As the empty bladder fills with urine and enlarges over a period of hours, it becomes impossible to replace it into the abdomen. This presents serious problems because the bladder is often unable to empty and the pressure within the bladder rises, causing the patient excruciating pain.

Strangulated rupture or hernia. This occurs if the arterial blood supply to the eviscerated organs is also reduced and the tissues start to die.

As the irreducible condition becomes strangulated, the viscera take on a blackened appearance and the arterial pulse becomes thin and weak before ceasing completely. If the wound is closed and no viscera can be seen, the skin overlying the area is often reddened and inflamed. The tense and painful nature of the swelling and its position (if a hernia) should lead the veterinary nurse to suspect the cause of the problem.

These animals are frequently toxic and collapse. If a loop of intestine is involved, there will also be vomiting because the bowel is obstructed as it passes into and out of the hernia or rupture.

Self-trauma. Animals with open eviscerated wounds are liable to damage the viscera when licking the wound. Sometimes, as with rectal and viscera prolapses, they may actually eat away the exposed organs in their desperation to clean the wound.

Trauma. Abdominal organs might also have been damaged in the accident which injured the abdominal wall. This can lead to peritonitis (if the bowel or bladder is perforated) or severe or even fatal haemorrhage (if the liver, kidney, spleen etc. are damaged). Eviscerated organs may have been so damaged in the course of the accident that they need to be surgically removed in order to save the life of the patient.

Collapsed lungs. In cases of diaphragmatic rupture, the lungs may be collapsed (see injuries to the respiratory tract).

Infection. As with any open wound, abdominal wounds are prone to infection, but the consequences are more severe if the abdominal cavity has been entered as peritonitis can develop.

Treatment

- **Clean the wound.** In cases where abdominal viscera protrude through an open wound, the hair should be clipped away in the normal manner, but antiseptics must *never* be used in case irritant chemicals penetrate the peritoneal cavity. The protruding viscera should be washed with warmed sterile saline to remove any grit or dirt.
- **Attempt to replace viscera into the abdominal cavity.** No force should be applied and it is easier to restrain the animal in such a position that the wounded side of the abdomen lies uppermost so that gravity assists the replacement. However, if there is any difficulty in breathing, the animal should not be forced to lie on its side or its back as this could prove fatal.
- **Prevent damage to exposed viscera.** If it is impossible to replace the viscera, they must be kept warm, moist and undamaged by a covering of sterile swabs soaked in sterile saline and bandaged firmly but gently in place, using a crepe bandage which encircles the abdomen or a many-tailed bandage. This is an important first aid measure that the owner should take at home to keep the exposed tissues viable during transport to the surgery. Sterile saline solutions, such as used in the care of contact lenses, are ideal to moisten the dressings, but cooled, boiled water may be used if no such solution is available. The viscera should be inspected every 15 minutes to renew the dampened swabs and check that the bandaging has not interfered with the circulation to the protruding viscera.
- **Observation and treatment for shock.** The animal must be constantly observed to prevent it tampering with the dressings and damaging the protruding viscera. All patients should be confined, made comfortable and treated for shock.
- **Prepare the theatre.** Veterinary assistance must be sought as soon as possible because irreducible ruptures or hernias may progress to strangulated conditions and these injuries, unless rapidly reduced, cause irreversible damage. Surgical interference is invariably necessary and the veterinary nurse should prepare the theatre accordingly.

Injuries to Abdominal Organs: Liver, Spleen, Pancreas

Signs of abdominal pain

Injury to any abdominal organ can cause acute abdominal pain and the symptoms displayed are the same, regardless of the cause or organ affected:

- **Body posture.** The animal stands with its back arched and its abdomen tightly 'tucked up' (Fig. 3.46(a)) or it may adopt the 'praying position', lying down on its sternum but with its hind legs still standing (Fig. 3.46(b)).
- **Abdominal boarding.** The slightest touch on the abdominal wall usually results in the abdominal muscles stiffening to become as hard as a board. This is also termed **guarding** of the abdomen.
- **Depression.** The patient is usually very ill and may even be collapsed. These animals are also commonly pyrexic.

Liver

Causes

- Trauma to the liver may occur in road accidents.
- Infectious canine hepatitis and *Leptospira ictero-haemorrhagica* can both severely injure the liver of the dog.
- Poisons (e.g. antifreeze) may cause acute liver damage in the dog and cat.
- Bile ducts or gall bladders, which become blocked or are ruptured in road accidents, also result in signs of liver damage as the irritant bile either cannot drain away and so causes liver inflammation or, in cases of rupture, drains into the abdominal cavity and collects there instead of being excreted into the lumen of the small intestine.

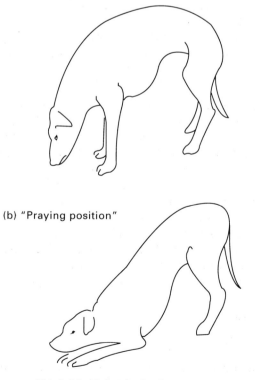

(a) Tucked-up abdomen

(b) "Praying position"

Fig. 3.46. Abdominal pain stance.

Signs

- **Pain**. Acute liver damage is usually accompanied by acute abdominal pain.
- **Vomiting**. Patients with liver problems are usually vomiting and there may be diarrhoea in cases of infection.
- **Jaundice**. Depending on the type, severity and duration of the injury, the patient's mucous membranes may also be jaundiced. Infections and poisons act directly to damage the liver tissues and so the signs are observed immediately, but it may be several days or weeks until a ruptured gall bladder or bile duct causes a problem. The bile which collects in the peritoneal cavity remains in the body instead of being excreted and is gradually absorbed back into the blood stream. The liver and kidneys are unable to cope with excreting this increased volume of bile salts and pigments and the levels in the blood stream steadily increase so that the animal becomes jaundiced and toxic.

Complications

- **Haemorrhage**. The liver is a very vascular organ and trauma may result in severe internal haemorrhage.
- **Diaphragmatic rupture**. Injuries which crush the anterior abdomen and damage the liver may also tear the diaphragm (see injuries to the respiratory tract).

Treatment. No specific first aid treatment is possible, but the veterinary nurse should remain alert to the possibility of infectious conditions in the unvaccinated animal and isolate the patient.

> WARNING
> It is also important to ensure rigorous hygiene precautions are enforced because leptospirosis is a zoonosis which can be fatal in humans.

Pending the attention of the veterinary surgeon, all patients should be made comfortable and treated for shock. It is generally not advisable to give fluids by mouth as this may provoke an attack of vomiting. If the animal does vomit, a sample should be kept in case the animal may have been poisoned.

Intravenous fluids may be required (e.g. Hartmann's solution) and plasma expanders (e.g. Haemaccel) or blood transfusions may be necessary in cases of internal haemorrhage. The veterinary nurse may also prepare for X-ray because it may be necessary to check for a ruptured diaphragm.

Spleen

Causes

- **Tumours**. Some dogs suffer from malignant tumours of the spleen, which can cause collapse

from a very sudden major internal haemorrhage if they erode through the splenic capsule.
- **Trauma**. The spleen may be ruptured following a crushing injury to the abdomen.
- **Torsion**. Very occasionally, the spleen rotates in the abdomen, twisting the loose gastrosplenic mesentry into a tight cord-like structure. This results in serious venous congestion of the spleen as the thin-walled veins collapse in the tightening gastrosplenic mesentry and the spleen can swell to enormous size.

Signs. Haemorrhage from the spleen, whether caused by an invading cancer or by external injury, is often severe and can be fatal. The animal is collapsed; it breathes rapidly and has a thin, rapid pulse and extremely pale mucous membranes. The sudden onset of collapse and circulatory shock is characteristic, there may have been a history of previous partial collapse with recovery once the bleeding stops.

Splenic torsions cause acute abdominal pain and sometimes it is possible to see the engorged spleen distending the anterior abdominal wall.

Complication. Severe internal haemorrhage and death.

Treatment. No specific first aid treatment is possible, though the abdomen may be firmly bandaged in cases of internal haemorrhage to attempt to increase the back pressure. The animal should be made as comfortable as possible and **treated for shock**. Surgical intervention may be necessary and plasma expanders or blood transfusions can be prepared for intravenous administration.

Pancreas

Cause. Acute pancreatitis can cause sudden death or acute illness in dogs. The problem arises because certain changes allow the trypsin in the pancreas to set off a chain reaction, which results in the digestion of the tissues of the pancreas—i.e. the animal starts to digest its own body. This digestion releases even more trypsin, which causes even more autodigestion. Once the process has started, it can rapidly escalate and bring about severe shock and the death of the patient, often in great pain.

Signs. The animal is extremely ill; it shows signs of acute abdominal pain and may vomit.

Treatment. There is little that can be done except to give fluids to correct the acid/base balance, give antibiotic cover and provide relief from pain by administering pain-killing drugs. The veterinary nurse should therefore treat the animal for shock and make it as comfortable as possible until the veterinary surgeon can give the necessary treatment. Lactated Ringer's solution may be warmed in readiness for intravenous administration and corticosteroid injections may be prepared for intravenous use.

Injuries to the Urogenital System

Definitions

- **Anuria** is the complete absence of passage of urine.
- **Oliguria** occurs when the animal only passes a very small volume of urine over a period of time.
- **Tachyuria** is the passing of small amounts of urine at very frequent intervals. A normal volume of urine is passed over a period of time, but as little-and-often dribbles rather than normal streams.
- **Dysuria** occurs when the patient has difficulty passing urine. This may be because it is too painful or because the outlet is obstructed.
- **Haematuria** is the passing of blood in the urine.

> WARNING
> Care must be taken when examining a bitch to ensure that the normal bleeding of the oestrous cycle is not confused with haematuria.

- **Cystitis** is the term given to inflammation of the bladder.

Kidney

Causes

- **Trauma**. Crushing or staking injuries of the abdomen which rupture the kidney result in instant death due to internal haemorrhage. The blood supply to the kidneys is extremely good and the effect of crushing the kidney is nearly as dramatic as severing the abdominal aorta. Less severe trauma may bruise the kidney tissue and result in haematuria.
- **Back pressure damage**. If the outflow of urine is obstructed at any point along the tract (e.g. by stones blocking the urethra), back pressure will build up in the kidney tissues as the urine continues to be produced but cannot drain away from the renal tubules. This pressure will eventually destroy the delicate filtration beds in the kidney.
- **Infection** with *Leptospira canicola* causes inflammation and destruction of the kidney tissues.
- **Ingestion of certain poisons** (e.g. antifreeze, chlorate herbicides, mercury compounds) can also cause acute kidney damage.

Signs

- **Abdominal pain**. Patients with kidney damage are frequently in severe pain and may stand with an arched back and be 'tucked up' in the abdomen or show signs of abdominal guarding when the abdomen is touched (Fig. 3.46).
- **Elevated temperature** in cases of infection.
- **Oliguria and haematuria**. The amount of urine which is produced by the kidney is reduced and often bloodstained.

Complications. Hypovolaemic shock and/or death may follow trauma to the kidney. Acute renal failure is always a risk following sudden damage to the renal tissues. The signs include vomiting, oliguria, dehydration, collapse and death.

Treatment. There are no specific first aid measures but the veterinary nurse should always be alert to the possibility of kidney damage if the abdomen has been crushed or poisons consumed. The volume and appearance of any urine passed should be recorded and the presence and extent of haematuria noted. **Samples should be kept for the veterinary surgeon to examine and for analysis in cases of suspected poisoning.**

These animals rapidly become acidotic and the setting up of a lactated Ringer's intravenous drip (e.g. Hartmann's solution) will greatly increase the chances of survival. The only contraindication for this treatment is an obstruction of the urinary tract, in which case it is best if the pressure is relieved before fluids are given.

Bladder

Causes

- **Trauma**. Rupture of the bladder may occur following crushing injuries to the abdomen if the bladder was full of urine. If the trauma is less severe, the bladder wall may simply be bruised and become inflamed. This is a common complication of pelvic fractures.
- **Irreducible hernias and ruptures**. If the bladder escapes from the abdominal cavity and then becomes trapped outside the body wall, the urethra may become obstructed. If this is not corrected, the pressure in the bladder may rise so dramatically that the bladder ruptures.
- **Bladder stones**. The presence of bladder stones inflames the mucosal lining of the bladder. If the urethra becomes obstructed, the bladder may rupture.
- **Infection**. Female patients are particularly prone to infection of the bladder, which can cause sudden and dramatic symptoms.

Signs of rupture of the bladder. Animals with ruptured bladders are pale and shocked and often collapsed. Occasionally a small drop of blood stained urine is seen at the vulva or prepuce. **No urine is passed** subsequently because the urine draining from the kidneys simply floods out through the ruptured wall of the bladder and collects in the abdominal cavity.

Signs of inflammation of the bladder (cystitis). If the bladder is simply bruised or inflamed, the animal shows dysuria, tachyuria and haematuria in many cases. These patients are not severely ill and may continue to eat normally, but are very restless and may cry continually, especially when straining to pass urine.

Complications. Uraemia and peritonitis follow bladder rupture. Bladder stones may pass into the urethra and obstruct it.

Treatment. No specific first aid measures are possible. The veterinary nurse must observe whether or not urine is passed and how frequently it is passed and must also note its appearance, smell and quantity.

If a rupture is suspected, the veterinary nurse should prepare catheters and X-ray plates so that a pneumocystogram can be performed to ascertain how severely the bladder is damaged. Emergency surgery will be necessary to repair the damaged wall.

Urethra

Causes

- **Trauma.** Fragments from pelvic fractures may pierce or bruise the urethra as it runs over the pubic symphysis. Occasionally the urethra may also be damaged in male animals if there are wounds to the perineum or penis.
- **Calculi.** The urethra of the male may become blocked by small stones which have been washed out of the bladder and may lodge firmly in the narrow part of the urethra as it passes through the os penis in the dog or just proximal to the tip of the penis in the cat. As this problem recurs in certain individuals, a good case history can be invaluable in reaching a correct diagnosis.

Signs of trauma. If the urethra is simply inflamed in the accident, urine will be passed normally but there may be some haematuria and dysuria, especially as the tissues start to swell in the hours following the accident. Occasionally, the lining of the urethra can swell so severely that it blocks the passage of urine and the animal really has to strain to pass anything at all.

If the urethra is ruptured, little or no urine will be passed through the penile opening, but some may leak out of the wound. Haemorrhage may be quite severe if the erectile tissue surrounding the urethra is damaged.

Signs of calculi. These patients are frequently anuric (i.e. do not pass urine). The animal will make many attempts to urinate and may succeed in passing a few drops. The bladder becomes distended as more urine is produced by the kidneys. The animal is very distressed and cries in pain. As the condition progresses, the patient will collapse and eventually the bladder may rupture. Palpation of the abdomen must not be attempted but the hard, spherical shape of the bladder is sometimes felt in the posterior abdomen whilst moving the patient.

Complications

- Haemorrhage if the wound damages the erectile tissues of the vascular penis.
- Rupture of the bladder.
- Kidney damage, leading to acute renal failure due to back pressure on the kidneys.

Treatment. There is no specific first aid treatment for any of the above conditions except if there are complications. Haemorrhage from erectile tissue is best controlled by digital pressure, pinching the tissues together. There is little force behind this haemorrhage and so constant pressure applied for 5 minutes should suffice to control it if the animal can be made to rest and does not interfere with the wound.

The animal should be made as comfortable as possible and treated for shock, pending the arrival of the veterinary surgeon. Catheterisation and surgical intervention are usually necessary and the theatre should be prepared accordingly.

Prostate Gland

Cause. Acute prostatitis in the dog is the only prostate condition which may present as an emergency. Any mature, entire dog can suffer from this problem, but it is more often a problem for the hypersexed animal. The cause is usually a bacterial infection.

Signs

- **Dysuria and possible haematuria.** The patient will strain to pass urine because the enlarged, inflamed prostate gland presses down on the urethra and partially occludes it.
- **Prepucial discharge.** The fluids from the infected gland drain into the urethra and out of the penis.
- **Vomiting** occurs in many cases, possibly because of endotoxaemia.
- **Pyrexia.** The temperature is usually markedly raised (104°F/40°C). Care must be taken when inserting the thermometer in small dogs because this procedure can be very painful if the thermometer should press into the gland (the prostate lies just ventral to the rectum and often bulges up, narrowing the rectum).

- **Abdominal pain** (Fig. 3.46). Typically, the patient is in acute pain and stands still, with the back arched high, refusing to walk. Any pressure on the abdominal wall results in groaning or the animal will turn and snap at the handler.
- **Depression**, followed by collapse in severe cases.

Treatment. There is no specific first aid treatment for this condition except general nursing care. Treatment usually consists of dosing with antibiotics and delmadinone acetate injections.

Penis

Causes

- **Trauma.** The tough fibrous coat of the penis may be damaged by self-inflicted injury in the over-sexed dog, exposing the cavernous tissues beneath.
- **Swelling.** The erect penis may become too engorged with blood to slide back into the prepuce and remains protruding. This is termed **paraphimosis**.
- **Foreign bodies.** Grass seeds etc. occasionally work their way up inside the prepuce.

Signs

- Trauma to the fibrous coat of the penis results in bouts of dramatic and copious haemorrhage every time the dog starts to get an erection. This is when the cavernous tissues fill with blood and, in cases of penile damage, the blood can flood out through the damaged fibrous coat.
- In cases of paraphimosis, the penis is very swollen and reddened and the prepucial opening appears to cut into the engorged tissues. The normally moist surface will dry out after a while, which makes replacing the protruding penis much more difficult.
- Foreign bodies inside the prepuce cause a heavy purulent discharge (which may be bloodstained) and irritation. The animal licks continually at the prepucial opening and is very restless, unable to settle comfortably. Palpation of the prepuce can be extremely painful. (Note that many hypersexed dogs normally have a thick green/yellow prepucial discharge but there is no pain or discomfort associated with the condition.)

Complication. The only complication to note is that of haemorrhage if the penis is traumatised.

Treatment for trauma cases. Veterinary assistance should be sought immediately in cases of penile haemorrhage but first aid can be given in the meantime. Cold compresses and ice packs will markedly decrease the blood flow to the penis and **pinching the skin just in front of the scrotum** further reduces the blood supply. These measures will help to control haemorrhage from the damaged penis.

The wound may be gently cleansed but great care should be taken to avoid disturbing the clots in the wound. Surgical repair is usually necessary.

Treatment for paraphimosis. Cold compresses and pinching the skin just in front of the scrotum will also decrease the size of the engorged penis sufficiently to allow it to slide back into the prepuce in many cases. However, if the tissues of the penis have become dry and tacky, liquid paraffin or KY jelly should be used to lubricate the tissues and aid reduction of the paraphimosis.

If these measures are not successful, the penis should be kept moist and **veterinary assistance must be sought** as it may be necessary to enlarge the prepucial opening surgically. Set out surgical instruments and prepare the theatre.

Treatment for foreign bodies. Foreign bodies can be removed if seen, but a general anaesthetic is often needed so that the penis can be fully extruded and the whole of the inside of the prepuce examined to ensure that all foreign bodies are removed and there is no other injury.

Vagina and Vulva

Causes. Most first aid situations in this area are associated with parturition (Chapter 19). Other conditions are:

- **Pyometra.** Owners may report that the bitch is 'bleeding' from the vulva, but this discharge usually turns out to be a reddish-brown purulent discharge from an open pyometra.
- **Vaginal polyps** and vaginal **prolapses** may occasionally be presented as an emergency.
- **Vaginal foreign bodies** do occasionally occur.
- **Trauma.** In some instances (e.g. road accidents), injuries to the perineum can affect the vulva.

Signs of open pyometra. Open pyometra cases are usually fairly bright and alert but there is much soiling of the fur around the vulva and the discharge is often unpleasantly smelly. The condition is classically seen in middle-aged animals (6–8 years old) and most bitches are midway between seasons, though these infections can occur immediately after a season. The patient is usually polydypsic.

Signs of polyps and prolapses. Vaginal polyps and prolapses are usually observed at the time of oestrus and appear as red, round, glistening masses which suddenly protrude from the vulva or are seen sitting between the lips of the vulva. The animal is well in herself and usually unconcerned about the problem, though she may strain occasionally, but the suddenness of the appearance of the prolapse worries the owner. Occasionally, protruding masses may become ulcerated and bleed but the haemorrhage, though messy, is not severe.

Signs of foreign bodies. Any foreign body in the vagina causes intense irritation, licking of the vulva and a purulent vaginal discharge if present for any length of time. The discharge is not as great as in the case of many open pyometras and can occur in any bitch, whether spayed or not.

Signs of wounds. Wounds to the vulva are usually lacerations or abrasions when the animal has been hit with force from the rear. There is usually much bruising.

Complications. Trauma to the perineum may also involve a fracture of the pelvis and damage to the urethra.

Treatment. Surgical intervention will usually be necessary in cases of open **pyometra** but rarely is emergency surgery necessary. **Vaginal polyps or prolapses** which protrude from the vulva should be replaced as soon as possible to prevent the surface from drying out and becoming damaged when the bitch sits down or licks the prolapsed tissues. Haemorrhage is not usually a problem in these cases, as any bleeding is normally capillary in nature. Gentle pressure applied to the prolapse is usually sufficient to replace it. If the surface has already become dry and sticky, it may also be necessary to lubricate the tissue with liquid paraffin or KY jelly. Where large polyps protrude, the lips of the vulva should be gently eased around the mass whilst applying pressure to replace it in the vagina. Prolapses which are impossible to reduce should be kept moist until the veterinary surgeon can attend the case. The patient should be kept under observation to ensure that she does not cause any damage to the prolapse. Haemorrhage may follow excessive licking of the polyp by the bitch. Fitting an Elizabethan collar will help to prevent self-trauma.

Foreign bodies may be removed if they can be seen easily but no undue force should be applied in case the foreign body is embedded in the wall of the vagina. A general anaesthetic is usually required. Any materials removed should be retained in case of possible litigation.

Wounds may be treated as described elsewhere in the text.

Injuries to the Eye
General Signs of Painful Injury to the Eye

Whatever the cause of pain in the eye, the clinical signs are similar:

- The eyelids are screwed up against the light (**blepharospasm**) and the patient may seek to hide away in dark corners because it dislikes bright light (**photophobia**) which causes the eyes to be even more painful.

- Tear production is increased and may overflow the eyelids (**epiphora**).
- The sclera and conjunctiva are often reddened and inflamed.
- Self-trauma: the animal may rub the eye with a forepaw, or rub its head against furniture etc.

Examination

The eye is a delicate and sensitive structure and should only be examined as described earlier. It is especially important to avoid touching the surface of the cornea with the finger as there will be a tendency to cause ulceration.

Eyelid
Causes

- **Wounds** to the eyelid are seen following road accidents, fights etc. or may be the result of self trauma.
- **Inflammatory reactions** occur as the result of allergic reactions, insect stings etc and may produce severe oedema of the eyelid conjunctiva.
- **Foreign bodies** (e.g. grass seeds) may become lodged under the eyelids or beneath the nictitating membrane. This is often a problem in rabbits and guinea pigs which are bedded on straw.

Signs of injury. Injuries to the eyelids are usually the most painless of all three conditions, unless due to self-trauma. There is rarely much swelling or bleeding and it can be quite difficult to see simple wounds.

If the injury was self-inflicted, the entire skin of the eyelids and adjoining area may be severely abraded, red raw and swollen. The cornea should always be carefully examined in any case of lid injury to check for signs of corneal damage.

Signs of inflammation. Inflammatory reactions are often very painful and may be so severe that the oedematous conjunctiva bulges up over the eyelid margin like a pink cushion (**chemosis**). If both upper and lower eyelids are affected, it may be difficult to see the eye itself because both upper and lower palpebral conjunctivae are so swollen (Fig. 3.47).

Signs of foreign bodies. The presence of foreign bodies is the most painful condition of all and it can be impossible even to examine the eye because the patient keeps it tightly shut. There may also be **corneal damage**, caused by the sharp foreign body scraping on the cornea every time the animal moves its eyeball.

If the object has been lodged in the eye for any length of time, it will cause a **purulent ocular discharge**.

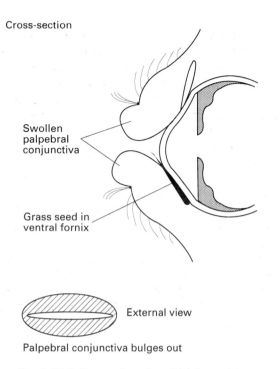

Cross-section

Swollen
palpebral
conjunctiva

Grass seed in
ventral fornix

External view

Palpebral conjunctiva bulges out

Fig. 3.47. Inflammation of eyelid (chemosis).

Occasionally, foreign bodies lie deep in the ventral or dorsal fornix (the pocket where the palpebral conjunctiva turns inwards to become the bulbar conjunctiva, Fig. 3.47) or become lodged behind the third eyelid so that they can easily be missed. Only the tip of the foreign body may protrude and the eye must be examined very thoroughly and carefully before deciding that there is no foreign body present.

Treatment. Any wounds should be cleansed with care to ensure that contamination (dirt, hair etc.) is not washed into the eye. Antiseptic solutions should not be used near the eye of the conscious animal.

The pain associated with inflammation, however caused, may be alleviated by the use of ice packs, applied gently to the area. The veterinary nurse may also apply 1–2 drops of an ophthalmic local anaesthetic preparation to the eye if these are available.

Non-penetrating foreign bodies should be removed wherever possible. It is best if local anaesthetic is administered as described above before the removal is attempted, as this is usually an acutely painful procedure. If the patient wriggles uncontrollably at the crucial moment, further damage may be done when implements accidentally jab into the eye.

Large foreign bodies (e.g. grass seeds) may be grasped manually and removed. No undue force must be used because part of the seed may break off and be left in the eye.

Smaller foreign bodies (e.g. grit) should be flushed into the corner of the eye using warmed sterile saline solution. Once lying on the sclera or lid conjunctiva, the culprit can be removed more easily and safely as the tissues are far less sensitive than the cornea, and

more robust. A piece of moistened lint or fine paint brush is used to lift the foreign body from the eye surface.

If the foreign body does not move when saline is flushed across the eye, it must be assumed to have penetrated the eyeball and should not be disturbed. Veterinary advice must be sought immediately.

Eyeball

Causes

- **Fractured skull.** The eyeball is well protected by the bony orbit and the eyelids. However, the force which fractures the orbital bones can produce severe bruising of the eye.
- **Blows to the eye.** Direct trauma to the eye can cause haemorrhage within the eye, despite the protective eyelids.
- In short-nosed breeds which have a very shallow bony orbit and protuberant eyes, injury to the orbital area (e.g. resulting from a road accident or a fight) can **prolapse** the eye.

Signs with skull fracture

- The eyeball often protrudes slightly from the socket because of a **retrobulbar haemorrhage** (bleeding into the soft tissues behind the eye in the orbit) and the eye may even prolapse.
- There is usually **bruising of the bulbar conjunctiva** (seen as a bright red blood blister on the white sclera).
- The **pupillary reflexes** may be decreased or absent and the pupil is constricted because the nerve supply to the iris is damaged.
- The animal may also be **concussed** and the signs of pain are variable, depending on its state of consciousness.

Signs of injury to the eyeball. Affected animals show signs of ocular pain but often the pain is duller and less acute than in cases of eyelid inflammation or foreign bodies. Bruising of the conjunctiva is commonly seen and the anterior chamber of the eye may look clouded with a red mist because the delicate iris haemorrhages and the blood swirls round in the aqueous humor.

Prolapse of the eyeball

The entire eyeball sits exposed on the side of the patient's face. It quickly becomes inflamed and congested as the eyelids close behind it and the cornea rapidly dries. Because the eyeball is now totally unprotected, other damage can occur.

Treatment. If any injury to the eyeball results in a protruding eye and loss of pupillary reflexes, the patient must be observed carefully in case this partial prolapse becomes a total prolapse.

The prolapsed eyeball is the only condition where specific first aid measures may be applied. **The eyeball must be replaced as soon as possible** because the dry cornea will soon ulcerate and the optic nerve may suffer permanent damage.

Liquid paraffin, olive oil or, preferably 'false tears' (e.g. methyl cellulose preparations) should be used to lubricate the eyeball, and a gentle attempt made to draw the lids out and over the eyeball. **The eyeball itself must never be pushed back in.** No force should be used and, if the attempt is unsuccessful, the cornea should be kept well moistened with a sterile saline or 'false tears' until a veterinary surgeon can attend the case.

If owners ring up and report that a pet's eye has prolapsed, they must be advised to keep the eyeball lubricated as described above so that the tissues do not dry out before the animal reaches the surgery. Contact lens saline is an ideal solution which may be available in the home; failing this, the eye may be kept moist with cold, boiled water.

The animal must be closely observed at all times to ensure that it does not cause further damage to the eye. It must also be treated for shock and made as comfortable as possible.

Cornea

Causes

- Non-penetrating wounds (ulcers) may be caused by foreign bodies in the eye, or sharp objects such as cats' claws or thorns. The surface of the cornea may also be damaged by splashes from scalding fluids, paint, acid or alkali.
- Penetrating wounds occur as the result of more serious injury received in fights, road accidents etc., and may be complicated by injury to, or prolapse of, the internal structures of the eye, particularly the vascular iris.

Signs of ulceration. The cornea is extremely sensitive and any injury causes pain. There is often a bluish or white tinge to the cornea at the site of the injury but otherwise the cornea looks normal.

Signs of penetrating wounds. Penetrating wounds result in a loss of pressure in the anterior chamber of the eye as the aqueous humor escapes through the wound. The cornea often appears wrinkled like the skin of a raisin instead of being smooth and rounded. Any pressure on the eyeball (as may be applied when parting the lids to examine the eye, for example) results in a gush of clear or bloodstained watery aqueous humor escaping from the eye.

Treatment. An eye splashed by chemicals or detergents should immediately be treated by repeated flushing of the eye surface. Sterile saline or contact lens solutions should be used, but tap water can be used in an emergency in the home.

Bicarbonate solutions may be applied to neutralise acid splashes and vinegar solutions for alkali damage, but **thorough flushing of the eye** is what really counts. Cold liquid paraffin should be used in the case of hot fat splashes to prevent the fat congealing on the cornea. The cornea may be cleansed by sterile saline and a sterile gauze pad fixed loosely in position over the eye with adhesive plaster, pending veterinary attendance.

Penetration wounds of the eyeball should be disturbed as little as possible to avoid loss of aqueous humor. Sometimes thorns may transfix the cornea but should be left for the veterinary surgeon to remove.

Following first aid measures, the animal should be confined in a darkened room or kennel to alleviate discomfort, but steps must be taken (e.g. by fitting an Elizabethan collar) to ensure that the wounded eye is not disturbed.

Injuries to the Ear

Injuries to the Ear Flap

Causes

- **Trauma.** The ears may be a site of injury following road accidents, or more often from fights and bites. Dogs exercised in dense undergrowth may catch the ear flap on thorns or barbed wire.
- **Insect stings and snake bites** can also affect the ear flap.
- **Aural haematomas** occur as a result of self-trauma or head shaking.

Signs. Open wounds of the ear bleed freely and may cause shaking of the head and irritation. Scratching at the ear will increase the haemorrhage, and may enlarge the wound.

Closed wounds result in swelling. If there is inflammation present (e.g. sting and snake bite injuries), this swelling is hot, hard and painful. Aural haematomas do not inflame and the swelling is cool and soft.

Treatment. Wounds to the ear flap should be treated by normal methods, but care must be taken when clipping the fur that the ear flap itself is not cut. Haemorrhage from ear flaps is not life-threatening but it is very messy. The haemorrhage constantly restarts as the animal shakes its head and blood will be splattered widely. It is usually necessary to bandage the ear flap by folding it back to lie over the top of the head, and fixing it with a wide bandage which encircles the head tightly. Large wounds may require surgical treatment later.

Stings and snake bites should be treated as described in the section on poisoning.

Aural haematomas should be treated as described in the wounds section (haematomas).

Foreign Bodies in the Ear

Signs. Grass seeds commonly gain access to the ear canal and travel downwards to lie in the horizontal ear canal, up against the ear drum. The animal will show intense irritation and pain, holding the head to one side, shaking its head violently and rubbing the ear with a forepaw, or along the ground. If the base of the vertical ear canal is palpated externally, the patient will often cry in pain.

Treatment. The foreign body, if visible, should be gently removed with forceps. If this is not possible, warmed olive oil or liquid paraffin may be poured into the ear to alleviate the discomfort. No attempt should be made to probe the ear, but veterinary attention should be sought. No food must be given because a general anaesthetic will usually be needed before any foreign body can be removed from the depths of the ear canal.

Vestibular Syndrome (Including 'Strokes')

Cause. This condition does not appear to be caused in the same way as human strokes, but the symptoms are so similar that it is often labelled as a stroke for convenience. (A true stroke is the result of cerebrovascular accident.) The symptoms result from injury to the vestibular system in the inner ear but the cause of injury is often unknown, although inflammation of the inner ear or inflammation of brain tissue itself (encephalitis) are responsible in certain cases.

Signs. The patient is usually an older dog but cats and rabbits with severe ear infections also suffer, as do the cage pets, hamsters, gerbils, rats and mice. The onset of the problem is sudden. The affected dog almost always has some degree of nystagmus but all patients will have marked head tilt and loss of balance.

Severe cases are unable to lie in sternal recumbency and stay collapsed on their sides. There may be reduced pain sensation in the feet of the affected side and pedal reflexes may be slowed but eye reflexes are usually unaffected. The patient may be depressed, but this is often largely due to the patient being unable to understand what is happening rather than true depression due to brain dysfunction. Many of these animals want to eat if they can get the food into their mouths.

Patients who are less affected are able to stand but show incoordination and a stumbling gait. They may walk in circles and fall over on the affected side. The animal is usually bright and appetite is unaffected if coordination permits prehension of food—it can be difficult to eat if the head is twisted on one side.

Treatment. There is little that a veterinary nurse can offer as first aid except to reassure the owner and patient. Owners are always fearful that a fatal 'stroke' may follow these symptoms and the patient may panic because it cannot coordinate its movements. Confine the animal to a small kennel or basket to restrict movement and to force it to rest. Once it stops falling over, it will feel more secure and settle down calmly.

Propentofylline is a very useful drug to try in these cases. Injections of diuretics and corticosteroids may also help, but complete recovery is rare and most patients are left with a varying degree of head tilt.

Death, Unconsciousness and Collapse

The first fact to establish when presented with an immobile, collapsed animal is whether the patient is alive or dead. Figure 3.48 gives the comparisons between flaccid, unconscious collapse and death.

Signs of Death

Signs of death include:

- Absence of heartbeat.
- Absence of respiratory movement.
- Dilation of the pupil and loss of light reflex.
- Loss of the corneal reflex.
- Glazing of the cornea.
- Body cooling and rigor mortis.

Absence of a heartbeat. Absence of the hearbeat for 3 minutes is detected by palpation of the chest for the apex beat, and listening to the chest with a stethoscope.

The heartbeat may be felt by placing one hand on either side of the chest wall so that the fingertips come to rest on the costal cartilages of ribs 3–6, i.e. at the bottom of the rib cage. This area would lie just under the elbow of the standing dog; in the collapsed patient it appears to be behind the elbow as the forelegs are usually extended when the animal lies on its side. Apply *gentle* pressure with the fingertips, pressing the costal cartilages inwards until the pulsations of the ventricles can be felt through the chest wall.

The procedure is easy in cats and dogs with deep, narrow chests but may be virtually impossible in barrel-chested breeds such as bulldogs.

The veterinary nurse should take every opportunity to practise feeling this apical heart beat in healthy, unconscious animals. Many opportunities arise in observing anaesthetised animals admitted for routine surgery and familiarity with techniques leads to confidence in assessing whether or not the heart of an emergency case is beating.

If no heartbeat is immediately obvious, a stethoscope must be used to detect any cardiac activity which may be impossible to feel by the above method, either because it is too faint or because the conformation of the chest is too broad. The head of

COMPARISON BETWEEN RECENT DEATH AND UNCONSCIOUSNESS		
Sign	**Death**	**Unconscious collapse**
Heart beat	Absent for more than 3 minutes	Regular, though slowed
Respiratory pattern	Absent, although occasionally Cheyne Stokes respiration is observed	Varies according to the depth of CNS depression (mimics anaesthesia)
Eyeball position	Central	Turned down or central, according to the depth of CNS depression
Cornea	Glazed	Normally moist
Corneal reflex	Absent	Present (unless eyelids paralysed)
Pupil size	Fully dilated	May vary in size, but are rarely fully dilated
Pupillary light reflex	Absent	Usually present unless iris paralysed
Movement	Absent, except Cheyne Stokes respiration Rigor mortis in a few hours	May be roused in stupor. Pedal reflexes present in mild cases of unconsciousness
Body temperature	Cools within 15 minutes	Remains constant

Fig. 3.48. Comparison between death and unconsciousness.

the stethoscope should be placed in the area of intercostal space 7–8. Again, the veterinary nurse should practise auscultating the heart of normal, unconscious animals to be confident of placing the stethoscope in the correct position for this emergency.

Absence of respiratory movement. The nurse should be familiar with shallow breathing and should watch closely for any breaths.

Dilation of the pupil and loss of light reflex. This is tested using a pen torch or auroscope head light source in a darkened room.

Loss of the corneal reflex. The cornea is easily damaged and so this reflex should only be tested by touching a wisp of moist cotton wool on to the cornea. This is sufficient to make the eyelids blink.

Glazing of the cornea. The surface of the eyeball lacks its usual lustre.

Body cooling and rigor mortis. After the muscles have relaxed, they gradually stiffen due to chemical changes in the muscle cells. Rigor mortis usually takes about 12 hours to set in throughout the body, but the rate is variable depending on the room temperature, cause of death and physical condition of the animal. The cooling of the body also takes several hours, again depending on the room temperature.

Rigor mortis will pass off after several days as decay sets in.

Unconsciousness

Loss of consciousness occurs when the brain is affected so that the animal is unable to respond normally to external stimuli.

In most cases, the brain is depressed and the patient becomes totally relaxed and comatose, but in other cases the brain is overactive and the body muscles are violently contracted as in epileptiform convulsions.

Signs of unconsciousness

Heart and pulse rates. The heart beat in the flaccid unconscious patient is usually regular but slowed. As the situation deteriorates, the rate slows further until cardiac arrest occurs.

Respiratory movements. The depth and rate of respiratory movements in the depressed unconscious patient mimic those seen in the different planes of anaesthesia. Deep, regular breathing may quicken as the animal regains consciousness or it may progress to rapid, shallow gasps as the brain becomes more and more depressed. **Cheyne Stokes** respiration (deep, convulsive gasps for breath at infrequent intervals) heralds the onset of death.

Position of the eyeball in the socket. In cases of epileptiform convulsions, the eyeball may stay in its usual position but remains in a fixed, unfocused stare. The eyes do not turn to follow movements or towards the owner in recognition.

In cases of flaccid unconsciousness (i.e. where the animal is totally relaxed) the eye positions often mimic those seen in the different levels of anaesthesia. Experience in judging the depth of anaesthesia may usually be applied to assess the degree of central nervous system depression of the unconscious patient. Evidence of **nystagmus** (rapid involuntary side-to-side or up and down movement of the eyeball) or **strabismus** (squint) should be noted.

Palpebral reflex. This should *not* be tested in the convulsing animal as the stimulus may worsen the convulsions. In the flaccid animal, the presence or absence of this reflex is another indication of the severity of brain depression. If the palpebral reflex is absent, the **corneal reflex** may be tested as described earlier for signs of death. The cornea is so sensitive that this is one of the last reflexes to be lost as the animal loses its fight for life. However, it should be remembered that, in some cases of head trauma where the motor nerves of the eyelid muscles are damaged, the animal will be unable to respond and may not necessarily be dying.

Pupil size. Compare the pupil size of each eye. Asymmetry of pupil size (**anisocoria**) can indicate unilateral brain damage.

Pupillary light reflex. This reflex should be tested in a darkened room, using a torch or auroscope head as a source of bright light. Both pupils should constrict equally as the light shines into the eye. Failure to do so indicates brain damage but, if the nerves to the pupil are damaged (e.g. by trauma as occurs in a prolapsed eyeball), the reflex may be absent in that eye because the reflex arc is unable to work. The unaffected eye should react normally.

Again, this test should not be carried out on the convulsing animal as it may make the situation worse.

Depth of unconsciousness. This is assessed by the various eye reflexes described above. The pedal reflexes are also a useful indication as to the depth of unconsciousness, since they are the first reflexes to be lost as brain activity becomes depressed and the last to return as the condition improves.

There are two terms used to describe the depth of unconsciousness:

- In **stupor**, the animal can be roused with difficulty and the pedal withdrawl reflex is still present, though the toes may need to be pinched quite hard. Pupillary and palpebral reflexes are also still present.
- In **coma**, the animal cannot be roused, the pedal reflexes are absent and the eye reflexes indicate a plane of surgical anaesthesia or deeper. The pupils become dilated as the condition deteriorates and death approaches.

Convulsions. Convulsions are violent, irregular, involuntary movements of the body. The time of onset and duration should be noted.

Incontinence. Urine or faeces may be passed by the unconscious animal either passively (a gradual seepage because the sphincter muscles relax) or actively (e.g. a pool of urine passed during an epileptiform fit).

Collapse

Collapse is said to have occurred when a conscious animal is unable or unwilling to stand up.

'Collapse' is the most common emergency reported by owners and covers a multitude of situations from an arthritic dog which is reluctant to get up and go for a walk to a deceased pet. The cause and severity of the 'collapse' must therefore first be discovered so that the correct first aid procedures may be carried out.

Signs of collapse

The difference between collapse and unconsciousness is whether the animal is still conscious or not. The conscious patient responds normally to sound, sight and touch. A dog will turn its eyes, if not its head, when its name is called. The conscious animal has all the normal eye reflexes and can focus on objects and follow movement with its eyes. The patient will respond to handling: either the animal will become calm or affectionate following gentle smoothing, or it may be aggressive to any handling. Beware: the response of the collapsed aggressive patient is coordinated and deliberate, so that the animal is well able to bite. If a patient has all these normal responses and yet is unwilling or unable to get up, it may be said to have collapsed.

The collapsed animal should always be treated with care because its condition may not be stable. In some cases, the patient may lapse into unconsciousness and die. In other cases, there may be a rapid improvement to normal health. As with cases of unconsciousness, a collapsed patient must be constantly observed and its reflexes assessed to ensure that the situation is not deteriorating.

Causes of collapse and unconsciousness

The causes of collapse and unconsciousness are listed in Fig. 3.49 but this is often not a clear-cut situation. It must be remembered that all the causes of unconsciousness may also cause the animal to collapse if the brain is only mildly depressed. Conversely, most causes of collapse may progress to unconsciousness if the situation deteriorates. Therefore, the categories indicated in Fig. 3.49 (i.e. whether a condition causes collapse or unconsciousness) simply reflect the most likely presenting symptom seen in day-to-day practice.

CAUSES OF COLLAPSE AND UNCONSCIOUSNESS			
Body system	**Cause**	**C**	**U**
CNS	Epilepsy	–	+
	Brain trauma e.g. blow to head	+	+
	Vestibular syndrome	+	–
	Disc protrusion	+	–
	Atlanto-axial subluxation	+	–
	Spinal fractures	+	–
Respiratory	Pharyngeal obstruction	–	+
	Lung collapse – Pneumothorax	+	–
	– Haemothorax	+	–
	Pyothorax	+	–
	Diaphragmatic rupture	+	–
	Lack of oxygenation of blood – Smoke inhalation	+	+
	– Drowning incident	+	+
	– Poisonings (CO, paraquat)	+	+
	– Lung haemorrhage	+	–
Circulatory	Cardiac failure	+	+
	Hypovolaemic shock – Acute haemorrhage	+	+
	– Severe fluid loss	+	–
	Traumatic shock e.g. RTAs	+	–
	Anaemia (long-term blood loss)	+	–
	Thrombosis – brachial or iliac	+	–
Abdominal catastrophy	Gastric torsion, bowel rupture	+	–
	Bladder rupture	+	–
	Urethral obstruction	+	–
	Acute prostatitis	+	–
	Acute hepatitis	+	–
	Splenic torsion	+	–
	Acute pancreatitis	+	–
Locomotor conditions	Dislocations and fractures of the limbs	+	–
	Arthritis, muscle wasting	+	–
Metabolic disturbances	Hyper/hypoglycaemia	+	+
	Hypocalcaemia	+	+
	Uraemic fits	+	+
	Toxaemia e.g. pyometra	+	–
Physical causes	Electrocution	–	+
	Hypothermia	+	+
	Hyperthermia	+	+
Drugs and Poisons	Any compound causing CNS depression	+	+

Key – C = Conscious collapse
     U = Unconscious collapse
     RTA = Road Traffic Accident
     CNS = Central Nervous System i.e. the brain and spinal cord

Fig. 3.49. Causes of collapse and unconsciousness.

Some conditions are placed in both categories. This is because that condition may be so acute in some accidents that the patient becomes unconscious almost immediately and the conscious collapse phase is scarcely noticeable. In other accidents, the situation may not be so severe and the patient is simply collapsed when presented. For example, hyperthermia (heatstroke) can present as either case, depending upon the vigilance of the owner. If an animal is confined to a car on a hot, humid day and left, it will be unconscious within an hour. If the same animal is left for 20 minutes in the same conditions, it will probably be collapsed but still conscious.

Treatment and Resuscitation Procedures

When an unconscious animal is first presented, the veterinary nurse should follow the treatment regime laid out in the first section of this chapter under 'Arrival at the Surgery'.

Maintaining the airway

The first action when presented with a collapsed unconscious patient is to clear an airway. Tight collars should be removed and the mouth examined as swiftly as possible to ensure that there is no obstruction at the back of the throat, e.g. blood, mucus etc. (the Heimlich manoeuvre to remove pharyngeal foreign bodies is described under specific treatments for asphyxia). If a foreign body cannot be removed, an endotracheal tube should be passed beside the obstruction or the object should be pushed to one side. Fluids should be swabbed away and the trachea intubated. The cuff should be inflated to avoid inhalation of fluids. The animal can then be connected to an oxygen-only anaesthetic machine and artificial respiration given if necessary. If the patient is breathing itself, it should be carefully observed as many of these cases regain consciousness rapidly. If no endotracheal tubes are available, the patient should be laid in the veterinary recovery position (Fig. 3.50).

Cardiac massage

The heart of an apparently dead animal may be stimulated by rhythmical compression of the lower rib cage over ribs 3–6. Cats' chests are easily compressed by placing the fingertips of both hands on either side of the thorax and applying gentle, firm pressure simultaneously to the rib cage. Large dogs need to be laid on their side in the recovery position (Fig. 3.50) and punched with a closed fist to stimulate the heart effectively.

Pressure should be applied at half-second intervals in the case of small animals. In larger patients, compressions at one-second intervals are sufficient.

Artificial respiration must be maintained at the same time as the cardiac massage is given and therefore it is best if two people cooperate in resuscitating the patient. If the veterinary nurse is alone, cardiac massage should be applied for 5 seconds, then the chest should be allowed to inflate with air; continue the cardiac massage for another 5 seconds before the chest is again inflated etc. In this way, there is oxygen available in the lungs as soon as the circulation restarts, but the cardiac massage is continued almost uninterrupted.

If the heart does not restart after 3 minutes of cardiac massage, the patient may be declared to be dead.

Artificial respiration

If respiratory movements have ceased, respiratory stimulant drugs may be used (e.g. doxapram hydrochloride) but, until the animal starts to breathe on its own, **the lungs must be mechanically inflated** if the patient is to continue to live.

The first task is to ensure a patent airway but subsequent action depends upon whether an endotracheal tube is available or not. It is *always* preferable to intubate these patients because:

- the tube ensures the airway remains patent;
- the inflated cuff avoids any inhalation of fluids;
- it is much more hygienic to give artificial respiration by giving gases or blowing down a clean tube than attempting mouth-to-nose resuscitation.

Non-intubated patients. Non-intubated patients should be placed in the recovery position (Fig. 3.50):

- The animal is laid on its side.
- The head and neck are extended.
- The tongue is pulled out to clear the airway.
- The front legs are pulled forwards so the upper leg does not rest on the chest, weighing it down and making inspiration more of an effort.
- Lay the palm of the hand flat in the middle of the chest wall, just behind the mass of the triceps muscle of the foreleg.
- Apply firm steady pressure and then release so that the elastic rib cage springs back, drawing air into the lungs. **Reapply the pressure every 1–2 seconds**.

This procedure must *not* be used in cases where any damage to the thoracic wall is suspected, as fractured ribs could easily pierce the lungs or heart during compression of the thorax. In such cases **mouth-to-nose resuscitation** should be used if no intubation facilities are to hand:

- The patient's tongue is first pulled forwards to ensure an unobstructed airway.
- Then the nose is grasped firmly but gently in the left hand so that the thumb and fingers curl round the snout to hold down the upper lip-folds and create an airtight seal. This is important because, if the mouth is not sealed, air blown into the nose simply takes the line of least resistance and escapes through the mouth instead of being forced into the lungs.
- The right hand is placed under the lower jaw to support the weight of the animal's head (Fig. 3.51).
- If the patient is a large dog, with lip margins too long for the left hand to cover so that the lips cannot be sealed effectively, the right hand should

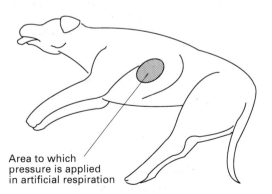

Fig. 3.50. Recovery position.

Area to which pressure is applied in artificial respiration

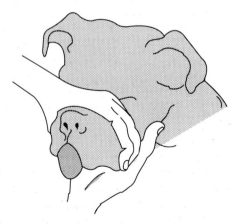

Fig. 3.51. Mouth-to-nose resuscitation: holding the nose.

also be used to seal the part of the lips which the left hand cannot reach.

- **Always wear a face mask when attempting this procedure** because of the risk to human health. Try to blow air away from your mouth, and do not inhale saliva or air from the patient.
- Care must also be taken not to overinflate the lungs or the delicate lung tissue may be damaged. Gentle puffs of sufficient force to cause the rib cage to lift just a little are best blown in at one-second intervals.

Intubated patients. Intubated patients should be connected to an oxygen supply from a closed-circuit anaesthetic machine and **the re-breathing bag used to inflate the lungs.** Only very gentle pressure may be needed at frequent intervals to mimic panting respiration, i.e. approximately 120 breaths per minute, 2 breaths a second. Massive inflation of the lungs (equivalent to drawing a deep breath) can overinflate them, causing damage to the lung alveoli and possibly driving the lungs against sharp fragments of broken ribs. This panting form of artificial respiration can be so effective that it is possible to 'rest' the respiration for 5 seconds in every 15 seconds to see if the breathing has restarted. However, if there is any sign of cyanosis, the respiration should be maintained continuously.

If no anaesthetic machine is available immediately, the animal should be intubated and the lungs inflated by blowing down the tube. The rate and force should be as for the mouth-to-nose resuscitation. Carbon dioxide in the nurse's exhaled breath may stimulate the animal to breathe.

Artificial respiration is continued until the animal starts to breathe on its own, (which may take up to an hour or more) or until death has intervened.

Prevention of hypoxia

Hypoxia occurs when the blood does not contain as much oxygen as normal.

Intubated unconscious patients can be connected to the oxygen supply of an anaesthetic machine.

If the animal is dyspnoeic but conscious, **it is most important that it is allowed to rest as much as possible.** Attempts to examine the mouth for obstructions should be abandoned if they cause distress. Struggling will only increase the body's demand for oxygen, so that the hypoxia becomes more severe and the patient's condition deteriorates. **The animal should be encouraged to breathe oxygen** or oxygen-enriched air to correct the hypoxia. Small dogs and cats can be placed in wire baskets, which in turn are placed in large plastic bags which may be inflated with oxygen to create a small oxygen tent. 'Gas out' boxes (used in some veterinary surgeries for anaesthetising recalcitrant cats) can be used as oxygen tents if connected to an oxygen-only anaesthetic machine.

Larger dogs must be encouraged to lie still while a stream of oxygen is directed at the nostrils.

Forcing a dog's head into a mask will only distress the animal and worsen the problem. However, a plastic bag may be used to create a light, flexible mask that funnels oxygen to the face. The bag should be large enough to fit comfortably over the entire head of the animal. Cut off one of the bottom corners and push the tube from the oxygen-only anaesthetic machine through the resulting hole. Adhesive tape may be used to attach the bag to the end of the tube. Gently draw the open end of the bag over the animal's face. Because the polyethylene is lightweight and transparent, the animal does not feel trapped and restricted and will often tolerate the arrangement very well (Fig. 3.52). The bag must hang freely ventrally to allow water vapour and expired air to escape. If the bag fits the face too tightly, a hot and humid atmosphere develops in the bag and distresses the patient.

Some animals may allow a nasal catheter to be inserted into the nostrils, especially if only semi-conscious.

Control of severe haemorrhage

This has already been described.

Conservation of heat

These animals are in a state of shock and should not be allowed to lose heat. The exception to this is, of course, the collapsed heatstroke patient. Rapid loss of heat from the body is essential if a heatstroke patient is to recover (see later).

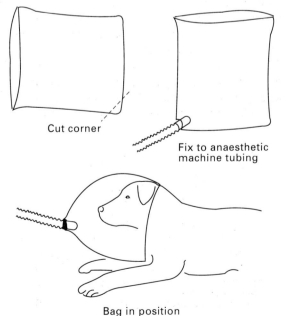

Cut corner

Fix to anaesthetic machine tubing

Bag in position

Fig. 3.52. Using a plastic bag as a face mask.

Administration of fluids

Fluids should never be given by mouth to an unconscious animal unless the trachea is intubated with an inflated cuffed tube and a stomach tube is passed. The only indication for such measures is the hypoglycaemic diabetic patient, when glucose solution should be given via the stomach tube.

Constant observation

When the patient has been stabilised and made comfortable, the most important point is to maintain constant, keen observation. The eye reflexes, breathing pattern and pulse rate of the unconscious patient should be checked at 10–15 minute intervals and the findings and time of testing recorded on a chart. Such charts enable the veterinary nurse to monitor the progress of the patient and are essential for the veterinary surgeon to estimate the rate of deterioration or improvement in the animal's condition. Evidence of rapid worsening of the situation may prompt surgical intervention in cases of head trauma or may mean that further drugs must be given in other cases. The charts also enable the veterinary surgeon to give a more accurate prognosis.

Specific Causes and Treatment of Unconsciousness

The causes of unconsciousness are shown in Figs 3.49, 3.53 and 3.54. Primary causes include those in which the patient becomes unconscious as an immediate result of injury or dysfunction of the nervous system itself. Secondary cases include those where the metabolism or function of the other body systems is upset, which then results in a loss of consciousness.

CLASSIFICATION OF CAUSES OF UNCONSCIOUSNESS

Primary causes	(a) Epilepsy (b) Direct trauma to the brain (c) Chemical causes – Poisons

Secondary causes	(a) Asphyxia
	(b) Metabolic disturbances
	   – ketoacidosis
	   – hypoglycaemia in diabetics
	   – hypocalcaemia in eclampsia
	   – uraemia in kidney failure
	(c) Circulatory disturbances
	   – cardiac failure
	   – hypovolaemic shock
	(d) Physical causes
	   – electrocution
	   – hyperthermia (heat stroke)
	   – hypothermia

Fig. 3.53. Classification of causes of unconsciousness.

CLASSIFICATION OF TYPES OF UNCONSCIOUSNESS

Spastic (rigid) unconsciousness	Primary epileptic convulsions Metabolic dysfunction Physical causes Chemical poisonings	– e.g. uraemic fits, eclampsia – electrocution – e.g. strychnine, slug bait
Flaccid (relaxed) unconsciousness	Oxygen deprivation Metabolic dysfunction Circulatory dysfunction Central nervous system injury Chemical poisoning	– asphyxia – e.g. diabetes mellitus – cardiac failure – severe haemorrhage – e.g. trauma following road accidents etc.
Death	Physical causes	– e.g. heat stroke

Fig. 3.54. Classification of types of unconsciousness.

Epileptiform fits

Cause. The condition is more common in dogs than in cats and is usually seen in animals 1–3 years old, especially if inclined to nervousness or over-excitability (**primary fits**). Older animals may suffer **secondary fits** which occur following brain damage by diseases (such as distemper), trauma (such as a blow to the head) or toxaemia (as seen in uraemic patients and poisoning cases).

Signs. Fits may be reported as the animal is waking up from sleep, but may also happen when it is fully conscious. In the latter case, the animal often becomes restless just before the fit commences and may be unusually affectionate, continually seeking reassurance from the owner. Occasionally the dog becomes hysterical, barking and rushing madly around before succumbing to the fit. The fit itself usually happens suddenly.

The animal having a fit collapses on to its side and goes into violent convulsions in what is known as the **ictal phase**. Its legs are extended, its head pulled back and neck extended; there is involuntary champing of the jaws, which churns saliva into a foaming froth around the lips. Its eyes are open and stare fixedly. The respiratory rate is much increased and defecation and urination are common during severe fits. Most convulsions subside after 5–10 minutes but occasionally the dog will remain in a fit for hours, relaxing from one attack only to start shaking with the next fit.

Following an attack, the dog usually rises and wanders about aimlessly and unsteadily, looking dazed and confused. Soon it recognises its owner and, although very tired, will be back to normal.

The 'petit mal' fit is often less dramatic: the animal simply wanders around, staring fixedly, unresponsive to the owner and unable to settle. This is the least severe form of fit and it is as well to remember that epileptic fits can vary in severity from this very mild form to the severe 'grand mal' fit.

Complications. The possibility of **rabies** must always be considered in cases of unusual nervous signs in the dog and cat, although the likelihood of this lethal disease manifesting itself in the household pet in the UK is still at present remote. In first aid history taking, the owners should be asked how long they have owned the pet and whether the animal has been abroad, especially within the past six months.

In the case of **secondary fits**, the underlying cause may make treatment impossible (see uraemia). Samples of urine, faeces and vomit should be saved in cases of suspected poisoning.

Fits are not fatal in most cases but, very rarely, the animal may have a **swallowed tongue** and start to choke. In these cases, the convulsive movements become weaker and the patient becomes cyanosed.

Treatment. Whatever the cause of the attack, the first aid treatment remains the same. These attacks represent gross overactivity of the central nervous system 'circuits' and any extra stimulus usually only worsens the situation and prolongs the fit.

- Owners should be advised to contain the dog in a darkened (no visual stimulus) quiet (no auditory stimulus) room.
- They should remain in the room with the dog but should **not touch it** (minimal tactile stimulus) unless the dog threatens to injure itself.
- Above all, **the owners must remain calm**, and any member of the family who threatens to become hysterical should not be allowed to stay with the dog.
- As the fits are often of short duration, it is best to leave the dog in the house to avoid stimulating it any further.
- Should the fit persist, or should the owner be unable to cope with the situation, the patient may be brought to the surgery.

At the surgery, the animal should be confined to a dark, quiet kennel for observation until the veterinary surgeon can attend to it. Injections of barbiturate or diazepam should be prepared because it may be necessary to anaesthetise or sedate the patient to control the fit.

When the dog is recovering from the fit and pacing around, reassurance may be given **if the dog seeks it**, but no attempt should be made to prevent the restlessness as this may simply spark off another fit. Similar advice should be given in the case of the very mild epileptic dog.

Should the patient show signs of **cyanosis**, it must be carefully observed and oxygen administered. If breathing ceases normal resuscitation procedures should follow.

> **WARNING**
> **Under no circumstances should the owner or veterinary nurse attempt to put a hand into the animal's mouth until the convulsions subside.** Such attempts are fruitless and can lead to severe bites being inflicted if the patient's jaws are still champing.

Direct trauma (concussion)

Causes. Any blow to the head, as sustained in a road accident or following a kick from a horse etc., may result in unconsciousness because pressure is exerted on the delicate cerebral hemispheres. Depressed fractures of the cranium will obviously cause such pressure and damage, but concussion is frequently seen without any fracture being present. In these cases it is due to intracranial haemorrhage or oedematous swelling in the meninges overlying the hemispheres, or in the nervous tissue itself. As the entire cranium is formed by bone, any swelling must press inwards on the brain itself (Fig. 3.55).

Signs. The signs of concussion are very variable, ranging from a slightly dazed animal to the comatose patient, depending on the degree of injury. The following signs may be seen:

- Shock.
- Haemorrhage from the nose, mouth or ears.
- Fracture of the cranium or hard palate also indicate trauma to the head. (Note that any palpation of the cranium must be carried out very gently for fear of depressing the fracture even deeper into the brain tissues.)
- The pupils may be unequally dilated, and vary in their reactions to light, indicating that one side of the brain is more affected than the other. The eyes may also show nystagmus or strabismus. In severe cases, the palpebral and corneal reflexes may be absent and the pupils dilated, but the veterinary nurse should test both eyes because of the likelihood of peripheral nerve damage in cases of head trauma. For example, paralysis of the facial nerve on one side of the face will mean that the

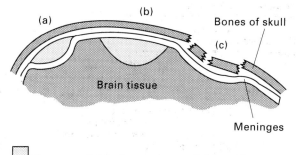

Tissues swollen by haemorrhage or inflammation

Fig. 3.55. Effects of direct trauma on the brain: (a) bleeding or oedema of meninges; (b) bleeding or oedema of brain tissue; (c) depressed skull fracture.

eyelid cannot blink as the palpebral reflex is tested but the other side of the face may be totally unaffected and react normally.

- Respiration is usually slow and shallow and the heart rate is depressed in severe cases.
- Movement in the conscious patient is often uncoordinated. The unconscious patient is flaccidly collapsed but occasionally there may be spasmodic muscular shivering.
- Conscious patients may vomit.
- In other cases, damage to certain areas of the brain leads to paralysis. Symptoms can be very variable depending upon the part of the brain injured and the extent of the injury.

Treatment. The most important first aid measures are to maintain the airway and to **constantly assess the eye reflexes and degree of depression of the nervous system**. Constant monitoring of these patients is an essential part of the veterinary nurse's duties. The reflexes should be checked every 10 minutes, noting the time and observations fully on the kennel chart. Otherwise, there is no specific treatment except to conserve heat and minimize the shock, by confining the animal to a quiet warm darkened kennel.

Spinal injury

Signs of spinal injury depend upon the place and degree of injury.

Cause. The causes of acute spinal injury fall into three categories:

- **Disc protrusion**, a problem seen in dogs, which usually affects the cervical region (e.g. poodle, spaniel) or the thoracolumbar region (e.g. dachshund, pekingese).
- **Spinal dislocation**, seen less commonly as an acute problem but which can cause sudden collapse in toy breeds with malformed atlantoaxial joints as the odontoid peg slips upwards to hit the spinal cord.
- **Spinal fractures**, which can occur in any animal following severe trauma.

Signs of cervical injury. These patients are usually in intense pain and lie still, reluctant to move, screaming whenever the spine twists. In severe cases, all four legs are paralysed (quadriplegia or tetraplegia) and the patient is incontinent. There may be withdrawal reflexes when the foot is pinched (a local reflex), but proprioception is reduced or absent because the nerve impulses cannot pass easily up to the brain as the pathways are damaged at the site of the trauma.

If the injury is less severe, the patient may appear uncoordinated, scuffing its toes as it walks, or it may appear lame in one leg if the injury affects one side of the spinal cord more than the other. It is reluctant to turn its head and it yelps every time it does so.

Signs of thoracolumbar injury. The patient shows pain and may cry out if the back is made to move suddenly. Intense trauma (usually seen as the result of a spinal fracture) may result in a collapsed patient with front legs rigidly extended and hind legs tightly flexed. Other severe injuries show paralysis of the hind legs (paraplegia) and incontinence. The animal may try to move around, walking normally with its front legs whilst the hind legs trail out behind. Withdrawal reflexes in the affected legs are normal but proprioception is reduced or absent for reasons explained above.

Patients able to stand do so with the back arched with less severe injury but will cry out if any force is applied to the midline of the back which pushes the arch downwards. The hind legs are often incoordinated if the animal tries to walk around. In many cases, the owner will report that the dog cried out in pain when trying to jump up, e.g. into a car, going upstairs etc.

Treatment. There is no specific first aid treatment for these cases. If spinal injury is suspected, the most important advice to owners over the telephone is:

- Move the animal as little as possible.
- Lift the animal as a unit so that the spine is *never* twisted.

Methods for transporting these animals are described at the beginning of this chapter. Upon arrival at the surgery and following a thorough examination, the patient should be confined to a kennel so that it moves as little as possible.

Radiographic examination will be necessary and the relevant preparations should be made.

Poisons

Poisoning should be considered in the case of unconscious animals if no other cause is apparent.

Asphyxia (suffocation)

Asphyxia or suffocation results from any failure to oxygenate the blood. **Partial asphyxia** occurs when small supplies of oxygen manage to reach the lungs, but the blood is only partially oxygenated and hypoxia results. **Hypoxia** occurs when there is an abnormally low level of oxygen in the tissues.

Causes

- **Partial or total airway obstruction**:
- Pharyngeal foreign bodies (Fig. 3.42).
- Swallowed tongue (Fig. 3.56).
- Swelling of the pharyngeal walls.
- Collapsed trachea as seen in cases of strangulation, choke chain injuries etc.

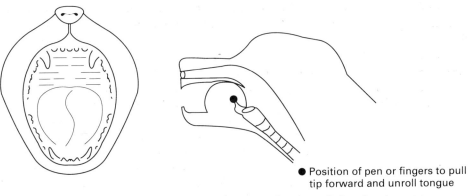

● Position of pen or fingers to pull
tip forward and unroll tongue

View of open mouth   Cross section through dogs head

Fig. 3.56. The 'swallowed' tongue.

- **Interference with respiratory movements**:
- Paralysis of the respiratory muscles by poisons such as strychnine, scoline, or nerve damage.
- Crushing injuries preventing normal respiratory movement.
- **Interference with oxygenation of the blood**
- Fluid in the alveolar spaces prevents the air entering these structures where the blood can be oxygenated. Drowning accidents, bleeding from the lungs, paraquat poisoning, congestive heart failure may all cause asphyxiation because of the effects they have on the alveolar spaces.
- Paracetamol and chlorate poisoning interferes with the oxygenation of red blood cells as it causes methaemoglobinaemia.
- Carbon monoxide poisoning from car exhaust fumes will also suffocate the animal as the red blood cells combine with the carbon monoxide in preference to oxygen, so that the oxygen content of the blood is severely reduced. Carbon monoxide poisoning in the home is often the result of badly ventilated gas heaters and closed fire-stoves.
- Inhalation of noxious fumes from house fires may result in oxygen starvation because there is little oxygen contained in the gases inhaled (most of the oxygen has been 'used up' by the flames) and the gases may be irritant which provokes inflammation of the respiratory tract and fluid release into the alveolar spaces. Animals that survive house fires but have inhaled smoke or fumes may be expected to develop bronchitis 48 hours after the incident. The nurse should anticipate this complication and advise the owner to bring the animal to the surgery for treatment even if it seems fine at the time of the accident.
- **Pleural cavity problems**:
- Pneumothorax, haemothorax and diaphragmatic hernia will all cause lung collapse.
- Fluid pleurisy is quite common in the cat and may produce collapse and asphyxia.

Signs. Signs include air hunger and cyanosis.

Air hunger: the animal will often lie in sternal recumbency with its neck extended and often mouth-breathing. Respiratory movements are strenuous and exaggerated, the animal literally gasping for breath, and the respiratory rate is increased (**tachypnoea**). These patients are always hypoxic, and often in great distress, especially if they struggle or try to move around too much. As the blood's oxygen levels fall still further, the animal becomes **hyperaesthetic** (excitable), reacting with abnormal violence to any stimulus and throwing itself around in an uncontrollable manner until unconsciousness intervenes. Death will soon follow.

Cyanosis occurs rapidly in cases of airway obstruction, but more slowly in other cases. The mucosa changes from pink to mauve and the animal will die unless rapid action is taken. Carbon monoxide poisoning is the exception to the cyanosis rule: the blood remains a brilliant cherry red despite the fact that there is very little oxygen in the blood stream. This is because the blood corpuscles carrying the carbon monoxide maintain the same colour as the corpuscles carrying oxygen.

General treatment. The mouth should be opened and the pharynx inspected for signs of obstruction. When the airway is cleared, the animal should be resuscitated as described earlier under artificial respiration and maintaining the airway.

Oxygenation is vital in all these cases, and providing pure oxygen for the animal to breathe means that the small volume of gas reaching the alveolar spaces is at least pure life-giving oxygen instead of the mere 20% present in inhaled air. If in doubt, the nurse should administer oxygen by face mask until the veterinary surgeon arrives.

Rest is also vital so that the body's demand for oxygen is kept to a minimum.

Treatments for obstruction by foreign bodies. Foreign bodies which obstruct the airway will kill animals very quickly, and **must be removed or held to one side to allow air to pass** down the trachea.

- Suspending the animal by its hind legs is an extremely simple and very valuable immediate treatment that encourages the foreign body to fall forwards in the pharynx, taking the pressure off the laryngeal opening and allowing air to pass through the nasal passages and into the trachea. If the animal coughs, the object may even dislodge and fall out of the mouth.

- Smooth, round-ended instruments may be used to hold the obstruction to one side. Whelping forceps are ideal, but fingers can be used in an emergency. However, great care is needed because these patients regain consciousness very rapidly and objects in the mouth could get badly chewed. This is no more than a temporary measure.
- A small endotracheal tube may be passed down the trachea beside the foreign body to maintain the airway in the asphyxiated unconscious patient. The animal must be very carefully observed for returning consciousness because the tube may need to be removed quickly to avoid complicating the situation with a chewed-off, inhaled endo-tracheal tube. Should unconsciousness return, the patient must be intubated again with all speed.
- A loose-fitting face mask may be improvised for cases of conscious, partial asphyxia (Fig. 3.52) in order to give the animal an oxygen-rich atmo-sphere to breathe. If this upsets the animal, do not persist in trying to use it.
- Removal of a smooth pharyngeal foreign body, such as a ball, should be possible using surgical instruments such as whelping forceps. However, this is usually impossible as the ball is tightly jammed in the pharynx and coated copiously with slippery saliva. Therefore other methods are needed and the Heimlich manoeuvre as applied to animals can be a life-saving procedure.

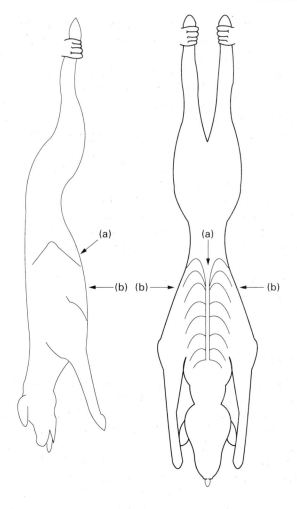

⟶ Direction and point of impact of blow.

Fig. 3.57. The Heimlich manoeuvre: (a) standard Heimlich manoeuvre; (b) modified version.

The Heimlich Manoeuvre

The principle is to administer a sharp punch to the abdominal wall just above the xiphisternum, angled downwards towards the diaphragm (Fig. 3.57(a)) so that the animal coughs and the smooth foreign body is dislodged. In order to get the object to fall out of the mouth, the procedure should be carried out with the patient suspended upside-down by the hind legs. A large dog may have to be suspended from a table edge or a wooden fence if out of doors. First aid workers also refer to this Heimlich manoeuvre as the 'abdominal thrust', which suggests the technique used in removing a foreign body.

The problem is that, once the animal is suspended in this way, it can be difficult to deliver an effective punch in narrow-chested patients because the weight of the body draws the costal arches even closer together at the xiphisternum and the abdominal muscles are stretched tight. If attempts prove useless, try placing the hands on either side of the suspended patient's chest wall (Fig. 3.57b) and delivering a sharp punch-like compression of the thorax. This usually has the desired effect. If a dog is too large to be suspended by its rear legs, its hindquarters should be raised as high as possible and its head allowed to

hang down before the blow is administered. The procedure may be repeated up to four times, but further attempts should be discontinued for fear of causing internal injury and the theatre should be prepared for an emergency tracheostomy. The ventral throat area should be clipped and scrubbed to save time. The patient should be kept alive using any of the other methods already described until the veterinary surgeon arrives.

Treatment for interference with respiratory move-ments. If the muscles are paralysed, the veterinary nurse should carry out artificial respiration. If it is impossible to pass an endotracheal tube, manual compression of the chest is the only way to draw air into the chest. However, this method of artificial respiration is not very efficient and the patient should be given oxygen to breathe through a face mask to ensure adequate oxygenation of the blood.

If respiration is painful because of chest wall trauma, the only useful first aid treatment is to give the animal oxygen to breathe through a loose-fitting face mask.

Treatment for fluid in the alveolar space. Where this is as the result of a drowning accident, the fluid must be drained out immediately. Any weed etc. in the mouth should be removed and the animal held up by its hind legs if possible and swung round in a circle or arc so that the centrifugal force encourages the fluid to drain out of the lungs. (This applies the same principle as used to revive puppies, only on a large scale.) If the animal is too big for this method, it must be laid on as steep a slope as possible and artificial respiration applied to encourage oxygenation and drainage of the chest. Once the animal has been resuscitated, it should be dried, and kept warm. Direct heat may be applied in these circumstances because these patients are often hypothermic.

Treatment for pleural cavity problems. This is described in the section about injuries to the respiratory tract.

Cardiac failure

Causes. Cardiac failure is usually seen in the older animal, often as a result of thickened heart valves which cannot close properly. These leaking valves decrease the efficiency of the heart as a pump and the rate at which the blood circulates around the body is slowed. If the right side of the heart is affected, the lung circulation is poor and the blood will not be oxygenated so efficiently. If the left side of the heart is affected, fluid may build up in the lungs because the left side of the heart cannot pump efficiently enough to move the venous blood from the lungs and around the systemic circulation. Inefficiency of the bicuspid valve may also lead to fainting fits as the heart is unable to pump sufficient oxygenated blood to the brain.

Acute heart failure can also occur in young animals if there is a heart defect which only becomes apparent as the animal matures and becomes more active. Parvovirus infection at a very young age can also damage the myocardium and cause heart failure in the young dog, but this is very rarely seen now as pups are protected by the immunity of the mother.

Signs. This condition is more often seen in dogs than in cats. The signs are as follows:

- Reluctance to exercise, which has gradually increased over a period of months in most cases.
- Coughing on exercise or exertion. The coughing fits become more prolonged and severe as the condition advances.
- Cyanosis as fluid builds up in the lungs and interferes with the oxygenation of blood. Patients collapse on exercise, showing signs of air hunger (see asphyxiation).
- Sudden collapse in acute heart failure or when the left side of the heart is affected. The animal may have suffered fainting fits in the past but these

were so brief, with the patient completely recovering after a few seconds, that the owner was not unduly worried. However, in acute heart failure, the animal does not revive spontaneously and there may be no heartbeat when it is presented at the surgery.

Dogs usually show all the above signs as they are inclined to try to carry on as normal despite coughing bouts and fainting fits. However, cats rarely show signs of cardiac failure until the condition is serious because they will rest sensibly if feeling short of breath. The owner may report that the cat has become lazier over a period of months, but rarely reports that the animal has been coughing. Therefore, the onset of signs may seem very acute and the animal is presented with a chest full of fluid, gasping for breath and going gently blue on the slightest exercise.

Treatment. If there is no heartbeat, cardiac massage should be applied as soon as possible. These cases rarely respond unless they are presented to the surgery within minutes of collapse.

If the heart is still beating, oxygen therapy should be given, for the animal is almost certainly hypoxic to some degree and must be made to rest.

Shock

Causes

- Acute haemorrhage.
- Severe fluid loss as in prolonged or severe bouts of vomiting and diarrhoea. There will also be dehydration in cases of renal failure, or in cases of water deprivation (e.g. a cat that has been trapped for days without access to water).
- Traumatic shock. The body's response to severe trauma is to shut down the non-essential circulation.

Signs and treatment for shock are given in the early section, Aims and Limitations.

Anaemia

Causes

- Flea infestation. Young, underweight kittens that have been rescued may be found to be collapsed because poor nourishment and a flea burden have caused severe anaemia.
- Feline infectious anaemia. This usually occurs in older cats and the onset is more gradual so that the animal is rarely presented as an emergency.

Signs

- Stupor.
- Extreme pallor of mucous membranes.
- Thin, very rapid pulse.

- Rapid shallow breathing.
- Depressed rectal temperature.

Treatment. Insulate, but do not warm the body because as much blood as possible must be kept flowing to the brain. Supply oxygen-enriched air to breathe so the little circulating blood available is rapidly oxygenated in the lungs. Deflea, preferably using a non-toxic preparation.

These cases usually carry a very poor prognosis.

Thromboses

Cause. The cause of this condition is a circulating clot (**embolus**) which lodges in the arteries supplying the hind or fore limbs so that the artery becomes blocked, denying the limb of its oxygenated blood supply. One or both back legs may be affected because the clot may lodge where the arteries branch from the aorta and cause both to be blocked. In the front leg, the blockage occurs at some distance from the aorta and therefore only one limb is affected.

Signs. This condition is more commonly seen in cats than in dogs. The animal is presented in extreme and acute pain, collapsed and howling. It frequently tries to drag itself around the table as if trying to escape from its own rear end. The distinctive signs are:

- Absence of pulse in the affected limb. No femoral or brachial pulse can be detected.
- Coldness of the limb. As no warm blood is flowing into the leg, the tissues of the leg cool rapidly and the foot feels ice-cold and clammy.
- Spastic contraction of the muscles. This tends to hold the leg in extension. Because of the lack of oxygen in the muscle tissue, the changes which occur are similar to those in rigor mortis.
- Decreased withdrawal reflexes. The leg is not rigid but the animal finds it difficult to move because of the muscular activity. The motivation to withdraw is not great because the animal is in such intense pain that a nip on the toe is insignificant.

Treatment. These animals are very shocked and in great pain. They need to be handled carefully.

Warm the limb, using a heat lamp, heated pads etc. Vasodilation is to be encouraged in these cases as it may enlarge the diameter of the affected artery at the site of the blockage so that the blood can once again flow past the obstruction.

Massage the limb. This may also help to dilate the blood vessel and stimulate the circulation down the leg. In practice this treatment is usually impossible because the patient is very likely to resent handling of its leg.

The animal should be encouraged to rest as much as possible because there is often an underlying heart condition.

Hypoglycaemic coma

Cause. Hypoglycaemia occurs in the diagnosed diabetic animal when there is an imbalance between the insulin given and the glucose available. Too much insulin removes the soluble circulating glucose and converts it to insoluble glycogen in the liver. The animal becomes hypoglycaemic (low levels of blood glucose) and the metabolism slows down. The causes of this condition are explained in Chapter 23 (Medical Nursing).

Signs. The time of onset depends upon the type of insulin used but usually the signs occur about 10 hours post injection:

- Dullness and lethargy.
- Ataxic (uncoordinated) movements.
- The mouth and body feel cold to the touch;
- Collapse—as the situation becomes more grave, the animal may start to twitch uncontrollably and may go into convulsions.
- Coma and death soon follow.

Treatment. **Glucose solution** should be administered immediately the first signs are seen. One or more tablespoonfuls should be given by mouth. If glucose is not available, honey should be used instead. If neither of these is available, sugar water can be given, but this has the disadvantage that the disaccharide of sugar must be digested first to release the glucose molecule, and this may not happen quickly enough to arrest the onset of the diabetic coma.

If the patient is unconscious, the owners should bring the animal to the surgery immediately for an intravenous injection of glucose. The injection should be prepared ready for administration by the veterinary surgeon and a glucose solution may also be prepared for oral administration by stomach tube.

Maintain the airway if unconscious.

Treat for shock.

Hypocalcaemia

Cause. Lack of circulating calcium ions causes malfunctions of the nervous and muscular tissue. The problem of eclampsia is usually seen in lactating bitches with large litters soon after birth when the pups are 2–3 or 5 weeks old. It has also been seen in cats nursing kittens. The demand by the rapidly growing offspring for milk is enormous and drains the calcium from the mother's body. To meet this demand, she must either take in calcium from the diet or reabsorb calcium from her bones. The latter is a slow process so that, unless enough calcium is given in the diet to cope with the demand, the mother will soon become deficient in circulating calcium ions and show signs of eclampsia.

Signs

- Restlessness and inability to settle to feed the litter.
- Panting respiration.
- Muscular tremors—the muscular tissue becomes unable to function normally as the calcium levels fall.
- Collapse and hyperaesthesia – the slightest sound now causes convulsive twitching.
- Unconsciousness. As the brain becomes more affected, the twitching lessens and ceases. Death will soon follow.

Treatment. Calcium given by mouth is not effective as it is poorly absorbed. Intravenous calcium must be injected, and syringes should be prepared (usually with 10% calcium solution) ready for injecting when the veterinary surgeon can attend the case.

No further sucking should be allowed by the pups as this will drain yet more calcium from the system.

Uraemia

Cause. Uraemic fits are usually seen in old dogs with chronic kidney failure and are due to a build-up of toxic substances (especially phosphates) in the bloodstream which would normally be excreted by the kidneys.

Signs. In most cases there is a long-standing history of polydypsia and weight loss, culminating in vomiting, anorexia and lethargy and, in the last stages, epileptiform convulsions. The breath may smell of urine.

Treatment. Euthanasia is usually necessary and the animal should be made comfortable and treated as an epileptic pending diagnosis by the veterinary surgeon.

Electrocution

Cause. Electrocution occurs when a high voltage passes through the animal's body. If the line of conduction passes through the animal's heart, the result is instantaneous cardiac arrest.

Signs. The animal is found collapsed by the source of the problem, but it may not be obvious exactly what has happened. Most cases occur because of electrical faults in everyday equipment and the most extraordinary things can happen. In one case the wire mesh of a kennel's exercise run became 'live' following an electrical fault and all the dogs in that block were electrocuted. In another case, a dog urinated on a lamppost and electrocuted himself because the lamppost was 'live'. (Water in any form is marvellous conductor of electricity.)

Treatment

> WARNING
> **SWITCH OFF THE ELECTRICITY SUPPLY** before touching the animal—the animal may well be electrically 'live' though clinically dead.
> If the mains switch cannot be located quickly, **use a dry wooden pole** (remember that water and metal both conduct electricity) to push the animal well away from any object which may be electrically active.

The animal should be given cardiac massage if no heartbeat can be felt, and the airway of an unconscious animal must be maintained, but these cases are usually hopeless.

Heatstroke

Cause. The cause is usually overexposure to heat, classically seen in short-nosed breeds left in a closed car in the full sun but it is also seen in hairy dogs that have undergone considerable exercise or have become very excited when the weather is warm and humid.

Signs. Initially, the animal is distressed, panting excessively and restless. As the situation worsens and the body temperature increases, the animal starts to become cyanosed, drools copiously with saliva and becomes unsteady on its feet. If the body temperature continues to climb, the animal will collapse; it becomes comatose and soon dies. The body feels burning hot and the rectal temperature is off the scale.

Treatment

- Cool the animal immediately using cold water baths, soaking the animal by running water from a hosepipe on it, covering the body with blankets and towels soaked in cold water, applying ice packs, etc. These measures have limited use as the sudden cooling will cause vasoconstriction in the skin, so that the blood arriving at the surface of the body to be cooled will be much reduced, but it is a valuable first step.
- As the blood is the body's transport system, cooling the blood is the most efficient way to cool the whole body and chilled intravenous drips may be set up as soon as possible. If no chilled drip is available, lay the giving set tube in a bed of crushed ice so that the intravenous fluid is chilled as it runs through the drip tubing.
- Confine the patient to a cool, airy kennel, preferably one with a concrete floor to encourage further heat loss by conduction. Lay a wet blanket over the animal to keep the coat wet and decrease its insulative properties.

- Maintain the airway. Swab saliva away from the unconscious patient, and give oxygen at the first signs of cyanosis.
- **Check the rectal temperature every 15 minutes** to avoid overdoing the cooling of the body. As soon as the temperature has fallen to 102°F, the animal should be dried off and placed in a cool kennel with access to cold drinking water. The temperature must then be checked every 30 minutes to ensure that it is not allowed to rise again.

Hypothermia

Cause. Hypothermia is a common problem of the very small and the very young and in victims of drowning accidents. Small mammals and birds readily suffer hypothermia; young puppies and kittens, with little or no temperature regulation, are helpless if warmth is not given.

Signs. The animal becomes sleepy and lethargic and does not bother to feed. Its movements become weaker and the patient becomes comatose. Its body feels cold to the touch and the rectal temperature is subnormal (around 98°F/38°C).

Treatment

- Massage with warm, rough towels to stimulate young neonates and to open up the cutaneous circulation so that the body is able to pick up radiant heat more efficiently. Towels also dry the fur of a patient suffering from exposure so that it regains its insulating cover.
- **Conserve heat** by laying the animal on thick bedding (e.g. Vetbed). Light coverings may be laid over the patient, but thick blankets should be avoided as they will prevent the animal from absorbing direct warmth.

- **Apply heat** by:
  - warmed intravenous drips (the most efficient method)
  - heat pads, hot water-bottles and avian hospitalisation cages (these are controlled forms of heating that are unlikely to overheat the patient
  - heat lamps for the mature animal, which can move away from the heat source when it becomes too hot.
- **Check the rectal temperature** every 15 minutes— or every 10 minutes with the young patient since these animals absorb the heat more quickly than the larger, adult animal. Recovery is usually rapid in the young and signs of returning consciousness and movement can also be used as a guide.
- **Maintain the temperature** by confining the patient to a warm box or kennel.

Further Reading

Andrews, A. H. and Humphries, D. J. (1982) *Poisoning in Veterinary Practice*, 2nd edn, National Office of Animal Health.

Edney, A. (1992) *The Complete Cat Care Manual*, Dorling Kindersley.

Fogle, B. (1993) *The Complete Dog Care Manual*, Dorling Kindersley.

Humphries, D. J. (1988) *Veterinary Toxicology*, 3rd edn, Balliere Tindall.

Marsden, A. K., Moffat, Sir C. and Scott, R. (1992) *First Aid Manual of the St John's Ambulance*, St Andrew's Ambulance Association and British Red Cross, 6th edn, Dorling Kindersley.

South West Oiled Seabird Group (1993) *First Aid for Oiled Seabirds* RSPCA, Horsham.

Taylor, D. T. (1992) *BVA Guide to Dog Care*, 2nd edn, Dorling Kindersley.

Turner, T. (1990) *Veterinary Notes for Dog Owners*, Stanley Paul.

4

Exotic Pets and Wildlife

J. E. COOPER and A. J. PEARSON

'Exotics', sometimes called the 'other' pets, are an important feature of veterinary practice in Britain and many other parts of the world. They include any small pet that is not a dog or a cat as well as wild animals brought in as casualties and they present an exciting challenge to the veterinary nurse, who is often the first and most immediate point of contact for the client.

Anatomy and Physiology

Many exotic pets are **vertebrates** and share various anatomical and physiological similarities. **Invertebrates** such as insects and spiders are substantially different. The main groups of exotic pets and their features are given in Fig. 4.1.

Mammals and birds are **endothermic**, or 'warm-blooded'. An endothermic animal is able to maintain its own body temperature above that of its surroundings, within certain limits, using internal (physiological) control mechanisms. Thus a rabbit's body temperature is likely to be 39.5°C in both summer and winter.

Reptiles, amphibians and invertebrates are **ectothermic**, or 'cold-blooded'. With very few exceptions they are unable to control their body temperature by intrinsic (internal) means and so it will fluctuate depending upon the ambient temperature. However, an ectothermic animal uses external or behavioural means to control its body temperature.

Mammals

The mammals that are most commonly kept as pets are set out in Fig. 4.2, which shows that they fall into three different groups (Orders): the Rodentia, the Lagomorpha and the Carnivora. Most of them can be considered domesticated species and many that have become popular as pets were first used as laboratory animals. Other species are sometimes encountered in veterinary practice, such as the diminutive Roborovski's hamster or the large Shaw's Jird, but knowledge of their close relatives means that they can be treated as if they were hamsters or gerbils although they are possibly a little less amenable to handling.

Although small mammals share many anatomical features, there are some differences that are relevant to the biology and veterinary care of these species (Figs 4.3 and 4.4). The veterinary nurse should take every opportunity to become familiar with the normal features, in order to be able to detect ill health or abnormalities more easily. Having once studied the anatomy and physiology of the dog and cat in detail (Chapter 14, Anatomy and Physiology), veterinary nurses should be able to note the external features of the herbivorous and omnivorous small mammals (i.e. excluding the carnivorous ferret) where they differ:

- Both the herbivorous and the omnivorous small mammals have chisel-shaped incisors for gnawing; they also have flat tables of cheek teeth for grinding coarse vegetable matter. The rodents have one pair of incisors in both upper and lower jaws. Rabbits have one pair in the lower jaw but two in the upper (one large pair and a smaller pair directly behind them). All the teeth of rabbits and herbivorous rodents are what is known as **open-rooted**: they grow continually throughout life.
- The joint surfaces of the tempero-mandibular joint are flat compared with those of the dog and cat, allowing both sideways and backwards-and-forwards movement of the lower jaw.
- Lower in the gastrointestinal tract they have a relatively large **caecum**, where bacteria break down the cellulose of plant cell walls to allow the animal to make use of this plant material as food.
- The rabbit and all the small rodents practise **coprophagia**, which is the eating of faeces. The rabbit passes two different types of faeces: the dry pellets that we consider 'normal'; and, at night, **caecal** pellets, which are dark in colour and covered with mucus so that they tend to stick together and emerge in a mass. These caecal pellets are eaten directly from the anus and complete a second passage of the gut so that all possible nutrients are extracted from the food.
- The hamsters have cheek pouches, used for carrying food back to the nest when on extensive foraging expeditions.
- The chinchillas and the small pet rodents tend to hold their food in their front paws while feeding. They are able to do this as they can pronate their front paws—rotating the radius to twist the carpus and manus, as can cats (but not dogs).

There are also certain features to note regarding skin and glands:

- Rabbits have no foot-pads: their feet are covered with hair.
- Female rabbits have a **dewlap** (a large fold of skin under the chin) from which they pluck fur to line the nest.

GROUPS OF EXOTIC ANIMALS AND THEIR MAIN FEATURES		
Group	**Features**	**Examples**
Mammals (Mammalia)	Internal skeleton Endothermic ('warm blooded') Skin bears hairs Lungs Bear live young Feed young on milk Internal fertilisation	Rat (*Rattus norvegicus*) Mouse (*Mus musculus*) Guinea pig (*Cavia porcellus*) Chinchilla (*Chinchilla laniger*) Syrian hamster (*Mesocricetus auratus*) Mongolian gerbil (*Meriones unguiculatus*) Ferret (*Mustela putorius furo*)
Birds (Aves)	Internal skeleton Endothermic Wings Skin bears feathers Scales on legs Lungs Eggs with hard shell Internal fertilisation	Budgerigar (*Melopsittacus undulatus*) African grey parrot (*Psittacus erithacus*) Amazon parrot (*Amazona* spp.) Canary (*Serinus canaria*) Cockatiel (*Nymphicus hollandicus*) Fowl (chicken) (*Gallus domesticus*) Pigeon (*Columba livia*)
Reptiles (Reptilia)	Internal skeleton Ectothermic ('cold-blooded') Dry skin with scales Lungs Oviparous (eggs with hard or soft shells) or ovoviviparous (live-bearing) Internal fertilisation	Common iguana (*Iguana iguana*) Mediterranean tortoise (*Testudo* spp.) Box tortoise (*Terrapene* spp.) Garter snake (*Thamnophis* spp.) Corn snake (*Elaphe guttata*) Leopard gecko (*Eublepharis macularius*)
Amphibians (Amphibia)	Internal skeleton Ectothermic Moist skin with mucus and sometimes poison glands Oviparous, occasionally ovoviviparous Lungs in adult, gills in larva (tadpole) Larval form External fertilisation	Common toad (*Bufo bufo*) Marine toad (*Bufo marinus*) European tree frog (*Hyla arborea*) Edible frog (*Rana esculenta*) Great-crested newt (*Triturus cristatus*) European salamander (*Salamandra salamandra*) Axolotl (*Ambystoma mexicanum*)
Fish (Pisces)	Internal skeleton Ectothermic Moist skin with scales Gills Oviparous (eggs without shells) or ovoviviparous (live-bearing) Sometimes larval form Usually external fertilisation	Goldfish (*Carassius auratus*) Koi carp (*Cyprinus carpio*) Guppy (*Lebistes reticulatus*) Angel fish (*Pterophyllum scalare*) Platies (*Xiphophorus* spp.) Siamese fighting fish (*Betta splendens*) Discus (*Symphysodon discus*) Oscar (*Astronotus ocellatus*) Seahorse (*Hippocampus* spp.)
Invertebrates Arthropods (Arthropoda)	External skeleton (cuticle) Paired jointed limbs Segmented Open vascular system Oviparous or viviparous	Indian stick insect (*Carausius morosus*) Red-kneed tarantula (*Euthalus smithii*) Tree bird spiders (*Avicularia* spp.) Tree crabs (*Coenobita* spp.) Emperor scorpion (*Pandinus imperator*)
Molluscs (Mollusca)	Shell but no cuticle Ventral muscular foot Unsegmented Open vascular system Oviparous or viviparous	African land snail (*Achatina* spp.) Garden snail (*Helix aspersa*)

Fig. 4.1. Main groups of exotic pets and their features.

- Gerbils have a large skin gland on the mid-ventral abdomen, which in old age may become hypertrophied.
- Syrian hamsters have glandular areas on their flanks, where the skin is darkly pigmented. Older hamsters often lose their hair in these areas.
- Guinea pigs have a greasy glandular area just above the tail, which is quite normal and should not be considered pathological.
- Chinchilla fur is very dense. These animals were originally imported to be bred for their pelts

(skins). The coat over the body has no guard hairs and there may be up to 70 fine downy hairs per skin follicle. The tail does have a covering of guard hairs and there are fewer downy hairs in this region.

Sexing small mammals

This is more difficult in some species than in others. In all female rodents, the genital and urinary orifices are separate so that there are three orifices (from the

SMALL MAMMAL SPECIES COMMONLY KEPT AS PETS				
Order	Sub-order	Family	Species	English name
Rodentia	Myomorpha	Muridae	*Rattus norvegicus*	Fancy rat
			Mus musculus	Mouse
		Cricetidae	*Meriones unguiculatus*	Mongolian gerbil
			Mesocricetus auratus	Syrian hamster
			Phodopus sungorus	Russian hamster [1]
			Cricetulus griseus	Chinese hamster [1]
	Hystricomorpha	Caviidae	*Cavia porcellus*	Guinea pig
		Chinchillidae	*Chinchilla laniger*	Chinchilla
	Sciuromorpha	Sciuridae	*Tamias sibiricus*	Siberian chipmunk
Lagomorpha		Leporidae	*Oryctolagus cuniculus*	Rabbit
Carnivora		Mustelidae	*Mustela putorius furo*	Ferret

1) The Russian and Chinese are the dwarf hamsters. Unlike the Syrian hamster they are social animals, living in family groups in the wild.
2) Note the division of the family 'Rodentia', the rodents. The 'Mouse-like' rodents are further divided into the rats and mice, and the gerbils and hamsters. All these small rodents are omnivorous. The Sciuromorphs, or squirrel-like rodents, are also omnivores, and the Siberian chipmunk has a lifestyle very like the squirrels of Europe and North America. Hystricomorphs are the third group of rodents; they are herbivores and come from South America.

Fig. 4.2. Small mammal species commonly kept as pets.

SMALL ANIMAL ANATOMY							
	Mouse	Rat	Syrian hamster	Gerbil	Guinea pig	Rabbit	Ferret
Teeth	Well developed incisors for gnawing (one upper pair – rodents, two upper pairs – one small – rabbit)						Well developed canines for tearing
Dental Formula	$\frac{1003}{1003}$	$\frac{1003}{1003}$	$\frac{1003}{1003}$	$\frac{1003}{1003}$	$\frac{1013}{1013}$	$\frac{1033}{1023}$	$\frac{3131}{3132}$
Ears	Hairless	Hairless	Sparse hair	Hairy	Sparse except tip	Hairy	Hairy
Cheek Pouches	Absent	Absent	Present	Absent	Absent	Absent	Absent
Stomach	Simple, two distinct regions	Simple, two distinct regions	Simple, two compartments	Simple, two distinct regions	Simple	Simple	Simple
Intestine	Long	Long	Long	Long	Long	Long	Short
Gall Bladder	Present	Absent	Present	Present	Present	Present	Present
Appendix	Small	Small	Small	Small	Large	Very large	No caecum or appendix
Mammary Glands	No teats in male	No teats in male	No teats in male	No teats in male	Teats in male	Teats in male	Teats in male
Testes	Retractable	Retractable	Retractable	Retractable	Retractable	Retractable	Not retractable
Scent Glands	None	None	On flanks	Ventral midline	Perineal	Perineal	Anal sacs
Tail	No hair, scales	No hair, scales	Hair	Hair	No tail	Hair	Hair

Fig. 4.3. Anatomical differences in small mammals.

most dorsal: anal, genital and urinary); in the male there are only two. However, the genital orifice is not patent much of the time and is often only to be seen as a patch or strip of naked skin. It becomes patent when the animal is in season, and prior to parturition. In any female rodent, the separate orifices make it easy to distinguish whether a discharge or bleeding is urinary or vaginal in origin.

Rabbits, and most rodents, have large, open inguinal rings which allow the testes to be retracted into the abdomen. In all the small pet mammals except the Russian hamster, the descended testes are obvious in the mature male. Otherwise the sexes can be distinguished by the presence of the vaginal membrane in the female, and the greater ano-genital distance in the male.

- *Rabbits* are not difficult to sex once the testes have descended, as they lie in scrotal sacs on either side of the penis, which is easily protruded in the adult rabbit, slightly less easily in the young. The vulva of the female is a slit, pointed at the front, whereas the prepuce is more circular.
- *Guinea pigs* are easy to sex from birth: the penis can be protruded with gentle pressure around the relevant orifice.
- *Chinchillas* can be difficult to sex unless one is aware that there is a significant urethral prominence in the female, which may be mistaken for a penis. Look for the ano-genital distance (greater in the male) and the vaginal membrane in the female.

BIOLOGICAL DATA FOR SMALL MAMMALS								
	Average life expectancy	Maturity	Oestrus	Gestation period	Size of litter	Age at weaning	Adult weight	Temperature °C
Rabbit	Male 8 yrs+ Female 6 yrs	3 mths+	Induced ovulation Oestrus Jan–Oct/Nov.	28–32 days	2–7	6 weeks	varies	38.5
Guinea Pig	4–7 yrs	M 8–10 wks F 4–5 wks	15–16 day cycle	60–72 days (avg 65)	2–6	3–3.5 wks	750–1000g	38–39
Rat	3 yrs	6 wks+	Every 4–5 days	20–22 days	6–12	21 days+	400–800g	38
Mouse	1–2.5 yrs	3–4 wks	Every 4–5 days	19–21 days	5–1	18 days+	20–40g	37.5
Gerbil	1.5–2.5 yrs	10–12 wks	Every 4–6 days	24–26 days	3–6	21–28 days	70–130g (M>F)	38
Syrian Hamster	1.5–2 yrs	6–10 wks	Every 4 days	15–18 days	3–7	21–28 days	85–150g	37–38
Russian Hamster	1.5–2 yrs	6–10 wks	Every 4 days	19–20 days	3–5	21–28 days		
Chinese Hamster	1.5–2 yrs	6–10 wks	Every 4 days	20–22 days	3–5	21–28 days		
Chinchilla	10 yrs (up to 15)	8 months	Seasonally polyoestrous. Cycle 30–35 days Nov–May	111 days	2 or 3 (1–4)	6–8 wks	Male 400g F 500g	38–39
Chipmunk	M 3 yrs F 5 yrs	1 year	Seasonally polyoestrous. Cycle 14 days Mar–Sep. 2 litters/yr	28–32 days	2–6	6–7 wks	80–130g	38 (N.B. hibernation)
Ferret	5–7 yrs	6–9 months	Induced ovulation. Oestrus Feb/Mar–Sept.	42 days	2–6 (up to 10)	8 wks	500–2000g	38.8

Fig. 4.4. General biology of small mammals.

- In the *ferret*, the opening of the prepuce is on the belly, near the umbilicus. The testes are only within the scrotum during the breeding season. The penis contains the os penis bone that can be easily palpated.

Birds

Birds may be kept either as pets (often individually, or in pairs, in cages indoors) or for breeding or exhibition. Larger species and most wild birds are bred in aviaries but the smaller domesticated species, such as budgerigars and canaries, are usually bred in custom-built bird-rooms.

Domesticated species are those that have been bred in captivity for long enough for significant genetic changes to be fixed in the species: such as the development of different breeds (in domestic fowl and canaries) or different colour mutations (in the budgerigar and the peach-faced lovebird, for example). There are 28 different orders of birds but most of those presented for veterinary attention are likely to fall into one of the following:

- Order Psittaciformes—budgerigar, parrots etc.
- Order Passeriformes—perching birds, including canary, finches.
- Order Falconiformes—diurnal (not nocturnal) birds of prey such as hawks, falcons.
- Order Strigiformes—owls.
- Order Galliformes—domestic fowl, pheasants, quail.
- Order Anseriformes—ducks, geese and swans.

Figure 4.5 describes some of the birds commonly kept in aviculture and also some of the different groups of non-domesticated species. Figure 4.6 shows the significance of some of the anatomical features of various species.

Although the anatomy of birds follows the basic vertebrate pattern, it also shows a number of important differences from mammals, including adaptations for flight—especially by keeping weight to a minimum.

Skeleton and muscles

- The bones have thin cortices and some of them are pneumatised: they contain an air sac as an extension of the respiratory system.
- Throughout the skeleton the number of joints (Fig. 4.7) is reduced to facilitate flying. The fusion of many of the vertebrae reduces mobility in the trunk region but a long, very flexible neck allows the bird to reach all parts of its body with its beak.
- An enlarged sternum, or keel bone, allows the attachment of very bulky flight muscles, which in some species may comprise up to one quarter of the body weight of the bird.
- The pelvis is modified to allow the passage of a large egg. This is achieved by having an open pubis rather than a symphysis.
- The weight of the skull is reduced by reduction of the maxillary region and there being no teeth.
- In many species the tongue is rigid, containing a lingual bone, whereas in many parrots the tongue is thick, fleshy and very mobile and is used to manipulate food.
- There is a **quadrate bone** lying between the maxilla and each dentary, producing two joints between upper and lower jaw. This allows a variable amount of backwards-and-forwards movement in

COMMONLY KEPT BIRDS IN AVICULTURE		
Name	**Origin**	**Description**
Domestic species		
Budgerigar (*Melopsittacus undulatus*)	Australia	Many colour varities. 'Show' budgies are much larger than the wild type.
Canary (*Canarius serinus*)	Canary Islands	Many different breeds, some judged on colour, some on colour and 'type' and some on their song.
Cockatiels (*Nymphicus hollandicus*)	Australia	Many colour varities.
Peach-faced Lovebirds	East Africa	In the wild a green bird with a pink/orange face and blue rump. Now in many colour varieties. An aggressive species.
Zebra Finches	Australia	A prolific breeder, now in many colour mutations.
Bengali	East Asia	A finch kept in its own right or as a foster parent for species unwilling to care for eggs or young in captivity.
Other species that may be considered by some to be domesticated are the Indian Ringneck Parakeet and the Australian Gouldian Finch, both of which are produced now in many colour mutations.		
Different groups of non-domesticated species commonly kept in aviculture.		
Foreign Finches		Commonly Australian, African or East Asian species.
Softbills		Such as Pekin Robins, Mynah birds, various starlings and thrushes.
British Birds		It is permitted to keep certain species of British Birds in captivity, but they must not be taken from the wild without a licence, and any young that are to be sold or exhibited must have been aviary-bred and close-ringed ('ABCR') during the first few days of life.
Grass parakeets		Small Australian parakeets related to the budgerigar. Examples are the Elegant, the Splendid, and Bourke's grass parakeet.
Parrots		Many species kept by enthusiasts and others by commercial breeders to supply the demand for English-bred, hand-reared (EBHR) parrots as pets.
Waterfowl and pheasants		Many species endangered in the wild and are kept successfully by aviculturlists. Birds that are to be kept 'free range' must not be allowed to escape into the wild and so must be pinioned.

Fig. 4.5. Bird species commonly kept.

ANATOMICAL FEATURES OF BIRDS	
Feature	**Significance**
Beak – variation in shape and size	Related to feeding habits, e.g. parrots open fruit and nuts, canaries and finches peck at seeds, raptors tear meat. Many psittacine birds also use beak for climbing.
Legs and feet – variation in appearance	Related to habits and habitat, e.g. parrots climb (two toes pointing forwards, two backwards), canaries and finches perch (three toes forwards, one backwards), raptors grasp prey with talons, ducks swim with webbed feet.
Wings – variation in shape and size	Related to flying, e.g. falcons have long pointed wings for hunting prey from a height, hawks have short rounded wings for quick dash through undergrowth. Some birds, e.g. penguin, ostrich, do not fly.
Plumage – variation in colour and structures (e.g. crests)	Related to behaviour, e.g. recognition of own species or a mate, threat or warning to predators. Some species show sexual dimorphism, i.e. plumage differs between male and female.

Fig. 4.6. Significance of anatomical features in birds.

different species (it is particularly well developed in the parrots). There is also a joint between the upper part of the beak and the rest of the skull—the **cranio-facial hinge**—and again the amount of movement varies from species to species.

- The number of digits in the forelimb (wing) is reduced to two: digit III, and a much reduced digit I which forms the **alula** or 'bastard wing' that carries a few feathers which are important for control at take-off and landing. In some birds there may be a claw on the alula.

Feathers

The plumage, composed of keratin, provides light-weight but strong feathers which also help to insulate the bird. The feathers are divided into several groups:

- **Flight feathers** of the wings and tail are long and rigid.

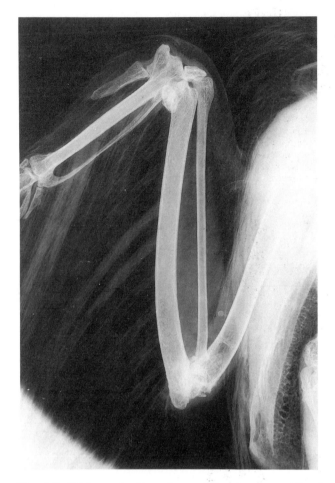

Fig. 4.7. Dislocated elbow in an injured raptor. (Good radiography facilitates diagnosis and treatment of skeletal problems in birds. Note that young growing feathers are visible on this radiograph—their vascular sheath is radiopaque.)

- **Contour feathers** are those that make up the outer layer of feathers over most of the body. They are shorter and more flexible than the flight feathers.
- **Down feathers** and **filoplumes** lie beneath the contour feathers and provide a layer of insulation. (Birds carry very little subcutaneous fat compared with mammals.)

All feathers have the same basic structure. In the majority of birds all the feathers are shed each year during the moulting season, which in most species occurs in late summer, at the end of the breeding season. The developing feather is covered by a keratin sheath; while it is growing, a blood vessel runs up the shaft, so that damage to a feather at this stage will result in haemorrhage.

Birds keep their feathers in good order by preening. Most birds use oil from the **preen gland** on the top of the tail to waterproof them although not all birds have a preen gland. Some birds (notably the cockatoos and cockatiel) produce a fine dust from their feathers which helps to keep the plumage in good order. Most birds in the wild bathe regularly and will do so in captivity as well.

It is important for all birds, but particularly for falconry birds and racing pigeons, to protect the feathers and minimise damage to the plumage when a bird is hospitalised.

The gastrointestinal tract

The gastrointestinal tract in birds follows the basic vertebrate pattern of foregut, midgut and hindgut but with certain modifications (Fig. 4.8):

- There are no teeth. Some birds hold food with their feet and tear it with their beaks; others swallow food whole.
- In most species there is a diverticulum of the oesophagus in the ventral neck—the **crop**. This is used as a storage organ. In pigeons and parrots it produces a secretion known as **crop milk** that is used to nourish the young in the nest. There is no crop in the owls or in many diving birds.
- The stomach in most species is divided into a **proventriculus**, which is the glandular stomach, and the **ventriculus** or **gizzard**, which is a thick-walled chamber where food can be ground up. There is no gizzard in birds that have a predominantly fluid diet, such as the nectar-eating sunbirds and hummingbirds.
- The small intestine is short but otherwise unremarkable.
- The large intestine may or may not sport two large **caeca** (sing. caecum) from the junction between large and small intestines. This is the site for bacterial digestion in herbivorous and omnivorous species. Caeca are reduced or absent in carnivorous and nectivorous species.
- The digestive, urinary and genital tracts all open to the outside through one orifice, the **cloaca** or **vent**.

The respiratory system

The respiratory system of the bird is very different from that of the mammal and these differences have implications for anaesthesia in birds.

- The bird has no diaphragm. The main muscles of respiration are the abdominal muscles, which should never be restricted during restraint of the animal.
- The lungs are small compared with those of the mammal, and they are non-distensible. They lie close to the dorsal body wall in the cranial part of the body cavity.
- The air is drawn into and expelled from the body by the expansion and contraction of thin-walled air sacs, which are lined with serous membrane and extend throughout the body, even into some of the bones (pneumatisation).
- Air circulates through the lungs continuously, during both inspiration and expiration. This means that changes in depth of anaesthesia are likely to

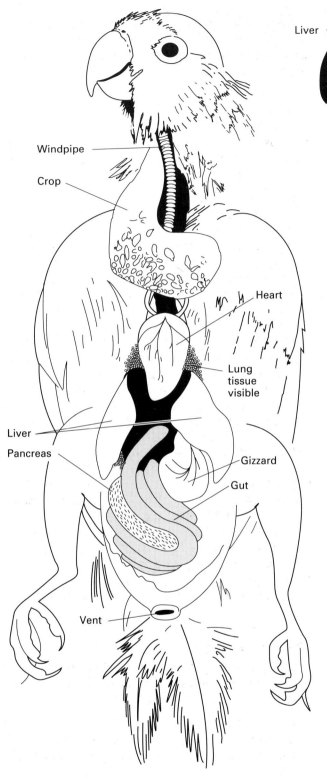

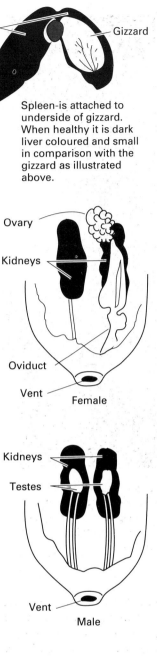

Spleen-is attached to underside of gizzard. When healthy it is dark liver coloured and small in comparison with the gizzard as illustrated above.

Lift out gut, etc., to reveal kidneys and sexual organs

Fig. 4.8. Internal organs of a parrot.

take place much faster in birds than in mammals of comparable size.

Reptiles and Amphibians

Figure 4.9 shows some of the species most commonly seen in veterinary practice. Reptiles and amphibians are ectothermic animals: although unable to control body temperature intrinsically, they can do so very effectively by behavioural means. For

example, a lizard basks in the sun in order to raise its body temperature but it hides under a log or seeks the shade in order to lower its body temperature.

Ectothermic animals have their own **preferred body temperature** (PBT), which is the temperature range at which they can move about and feed and at which their digestive enzymes etc. are able to act. Some species are tolerant of wide ranges of temperature; others come from very stable environments in the wild, where there is very little

SOME SPECIES OF REPTILE AND AMPHIBIAN SEEN IN VETERINARY PRACTICES

	Type	Species	
Class Reptilia	Order Chelonia (tortoises and turtles)	*Testudo hermanni*	Hermann's tortoise
		Testudo graeca	Spur-thighed tortoise
		Terrapene spp.	American box tortoise/'turtle'
		Pseudemys scripta elegans	Red-eared terrapin
	Order Squamata (snakes and lizards)	*Natrix natrix*	Grass snake
		Thamnophis spp.	Garter snake
		Elaphe guttata	Corn snake
		Elaphe obsoleta	Black rat snake
		Lampropeltis spp.	King snake
		Python sebae	African rock python
		P. regius	Royal python
		P. molurus	Indian python
		P. reticulatus	Reticulated python
		Lacerta vivipara	Common lizard
		Anguis fragilis	Slow-worm
		Iguana iguana	Common or green iguana
Class Amphibia	Order Anura (frogs and toads)	*Bufo bufo*	Common toad
		Bufo marinus	Marine toad
		Xenopus spp.	Clawed toad
		Rana esculenta	Edible frog
		Rana pipiens	Leopard frog
		Hyla arborea	European tree frog
	Order Urodela (newts and salamanders)	*Triturus cristatus*	Great-crested newt
		Salamandra salamandra	European salamander
		Ambystoma mexicanum	Axolotl

Fig. 4.9. Reptiles and amphibians kept as pets.

temperature variation. Examples of PBT for different reptiles are given in Fig. 4.10.

Some reptiles **hibernate** in cold weather. This is a complex physiological process and should not be confused with torpor induced by a sudden temperature drop. Other species **aestivate**: that is, they become lethargic and they sleep because the temperature is too high and/or environmental conditions are too dry.

All reptiles have a dry skin, impervious to water and usually covered with scales. All of them shed (slough) their skins as they grow. Some, such as the tortoises, shed it in small parts; others, such as the snakes and some lizards, shed their skins at one time, often in one piece.

Some lizards can shed their tails (**autotomy**) if they are handled incorrectly—for example, if the tail is grasped. This is a defence mechanism when it occurs in the wild: a predator's attention may be attracted to the discarded tail, allowing the lizard itself to escape unscathed. A new tail will grow but it is a poor replica of the original, supported by cartilage and not bone.

Although the basic anatomy of reptiles is similar to that of other vertebrates, the following special points should be noted:

- **Tortoises** and other chelonians have a modified skeleton: a bony 'box' composed of an upper part (**carapace**) and lower part (**plastron**), fused at the sides. The box consists of modified vertebral column, ribs and sternum.
- Snakes and certain snake-like lizards have modifications related to their elongated shape: they have no limbs, or only vestigial limbs, and they have elongated lungs (only one functional in snakes), liver and intestine.

EXAMPLES OF PREFERRED BODY TEMPERATURE (PBT) FOR REPTILES

Species	Activity range (°C)	PBC (°C)
Box turtle (*Terrapene ornata*)	22–35	27
Greek tortoise (*Testudo graeca*)	15–30	24
Green anole (*Anolis carolinensis*)	30–36	34
Green (common) iguana (*Iguana iguana*)	26–42	33
Flap-necked chameleon (*Chamaeleo dilepis*)	21–36	31
Slow-worm (*Anguis fragilis*)	14–29	22
Boa constrictor (*Constrictor constrictor*)	26–37	32
Garter snake (*Thamnophis sirtalis*)	20–35	29

Fig. 4.10. Preferred body temperatures of some reptile species. Adapted from Cooper and Jackson (1981).

Reproduction

Reptiles produce eggs and they are either oviparous or ovo-viviparous:

- **Oviparous** reptiles lay their eggs within a calcareous shell (some are almost as rigid as a bird's egg but others are little more than a parchment-like membrane).
- **Ovo-viviparous** reptiles retain their eggs within the body of the female until the young are fully developed and capable of independent life.

This retention of the egg until hatching is not the same as true **viviparity**, because the developing reptile embryo is nourished only by the yolk of the

WATER TEMPERATURES FOR FISH		
Type	**Cold (up to 21°C)**	**Warm (21°–29°C)**
Freshwater	Goldfish	Guppy
Saltwater	Herring	Seahorse

Fig. 4.11. Water temperatures for fish.

egg, rather than by the mother via a placenta as is the case with viviparous mammals.

The young reptiles, whether hatched or born, emerge as small replicas of the adult and are immediately capable of feeding themselves.

Amphibians

Amphibians are often grouped and discussed with reptiles but they show many differences. In particular their skin is generally thin, mucous and permeable. Many amphibians can respire through their skin as well as using lungs (adults) or gills (larvae). The larvae metamorphose into adults.

Fish

There are three main groups of fish: the primitive Placoderms, the huge group of Osteichthyes (bony fish) and the Chondrichthyes (cartilaginous fish). Those of most relevance to veterinary practice are the bony fish (e.g. goldfish). Cartilaginous fish, such as sharks, are sometimes kept in captivity.

The type and temperature of water in which fish live are very relevant to their physiology and health, and Fig. 4.11 gives some examples.

Management and Nutrition

Veterinary nurses are often asked for advice on the management of exotic pets, including suitable housing, feeding and general husbandry and perhaps breeding. They are also asked which pets might be suitable in various circumstances. It is therefore important to have a good background knowledge on all aspects of pet care, as well as knowing how to handle the animals when they are brought into the practice and how to look after those that become hospitalised.

Choosing a Pet

The choice of pet depends upon many factors and Fig. 4.12 suggests the main questions that should be asked of a potential owner who is considering an exotic as a pet. Clients may want pets for various purposes and these requirements have to be taken into consideration when making a choice. In all cases the animal must be easily handled and managed, relatively robust and unlikely to transmit disease. Examples of specific circumstances are given in Fig. 4.13.

ADVISING ON CHOICE OF PET: QUESTIONS TO ASK	
Question	**Explanation**
Are financial considerations important?	Some species are expensive to keep.
What facilities do you have?	Avoid large pets such as rabbits and parrots if the owner has no garden or lives in a flat.
How much spare time do you have?	Some pets, such as parrots, need considerable attention if they are not to become bored. Others, such as fish and invertebrates, need relatively little attention.
What are your domestic arrangements?	Some pets are unsuitable for young children or elderly persons. Some animals are active at night, others by day.
Are there any significant human health consequences?	People who are sensitive to fur or feathers should be wary of mammals and birds. Immuno-suppressed persons should only have contact with pets of known health status.
What other animals do you keep?	Some species may be incompatible or difficult to keep together, e.g. small birds and cats. Commensal bacterial and other organisms of some species may cause clinical disease in others.

Fig. 4.12. Advising on choice of pet: questions to ask.

ADVISING ON CHOICE OF PET: CONSIDERATIONS	
Requirement	**Considerations**
A pet for children	Diurnal.
A pet (companion) for elderly people	Easy to feed. Food readily obtained and affordable. Temperature needs compatible with those of owner(s).
A family pet	No risk to babies. Compatible with family's lifestyle.
For educational studies in the classroom	Weekend and holiday care need consideration. Heating may be switched off. Food supply must be reliable. Continuity in terms of care.
Pets for education talks and visits	Portability. Resilient to repeated handling. No special legal requirements.

Fig. 4.13. Advising on choice of pet: considerations.

Mammals

The housing, nutrition, general management and breeding of rodents, rabbits and ferrets are summarised in Fig. 4.14, and the species are looked at in more detail below. There is also useful information on cages for small mammals in the *How to Choose . . .* leaflets produced by the Universities Federation for Animal Welfare (UFAW), copies of which can be given to clients—preferably before they acquire a new pet. Much useful information on the management of small mammals has resulted from their use in laboratories and contacts with these establishments can prove beneficial.

Rabbits and guinea pigs

Husbandry and housing. Rabbits and guinea pigs are usually kept out of doors, although many people now also keep them as indoor pets. The standard housing for the rabbit or guinea pig is a hutch, with a covered sleeping area and a wire-fronted 'living' area. Owners should be encouraged to view a grassy outdoor run as essential for these species, or to allow regular 'free-ranging' in the garden.

Rabbits are hardy in the British climate and suffer only if they are unable to keep dry, or from excessively high temperatures. With an underground burrow in the wild, they are always able to escape from the rain and from the heat of the summer sun.

Guinea pigs also dislike very hot weather and may suffer if they cannot stay dry.

Rabbits and guinea pigs may (but by no means must) be taken indoors during the winter, but care should be taken that the winter accommodation is well-ventilated and not overheated, as poor ventilation and overheating may predispose to respiratory disease, particularly in rabbits.

Both species are social animals, living in colonies in the wild. Rabbits and guinea pigs can sometimes be kept together, although in some cases problems are encountered such as rabbits mounting cavies, or the cavies chewing a rabbit's fur. Owners should be encouraged to keep rabbits together, and to keep guinea pigs together, but with certain precautions:

- Two male rabbits will fight.
- Two female rabbits may live in harmony, or one may start to exert dominance over the other when she comes into season and starts to defend the 'nest burrow' as her own.
- A male and a female rabbit will live together, and either (or preferably both) can be neutered to prevent unwanted offspring. Rabbits in the wild will form pair bonds and so obviously this is the best and most natural arrangement for them in captivity.
- A group of female guinea pigs will live together without fighting.
- Male guinea pigs will live together without fighting if there are no females within sight, sound or smell.

Feeding. As rabbits and guinea pigs are grazing animals, the most important part of their diet is good quality *roughage*—either hay or grazing. In the absence of sufficient roughage, both species (but particularly the guinea pig) may chew the fur of companions to make up the deficiency.

In the same way that puppies, kittens or breeding or working dogs are fed differently compared with a sedentary pet, so too a young or breeding rabbit or guinea pig requires a different diet from that of a sedentary adult animal. The amount of *protein* in the diet is as important for a young rabbit or guinea pig as it is for a young dog. The pellets used by rabbit breeders usually contain approximately 18% protein; commercial rabbit and guinea pig mixes vary in protein between 12.5% and 16.5%, and the higher level should be regarded as optimum for young and breeding rabbits.

Free access to good quality grazing can make up a shortfall in the quality of the dry feed. Remember that during the winter the food value and certainly the *vitamin* content in greens that have been standing without growing for months are quite low.

Guinea pigs have a specific requirement for dietary **vitamin C**: animals on free range, especially during the spring, summer and autumn, usually find enough vitamin C in the growing grass but otherwise the diet should be supplemented at the rate of 50 mg per guinea pig per day (more for pregnant and lactating animals). Some guinea pig mixes now contain this vitamin but otherwise it can be given in water, although this poses two possible problems:

- If given in a water bottle, it should be in one with a stainless steel spout, as the soft metal of many drinking bottles will inactivate vitamin C.
- If given in a drinking bowl, remember that vitamin C is inactivated by organic matter—and that guinea pigs are known to deposit their faeces in the bowls.

Some rabbit pellets and mixes contain **coccidiostats** and these should *not* be fed to guinea pigs due to the risks of toxicity. Coccidiosis is not a major problem in guinea-pigs (though it can occur) and coccidiostats tend to reduce the efficiency of the gut, and cause poor growth in young animals.

Handling rabbits. Rabbits can be picked up by the scruff and supported under the rump. If they are then tucked under the arm, so that the eyes are covered, they can be carried safely using only one arm and (usually) without any struggling (Fig. 4.15).

Handling guinea pigs. Guinea pigs can be picked up with a hand around the shoulders. They should also be supported under the rump, especially in the case of large or pregnant animals.

Breeding rabbits. Rabbits are seasonally poly-oestrous and are induced ovulators. They are mated by taking the female (doe) to the male (buck). She is then removed after mating, which takes place almost

CARE OF SMALL MAMMALS				
	Rabbits and Guinea pigs	**Rats and Mice**	**Gerbils and Hamsters***	**Ferrets**
Housing	Hutches or floor pens or outside runs	Cages or mouse/rat houses with opportunity to climb	Cages with deep bedding for tunnelling	As rabbit and guinea pig
Bedding	Newspaper plus sawdust or woodchips and hay/straw	Sawdust, shavings, woodchips, well shredded paper	As rats and mice	As rabbit and guinea pig
	(Avoid synthetic fibres which can wrap around limbs or cause impaction of stomach)			
Diet	Pelleted diets are available for all species but are best supplemented with: Vegetables, fruit, seeds. Some rodents will eat and apparently benefit from live invertebrates Rabbits and guinea pigs need hay			Meat and eggs
Special care	All species should be kept dry in a draught-free environment. A warm area is needed if rabbits, guinea pigs or ferrets are kept out-of-doors. Hygiene is important: cages should be cleaned thoroughly at least once a week.			
Vaccines, medicines	Myxomatosis vaccine may be advisable for rabbits	—	—	Distemper vaccine may be advisable
	Avoid unnecessary use of antimicrobial agents in all species but especially rabbits and rodents			

Fig. 4.14. Small mammal husbandry: a summary.

(a)

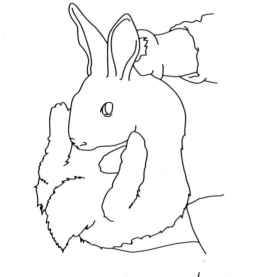

(b)

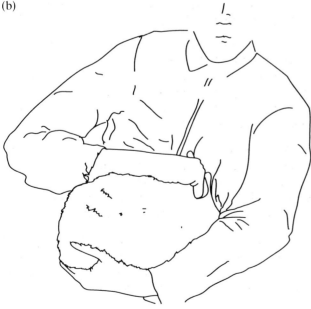

Fig. 4.15. Handling a rabbit: (a) lifting by holding the scruff in one hand and using the other hand to support the body; (b) carrying safely under the arm so that the rabbit's head is covered, leaving one hand free to open doors etc.

immediately. Pregnancy diagnosis by abdominal palpation can be performed at about 14 days. The gestation period is 28–32 days; the larger breeds take longer and have larger litters.

The doe spends very little time with her young, leaving them covered up in the nest and returning only once or twice every 24 hours to feed them. Owners may become anxious at the doe's apparent lack of interest in her litter and have to be reassured that this is normal. In the wild, the young are in danger every time the doe goes to them, possibly showing predators the way to the nest.

Young rabbits may be weaned from 6 weeks of age, preferably by removing the doe. The litter should then be kept together in the familiar surroundings for a further week before they are sold.

Breeding guinea pigs. Guinea pigs have a long gestation period (63 days or more) and give birth to precocious young. Guinea pigs should be bred for the first time before they are a year old, as the large size of the young means that the pubic symphysis must open to allow them to be born. If the sow is too old before her first litter, the symphysis may not open and a caesarian section may be required. The opening of the symphysis indicates that she is likely to give birth within a couple of days.

Note that the age of puberty in the female guinea pig is only 4–5 weeks. The male should be removed in good time so that young females in the litter are not already pregnant by the time they are weaned.

Chinchillas

Husbandry and housing. Chinchillas are native to the Andes mountains in South America but there are very few left in the wild. They were first imported for their skins but are now mainly bred as pets. The wild chinchilla is grey but many other colours have been developed by selective breeding.

Chinchillas are social animals and so are best kept in pairs. Ideally the pairs should be established while the animals are young. Females are more aggressive than males: if adults are to be introduced to one another, they should be kept in adjoining cages for a while and then the female should be introduced into the male's cage.

Although chinchillas can be recommended as pets for older children, they are nocturnal animals and are very agile and active after dark. It is better not to house them in bedrooms where people are trying to sleep. They are normally kept indoors and so do not suffer extremes of cold, but with their very dense coats they are susceptible to heat.

They are usually kept in all-wire cages, which should be as large as possible to allow for plenty of exercise, and should include ledges and branches to climb on and chew and a nest-box for sleeping. They are very destructive animals and all the food and water containers should be of earthenware or metal, as plastic will be chewed.

They keep their fur in order by dust-bathing. A shallow, non-chewable pan of commercial 'chinchilla dust/sand' should be put into the cage each day but should not be left there permanently as the animals tend to use it as a litter tray once they have dust-bathed.

Feeding. A commercial chinchilla pellet contains about 18% protein. The animals must also be given good quality hay; and treats such as apple and carrot are acceptable, as are raisins and the occasional peanut. Too much of any high-fat foods such as peanuts or sunflower seeds may dull the coat and, if given to excess, may lead to fatty changes in the liver.

Handling. Chinchillas should be picked up gently around the shoulders, if necessary using the base of the tail as further support. Breeders who show their animals do not appreciate greasy hands spoiling the fur, and a pair of light cotton gloves, a scarf or a towel can be used when handling such animals.

Breeding. The breeding season is from November to May in the northern hemisphere. The gestation period is 111–114 days and up to three precocious young are born. Owners sometimes ask whether to remove the male or leave him in with the female and the litter. In most cases the male is very caring and protective but may tread on the young accidentally as he runs around the cage, particularly if no nest-box is provided.

Chipmunks

Husbandry and housing. The Siberian chipmunk has become popular as a pet in recent years. Because the animals can become very stressed in the presence of electrical equipment such as televisions, videos and computers, they should be kept out of doors.

They will live outside happily all the year round, as long as they have weatherproof nest-boxes and their enclosure is shaded to protect them from very hot weather. They do not hibernate for long periods but will sleep for short periods during very cold weather, becoming active again on warmer days.

They are usually kept in aviary-like accommodation, built with security in mind and always with a safety door. A weatherproof nest-box stuffed with hay should be provided for each adult, as they prefer not to share sleeping-quarters. They can be kept as a pair or, if the aviary is large enough, as a group although there may be aggression between males or between females, particularly during the breeding season. They usually have two litters a year, in about April and again in August. The young leave the nest-box at about 6 weeks of age but should be left with the parents for at least another 2 weeks.

Feeding. Chipmunks are omnivorous and should be fed a diet that contains meat protein, fresh fruit and vegetables and a seed-and-nut mix. The animal protein can be provided by a complete cat food; the seed-and-nut mix can be a combination of birdseed with a commercial small rodent mix.

Handling. Unless they have been hand-reared, chipmunks are not easy to handle and are best captured using a light net or trapped inside a nest-box and moved with the nest-box. If hospitalisation becomes necessary it should be for the minimum time possible: the veterinary surgery is likely to be a very stressful environment for them.

Small mammals (rats, mice, gerbils and hamsters)

The veterinary nurse is sometimes asked for advice about choosing small mammal pets for children and the following facts are worth bearing in mind:

- Hamsters are nocturnal; gerbils are diurnal; rats and mice are happy to be active at any time.
- All small mammals need to be handled regularly to keep them tame.
- Gerbils, when alarmed, leap in the air—and out of the owner's hands.
- Hamsters and gerbils are easily injured by falling.
- Rats and mice are climbers; they cling on to clothing etc. and are less likely to injure themselves if they fall.
- Rats are probably the quickest learning of the small mammal pets. They are more likely to form attachments to their owners. Fancy rats, handled regularly from weaning, are very unlikely to bite.

Husbandry and housing. Syrian hamsters are solitary by nature. Dwarf hamsters will usually agree to live in a pair if put together when young but it is unwise to attempt to introduce two adults to each other. Gerbils are social animals and live in extended family groups—do not attempt to introduce a non-family gerbil to a group but make up pairs at weaning. Rats and mice are loosely social and very tolerant: two or more female rats or mice will live satisfactorily together; males will tend to fight but sometimes two or more males will live together if there are no females within sight, sound or smell.

Feeding. All these small mammals are omnivores, thriving on a diet containing a proportion of animal-based protein. In the wild, hamsters and gerbils in particular will catch and eat invertebrates, while wild rats and mice will also eat carrion. A comparison of the nutritional content of most commercial 'hamster mixes' with that of a commercial laboratory animal pellet shows how poor the diet is on which these pets live. The diet, and thus their general health, can be improved by giving a daily helping of table scraps plus small pieces of fruit and vegetable.

Handling. Tame hamsters and gerbils can be scooped up into two cupped hands, but be sure to support a gerbil so that it cannot leap away. Gerbils should never be picked up by the tail, as the skin may peel off.

In the case of aggressive small mammals, some authorities recommend scruffing but this can be distressing for the watching owner and is none too easy to accomplish without being bitten. It may also be positively injurious for the Syrian hamster, with its protuberant eyes (the problems are similar, when handling a Pekingese dog). It is best to pick up potentially aggressive small mammals with the aid of a small net or a towel: they can then be manipulated within the towel to expose the part required for examination or injection.

Mice may be picked up around the shoulders, or by the base of the tail, and then placed on a surface such as a rough towel. Pet fancy rats accustomed to being handled may also be picked up round the shoulders (Fig. 4.16(a)); a more anxious handler can put a thumb under the animal's lower jaw to hold the mouth gently closed. Awkward animals are best handled using a towel, after initially taking hold of the base of the tail. Rats may be scruffed to restrain them for injections but being rolled up in a light towel (Fig. 4.16(b)) is less stressful for an animal that is used to only gentle handling at home.

Breeding. Most small mammals can be induced to breed all the year round but in practice they tend to stop breeding during periods of decreasing day length, from late summer to the turn of the year. They all have a post-partum oestrus, which means that if male and female are kept together or have brief contact after parturition the litters may be born every few weeks, depending on the gestation period.

The solitary Syrian hamster female will usually be aggressive towards a male except when she is in oestrus, which occurs every 4 days. When ready to

(a)

(b)

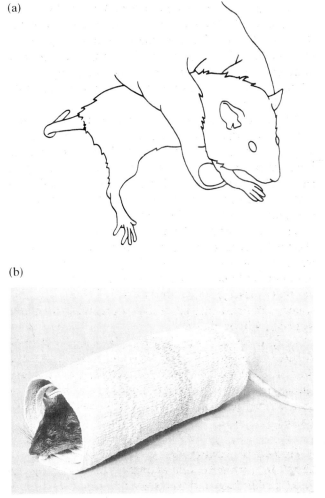

Fig. 4.16. Handling a pet rat: (a) holding by grasping the shoulders; (b) wrapped in a towel while recovering from anaesthesia (in this case, the towel is important in post-anaesthetic nursing care as small animals can quickly become hypothermic, but towel-wrapping is also useful as a restraint for an active rat).

mate she exhibits lordosis (ventral curvature of the lower spine), like most of the small mammals.

The young of most small mammals commonly kept as pets are born naked and blind. Many books, and folklore in general, claim that the young should not be handled for, say, a week after birth because it would induce the mother to eat her young. In practice this depends on such things as the tameness of the mother and her confidence in her usual handler. Many breeders handle young from birth.

Pet owners should be reminded that the mother will require several times as much food as usual while raising a litter, particularly a large litter. The usual diet can be supplemented with dry complete cat or dog foods and baby-weaning foods.

Weaning should not be carried out too early. The young will start to eat solid food some time before they are ready to be weaned. To avoid stress at weaning, the female should be removed and the litter left together in the familiar environment for a few days before being sold or rehoused. In this way they lose their mother, siblings and familiar environment in easy stages rather than all at once.

Ferrets

Housing. For at least two thousand years ferrets have been kept for hunting. Working ferrets are often kept in hutches or in a 'ferret court' which may be an outdoor enclosure with a shelter, or an indoor area in a shed or barn where a number of ferrets live together.

Pet ferrets may live indoors or in a hutch outside. It is important to remember that ferrets are highly active carnivores and supreme escapologists, with an intelligence comparable to that of a cat. All pet ferrets should have regular exercise (mental as well as physical) in a stimulating environment and they have a great capacity for 'play'. Although solitary in the wild, they enjoy company and two or more will usually live together though two males are likely to fight.

Feeding. Working ferrets are often fed on their prey. The ferret's nutritional requirements are similar to those of cats but tinned cat foods tend to produce foul-smelling faeces (complete cat foods make them more acceptable). All ferrets, working or not, enjoy whole carcases occasionally, such as are sold frozen for feeding to snakes and birds of prey. On no account should ferrets be restricted to the traditional diet of bread and milk but milk alone will often be useful to tempt a sick or anorexic ferret to feed.

Handling. Ferrets can be picked up around the shoulders, with a thumb placed under the lower jaw if there is any suspicion that the animal might attempt to bite (Fig. 4.17). Biting is more often through surprise than aggression, and it should also be remembered that ferrets have very poor eyesight but are highly efficient predators: a tentative finger is

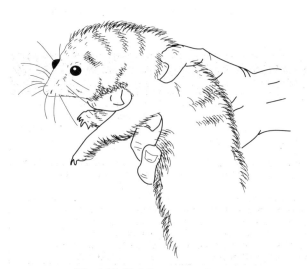

Fig. 4.17. Holding a tame ferret.

assumed to be edible prey. If a ferret does bite, its jaws tend to 'lock' and it can be difficult to remove though there are one or two tricks (including simply letting the animal find its feet if it is dangling in mid-air or immersing the ferret in water).

Breeding. The breeding season for ferrets lasts from spring to autumn in the Northern hemisphere. The testes of the male (hob) are withdrawn into the abdomen during winter and descend into the scrotum at the onset of the breeding season. When the female (jill) comes into season her vulva swells. She is an induced ovulator and is seasonally polyoestrus (like the cat—Chapter 19); if she is not mated she can remain in season until the autumn, which can be dangerous for her and can produce a sometimes fatal anaemia. Unless jills are required for breeding, spaying is recommended or the use of a 'jill jab' as a stimulant probe. Some ferret keepers who want to postpone breeding in a young jill will 'mate' her with a vasectomised hob to take her out of season and into a pseudopregnancy.

Birds

An understanding of the biology and natural history of birds is important if one is to deal adequately with them in captivity and, particularly, to provide them with optimum conditions when they are unwell. Some key points for hospitalised birds are as follows.

- *Birds are easily stressed,* especially by close proximity of people, by loud noises and by violent movements:
  —Reduce close contact by keeping birds some distance from people and other animals. An elevated position for the cage is ideal: most birds like to be in a high commanding position with a good view of their environment. Observe the bird from a distance before approaching it.
  —Further reduce the stress of proximity by covering part of the cage or providing vegetation behind which the bird can hide.
  —Reduce light intensity if a bird is frightened but remember that most birds must be able to see in order to feed.
  —Avoid excess noises, including rattling of keys, banging of doors, barking of dogs. Avoid unnecessary visitors.
- *Birds must feed regularly,* especially if they are small species with a high metabolic rate:
  —Encourage feeding by providing the company of other birds or by offering moving or colourful food items such as mealworms, egg or berries (depending upon species).
  —Acceptability may be enhanced if seeds are soaked before being offered, or if novelties are provided, e.g. teasel head containing seeds.
  —Food and water containers must be the correct shape; for instance, a heron needs a deep water container, not a shallow bowl.

- *Encourage normal behaviour* to promote recovery from illness. For example:
  —Social species will benefit from company.
  —Preening behaviour may be stimulated if the bird's plumage is sprayed.
- *High standards* of hospitalisation facilities promote better care of avian patients. Examples of good features include:
  —Elevated cages.
  —Dimmer switches to alter light intensity.
  —A door that opens inwards (to discourage escapees from coming out) but that also closes naturally.

Choosing birds as pets

A veterinary nurse who is asked to give advice to novice bird-keepers should encourage them in the right direction (for the sake of the birds) with the following suggestions:

- Gain experience by keeping domesticated rather than wild species in the first instance.
- Those who would like a pet parrot but have never kept birds before: start with, perhaps, a pair of hand-reared cockatiels before attempting to keep the larger, non-domesticated species.
- Those who are determined to acquire large parrots as pets: spend a little more and acquire an English-bred, hand-reared parrot rather than an imported, wild-caught bird.
- Bear in mind that each species of large parrot has different inherent characteristics—in exactly the same way that different breeds of dog have different characteristics.
- Consult library books on the subject and talk to experienced bird keepers before deciding to acquire a bird.
- Remember that a parrot might live for 40 or 50 years, or more.
- The young English-bred parrot that is sold just after weaning is a particularly demanding pet; it requires as much of its owner's time as would a new puppy.
- Most birds, and particularly the parrot species, are social and do much better when they have the company of their own species as well as that of humans.

Cages and aviaries

Accommodation for pet birds can be divided into cages and the larger aviaries. In addition some tame birds may be allowed the freedom of the house, a practice that appeals to many people but the bird may damage furniture or other objects and can expose itself to hazards such as electric wires, ovens, poisonous chemicals and perhaps lead pecked from leaded-light windows or old paint.

Cages. The two main groups of cage are the all-wire type or the box cage (with wire at the front but solid sides, roof and back wall). Their features are described in Fig. 4.18.

All-wire cages are acceptable for tame birds but they should always be placed at the side of the room or in a corner, reasonably high up, to give the bird a sense of security. Box cages are more suitable for wild and more nervous species, which feel less stressed when they cannot be viewed from all sides.

In the UK, any cage used for a captive bird (except poultry) should by law be large enough for the bird to stretch both wings fully. There is an exemption for birds that are being transported (e.g. to the surgery) or are under treatment by a veterinary surgeon but this does not necessarily apply to any bird in a veterinary practice or under the care of a non-veterinarian.

Cages for pet birds should be as large as possible, allowing room for parrots to climb and for canaries or finches to have a short flight between perches. Most commercial cages are fitted with ridged, plastic perches, which should be replaced by natural perching in several different diameters for the sake of the bird's feet. Fruit trees (unsprayed) and willows are reliable sources of non-poisonous wood but the branches should be scrubbed to remove any wild-bird droppings before they are placed in the cage.

Food and water receptacles should be placed where the bird can reach them easily (bearing in mind whether the bird normally feeds on or off the ground) but cannot defecate into them. Most parrots, whether large or small, appreciate 'toys' in the form of things to investigate, chew and destroy but there should not be so many toys that there is no room for movement.

Hygiene is most important. Food and water containers should be cleaned daily. Cages should be emptied and thoroughly cleaned at least once a week.

Aviaries. Many people choose to keep birds in aviaries. They may have only one aviary as an

TYPES OF BIRD CAGE	
Box	**Wire**
Open on only one side (front).	Open on all sides, unless covered.
Often made of wood, not easily disinfected, subject to chewing.	Easily disinfected, not likely to be chewed.
Bird usually less easily frightened as it feels secure.	Bird easily frightened unless one or more sides are covered.
If illumination poor, inner recesses of cage may be too dark for feeding and other normal behaviour.	Illumination good: facilitates clinical observation and encourages normal behaviour.
Not liable to draughts but ventilation often poor.	Liable to draughts but ventilation good.

Fig. 4.18. Cage design: box cages and all-wire cages.

ornament in the garden; or they may have a number and be keen aviculturists who try to breed birds in captivity. Most serious aviculturists are well aware of how to build and maintain an aviary but the amateur wishing to have one in the garden may ask for advice at the veterinary practice.

There are two components to an aviary:

- The mesh flight area—open to the air, wind, rain, snow and sun.
- The sheltered area—enclosed (other than an entrance), windproof, warmer, probably with windows to allow some sun to enter.

Each design should suit the intended occupants but the main points to be considered are as follows:

- Is planning permission necessary? In any case, as a courtesy, inform neighbours, and do not keep noisy species if the neighbours are close by or the garden is small.
- Avoid overhanging trees and strong winds.
- Try to position the aviary away from the road where disturbance and theft may prove a problem. Bird theft is big business: keep only low-value species or invest in proper security.
- The smallest viable aviary is about 1.8m × 0.9m (say 6ft × 3ft) but at this size it will be very difficult to keep clean.
- All aviaries should be protected against rats and mice by having deep foundations or a solid concrete base and also suitable wire around the room to exclude the rodents (e.g. $\frac{1}{2}$ inch × $\frac{1}{2}$ inch weld mesh).
- A frost-free shelter should be provided for all but the hardiest species. The shelter should have heat and light for any species likely to suffer during the winter without them.
- Roofing over the flight area will reduce the possibility of disease spreading from wild birds.
- Human entrance to the aviary is likely to be through a door. This should always open inwards (to discourage birds from flying out) and it is wise to have a double-door safety porch to minimise escape. At no time should both doors be open simultaneously.
- Seek advice about stocking densities and compatible species. Usually, only one pair of parrots can be kept in each aviary.
- Large parrot species may require heavy gauge wire to keep them contained (up to 14 or 12g).

Disease control can be a problem in aviaries, especially if they cannot be fully cleaned because of the presence of soil, plants etc. The following routines are important:

- Remove as much faeces, uneaten food, old feathers, soiled leaves and other debris as possible, preferably once a week.
- Ensure that the aviary is well-watered and receives ample sunshine.

- At least twice a year turn over or replace soil and have faeces of birds checked for endoparasites.
- Ensure that aviary birds are kept under careful observation and can easily be caught or isolated if they appear to be unwell.

Handling birds

> All birds, except nocturnal species such as owls, are more easily caught and handled in the dark or in subdued light, which calms them.

Before removing a bird from a cage, always check that no doors or windows are open and no fans are in operation. Always transport birds in a secure box or basket, even over very short distances.

Small cage birds should be caught within their cage with as little chasing about as possible. Quietly remove toys and perches first.

Large birds, and those inclined to bite, can be caught using a towel or gloves—a towel is often preferable as it gives better control and does not restrict the use of the handler's fingers once the bird has been caught. The large parrots should be grasped gently at the base of the skull with one hand, the other being used to support body and legs. A bird that clings to the bars of the cage with beak or feet should be detached gently by an assistant, not just pulled away. Pecking can be discouraged by putting an elastic band over the beak (but remember to remove it!) or by covering the bird's head with a light cloth bag.

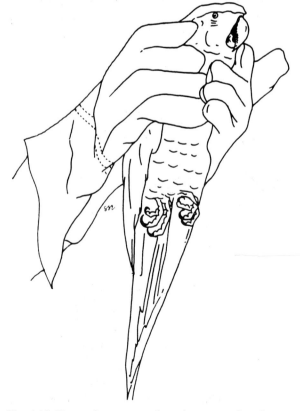

Fig. 4.19. Removing a parrot from its cage, using gloves.

Whatever the species, the aim when handling a bird should be to restrain its wings so that it can neither fly nor flap. Small birds can be held in one hand, with fingers around the neck, while larger birds are best grasped round the body (Figs 4.20 and 4.21).

Most pet birds are tame. This must be distinguished from **imprinting**, whereby a bird that has been hand-reared becomes imprinted upon humans rather than birds of its own species. Such individuals usually make affectionate and trusting pets but may react adversely to other birds and can develop other behavioural problems.

Feeding

The nutrition of birds is an important subject. Many non-specific diseases are due to or are exacerbated by nutritional deficiencies. Birds may be predominantly vegetarian, predominantly carnivorous or omnivorous (taking a mixture of foods). In practical terms several feeding groups of birds are recognised (Fig. 4.22).

In the wild, most birds have seasonal changes in their diet. Typical garden 'seed-eaters' often become almost entirely insectivorous during spring and summer and might enjoy a late summer/autumn glut of fruit before the leaner days of winter. Throughout the world, most birds time their breeding season to coincide with peak food availability to rear their young, be it the onset of warmer weather or the rainy season.

For captive birds, food should be fresh and of good quality and should be replaced regularly. Small birds (e.g. canaries) require ad lib feeding; they may eat 25% or more of their body weight per day. Large birds (e.g. owls) may need feeding only once a day.

All captive birds should have a constant supply of clean drinking-water, though some species (e.g. raptors) will only drink infrequently or during certain periods such as egg-laying.

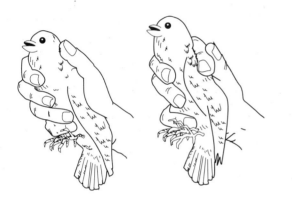

Fig. 4.20. Holding a small bird. Great care must be taken with these delicate animals, and no pressure should be placed on the abdomen.

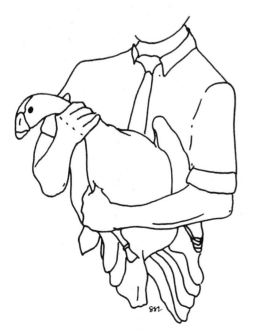

Fig. 4.21. Restraining a large bird: its neck is supported and it is unable to flap its wings.

Seed-eaters (Hardbills). Dry seeds are a convenient way to supply a very basic diet but there are very few birds that eat only dry seeds in the wild. No bird should be fed on dry seeds alone. However, birds that have been fed on one diet for a long time may be very reluctant to change, so that patience and determination are required. As with all animals, diet changes should be introduced gradually.

The veterinary nurse should be aware of the different seed mixes that are available for cage birds and should be able to distinguish between mixes for budgerigars, canaries, parakeets and finches and be able to identify the seeds in them. The different types of seed have different food values, so that birds fed on one mix may be deficient in different nutrients from those fed on another mix.

Basic seed diets for small cage birds may be supplemented with:

- **Soft-foods**—egg-based foods that can be fed all the year round but particularly during the breeding season and moult or during convalescence.
- **Tonic mixes**—seed mixes giving a greater variety and more fat-rich seeds (useful during the winter when the need is for energy to keep warm, but feeding an excess of fat-rich seeds can lead to problems).
- **Greenstuff**—chemical-free weeds and vegetables from the garden increase the level of fat-soluble vitamins in the diet (always deficient in a seed-only diet).
- **Fruit**.
- **Vitamin/mineral supplements**—if the adequacy of the diet is in doubt.
- **Grit and cuttlefish bone**—essential for budgerigars that are not given iodine-supplemented seed; for other birds they can be another way of supplementing minerals in the diet.

FEATURES OF BIRDS AFFECTING FEEDING PREFERENCES			
Group	Predominant food	Characteristic features	Examples
Hardbills	Seed	Strong broad beaks	Finches
Softbills	Fruit and/or insects	Pointed beaks	Thrushes, whydahs
Birds of prey	Dead animals (meat)	Hooked beaks	Falcons, hawks, owls
Nectar-feeding	Nectar, sometimes fruit	Long thin beaks and/or specialised tongues	Sunbirds, hummingbirds, lories, lorikeets

Fig. 4.22. Features of birds affecting feeding preferences.

Softbills. The softbills are birds that feed naturally on 'soft' foods such as insects and fruit, in contrast to the hardbills that have beaks adapted to feeding on grain, seeds and nuts. Softbills commonly kept as pets include the Great Hill Mynah and the Pekin Robin as well as various indigenous aviary species. They are fed on proprietary softbill foods supplemented with fruit, vegetables, cheese, meat, insects etc., according to the natural diet of the species in the wild. Those who care for wild bird casualties sometimes breed suitable insects (such as grasshoppers and maggots) to provide a ready supply of fresh food for softbills.

Parrots and parakeets. Different parrot species are adapted to different habitats in the wild and so have different dietary preferences. None of them eat exclusively dry seeds. Some are nectar feeders (lories and lorikeets) and in captivity they are fed on a variety of commercial and home-made nectar substitutes with the addition of fruit. Most of the large parrots are omnivorous in the wild, eating a mixture of fruit, vegetables and seeds, plus insects and carrion to provide extra protein. A good diet for captive large parrots may include a good-quality parrot mix—but only up to about 20% of the total bulk of the diet. The rest will be made up of fruit, all sorts of vegetables and perhaps meat, dairy produce (yogurt, fromage frais, cheese), brown bread etc. Any bird that is not eating a very mixed diet will need a vitamin/mineral supplement.

Some pet parrots are encouraged to eat whatever the rest of the household is eating and, depending on that household's dietary habits, this can result in a well-nourished parrot. Parrots can be resistant to dietary change but are often willing to try foods if they see someone else enjoying them—either another parrot or the owner.

The birds tend to be wasteful feeders, taking one or two bites from a piece of fruit and then discarding the rest. This is sometimes interpreted by the owner as a dislike of a certain food. To minimise waste, it may be best to cut the food into small pieces before offering it.

Raptors

The diurnal birds of prey and owls are often brought into veterinary practices, perhaps as wild casualties or as birds belonging to falconers (either for hunting or for breeding). Falconry has become increasingly popular and while many people take a great deal of trouble to gain knowledge before acquiring a bird, others do not. Those who do show an interest should be encouraged by the veterinary nurse to go on a reputable falconry course before acquiring their own birds.

Raptors brought into the practice have special requirements that concern legislation as well as general handling and husbandry.

Legal position. In the UK, the Wildlife and Countryside Act 1981 makes it an offence to have in captivity a falconiform bird of prey (hawk, eagle, falcon etc.) unless the bird has been ringed and registered. There is **an exemption for up to 6 weeks** for birds that are under the care of a veterinary surgeon, as long as proper records are kept.

Handling raptors. The general rules of handling are as for other birds but owls are usually quieter in bright light rather than darkness. Gloves will protect the handler; alternatively, the bird can be wrapped in a towel. Falconers' birds are often relatively easy to handle, especially if they wear a hood; advantage can also be taken of their jesses and leash, which can be held or pulled tight.

Falconry birds that come to the surgery on the falconer's fist can be restrained for examination by being 'cast'—catching them by both hands around the body from behind, holding the wings against the body. The bird can then be laid on its sternum, preferably on a towel. Cover the bird's head if it is not already hooded, so that it becomes quieter and more amenable.

Feeding raptors. The majority of birds of prey are wholly carnivorous but the preferred diet depends upon the species. Live food is not needed in captivity. Most species will take butcher's meat, dead mice or dead day-old chicks (hatchery waste) or quail. A regular supply of bone is important as a mineral source, especially for young birds. Feathers, fur and roughage will be regularly regurgitated as a pellet.

Water must be provided but is rarely taken, as the birds obtain moisture from their diet.

Reptiles and Amphibians

Housing

Reptiles and amphibians vary greatly in their requirements but the main features of a captive environment are common to all and involve the following considerations:

- Provide ample *space* for normal behaviour including moving, climbing, swimming as appropriate.
- Ensure that the *type* of environment matches that of the animal in the wild, e.g. damp areas for toads, pieces of bark (or artifical material) under which lizards can hide. Provide choices.
- Have a *temperature gradient* (warmer at one end) so that the animal can select the temperature it favours. The heating element should be attached to a thermostat and monitored with a thermometer (ideally a maximum/minimum thermometer). The vivaria should be maintained at the inhabitant's PBT.
- Although some snakes can cope with poorer *lighting* conditions, lizards and land chelonia require good lighting for activity and foraging. Various fluorescent tubes are made specifically for vivariums and will provide a good daylight spectrum, including some ultraviolet light.
- *Humidity* is important. Powerful heaters tend to dry the atmosphere. Regular water-spraying from a plant mister will maintain a reasonable degree of humidity and this should be done regularly, even for desert species and of course very often for rainforest species.
- *Drinking-water* must be provided, though some species (e.g. chameleons) will only drink drops from moist foliage.
- *Ventilation* is important for maintaining health in the vivarium. If it is poor, it can be improved by introducing an airline powered by a small aquarium pump to encourage the circulation of fresh air, but this should be placed with care so that it does not cause draughts.

Vivariums may be glass aquarium tanks or they may be custom-built, often made from chipboard covered with melamine, the corners sealed with an aquarium sealant. Glass tanks are much harder to maintain at a reasonable temperature and are more difficult to service because the only access is from the top.

The furnishings of a vivarium will vary. Some herpetologists favour a clinically hygienic environment for snakes, with paper on the floor, a hide-box and a climbing branch for arboreal species. Others prefer a more natural design. Common substrates include bark chippings, peat, aquarium gravel and sand; the latter tends to be used only for desert species of lizard but not for snakes as it can cause scale abrasions. Arboreal species should be allowed branches for climbing; burrowing species need sufficient depth of substrate for hiding. All species should have hiding areas or hide-boxes.

Hygiene is essential. Faeces should be removed as soon as possible, along with soiled areas of substrate. This is not easy in the 'natural' type of vivarium and tends to be done infrequently. Hypochlorite is a suitable disinfectant for the stripped-down vivarium, which must then be thoroughly rinsed and dried before being refurnished and its inhabitants returned.

Nutrition

Reptiles range from total herbivores (eating only plants) through omnivores (taking a mixture of plants and animals) to total carnivores (eating only animals). Some general guidelines are given in Fig. 4.23.

Rodent-eating snakes. These include corn snakes, rat snakes and all the commonly kept pythons and boas. They should be fed on whole dead rodents—it is inadvisable in the UK to feed live vertebrate prey as it may make one liable to be prosecuted under the Protection of Animals Act 1911. As a general rule, feed as much food as the snake will take at a sitting

FEEDING REPTILES	
Order	
Order Crocodilia	Crocodiles, alligators and caimans: predominantly carnivorous.
Order Chelonia	Land tortoises: predominantly herbivorous but a number of species (e.g. box turtles) take food of animal origin. Freshwater terrapins: predominantly carnivorous. Marine turtles: predominantly carnivorous.
Order Squamata	Snakes: predominantly carnivorous. Lizards: predominantly carnivorous but a few species (e.g. iguanas) take food of plant origin.
EXAMPLES OF DIETS ARE:	
Species	**Staple diet**
Greek (spur-thighed) tortoise (*Testudo graeca*)	Vegetable material.
Garter snake (*Thamnophis* spp.)	Fish, amphibians, earthworms.

Fig. 4.23. Feeding reptiles.

and then do not feed again until that meal has been digested and faeces passed. Captive-bred snakes are accustomed to feeding on dead prey; wild-caught snakes are sometimes more difficult to feed.

Fish-eating and invertebrate-eating snakes. These include garter snakes and they can be fed on earthworms, small mice and pieces of fish. To destroy thiaminase before being fed, frozen fish such as whitebait should be heat-treated in water at 80°C for 10 minutes.

Insectivorous lizards. These can be fed on commercially produced insects such as crickets and locusts. It is important to dust the insects with a vitamin/mineral supplement first and to feed the correct size of insect for the animal. Lizards fed an unsupplemented diet tend to suffer from vitamin A deficiency and from osteodystrophy caused by the poor Ca:P ratio in insects. Many insectivorous lizards in the wild also consume pollen, nectar and some fruit. Sweet, fruity substitutes should be offered from time to time.

Large omnivorous lizards. Lizards such as green iguanas are mainly insectivorous when young, becoming omnivorous as they grow. Their diet should contain a good amount of animal protein, as well as a good mixture of fruit and vegetables, and should be supplemented with calcium and vitamin D_3.

Basic husbandry

Mediterranean tortoises. Of the two common Mediterranean species, Hermann's tortoise (*Testudo hermanni*) has a horny spur on the end of its tail whereas the spur-thighed or Greek tortoise (*T. graeca*) has a short spur on the caudal aspect of each thigh.

Mediterranean tortoises can spend most of the spring and summer outside, with a shelter to sleep in at night. Indoor heated accommodation should be available for days when it is too cold for the tortoises to be active and feeding out of doors. Some people uses greenhouses (heated or unheated) for this purpose.

Tortoises are herbivorous and the best diet for them is what they can find free-ranging over a large garden. If confined to a small pen, more food will have to be provided. Those that are kept over a period on one patch of ground may suffer from high levels of roundworm infestation and need regular worming.

Male Mediterranean tortoises are most persistent in their pursuit of females (other species are not). Courtship consists of butting the shell of the female and biting at her legs. Confined together in a small pen, a great deal of damage can be done to both animals if the female cannot escape from the male. It is best to keep males and females separate except when mating is required.

Mediterranean tortoises hibernate during the winter (and only those clearly unfit to do so should be kept awake). They should not be offered food for 3–4 weeks prior to hibernation, so that the intestines are empty before the animal becomes torpid. It is very difficult to keep a tortoise awake once day length starts to decrease; to keep it awake and feeding it is necessary to maintain artificial heat and also an artificial day length of 12 hours, with 'daylight' quality lighting.

Hibernation should be in a frost-proof and rodent-proof environment with good ventilation. The choice of insulation (for example hay, leafmould or shredded paper) does not matter as long as the tortoise is well protected. A healthy tortoise can lose up to 1% of its body weight per month in hibernation and anxious owners are known to weigh their pets regularly throughout the winter to monitor health. A sudden drop in weight indicates that something may be amiss and the tortoise should be awoken.

Young tortoises. Since import controls were applied, the average age of pet tortoises in the UK has been increasing steadily but many people now successfully produce hatchling tortoises. However, these enchanting little animals are very difficult to rear. They should be treated as adults as far as possible, i.e. they should graze outside and have access to sunlight, preferably in a cold-frame without its top to provide a draughtproof grazing area. On cold days they can be kept indoors in a vivarium. They should never be overfed: in the wild they would be active for much of the day in search of food, but in captivity they are inevitably less active and need less food to maintain optimum growth rate. Overfeeding and lack of supplementation of the diet lead to gross shell deformities in young tortoises that have grown much too fast.

Young tortoises would hibernate in the wild and should be allowed do so in captivity.

Box 'turtles'. In the past the majority of land tortoises kept in the UK and other European countries were of the Mediterranean species. Large numbers were imported, often under unhygienic and inhumane conditions, and the mortality rate was very high.

Tighter controls on the capture and sale of Mediterranean tortoises has led to other species being imported and finding their way into homes and collections. These include the hinge-backed tortoises, *Kinixys* spp., from Africa and the box 'turtles', *Terrapene* spp., from North America. The veterinary nurse should be familiar with the needs of box turtles (or tortoises), of which there are several species and subspecies, some of the latter being difficult to differentiate. It should be noted that their requirements in captivity are very different from those of the Mediterranean tortoises.

There are two main groups of these American tortoises. The Eastern usually has a uniformly dull brown plastron, sometimes smudged with darker brown; the Western has an intricate pattern of dark brown and yellow stripes on the plastron. The Eastern Box comes from the south-eastern states such as Florida and is adapted to a warm climate with a high relative humidity; the Western comes from the more arid states of New Mexico and Arizona and so prefers a drier climate.

In general box tortoises should be kept all the year round in an indoor vivarium, in a warm environment and moist atmosphere but with good ventilation so that it never becomes stuffy. Species and subspecies vary in their temperature requirements and it is best to provide a temperature gradient of 20–30°C. During the summer, when the temperature is over 21°C, they enjoy being out of doors in a planted enclosure where they have access to water and shade—they do not appreciate being left in the full sun.

The box tortoises are more closely related to freshwater terrapins than to true land tortoises. Most of them are omnivores, although youngsters may be largely carnivorous and some subspecies prefer insects. Many captive box turtles are not given an adequate diet. Only one third of the diet should consist of plant material, and of that 75% should be vegetable and 25% fruit. The remaining two-thirds of the diet should be of animal material and examples of good sources of animal protein include crickets, grasshoppers, slugs, caterpillars, mealworms and sardines. Invertebrate food should be dusted with a calcium supplement to minimise the risk of metabolic bone disease. Small amounts of dog or cat food can be given but large quantities may cause nutritional disorders as they are not formulated for these species.

Most (but not all) box tortoises hibernate in the winter, though some can be kept awake in a warm cage with ample lighting. As with Mediterranean species, only healthy box tortoises should be allowed to hibernate. The optimum conditions for hibernation are a temperature of 7–17°C, a draught-free and rodent-proof box and at least 40cm depth of bedding—dry leaves, good quality hay or shredded paper.

Health care of box turtles is important and follows the general guidelines for captive chelonians. However, these animals can prove difficult to examine if they withdraw their head and all four limbs and close the shell.

Terrapins. The terrapin most commonly seen in captivity in this country is the red-eared terrapin of North America. Hatchlings are sold at 3–5 cm long. The adult male is approximately 17–18 cm long and the female can grow to 28–30 cm.

Young terrapins require a vivarium with heated water and a basking area, with a basking spotlight, to help them dry out and to shed their scutes as they grow. They can be fed on a mixture of trout pellets, complete cat food, meat and fish. The latter should be supplemented with vitamins and minerals before feeding, and frozen fish such as whitebait should be heat-treated (as described for garter snakes). To minimise fouling of the water, it is best not to feed terrapins in their tank but in a separate container.

Large terrapins do well in an outdoor pond during the summer but it should be enclosed so that they cannot escape.

Mature males can be very aggressive and will attack other males (and sometimes females) if they are kept together in a small tank where the subordinate animal cannot escape.

Snakes. The detailed requirements of snakes in captivity depend on the species. The North American group includes corn snakes, rat snakes, garter snakes and king snakes.

- Corn snakes and rat snakes are generally easy to maintain in captivity and easy to handle (particularly the corn snake). Captive-bred young of these rodent-eaters are commonly available and there are several colour mutations in the corn snake.
- Garter snakes are relatively small and are good first snakes for well-informed children. In the wild they live in woodland and by watercourses, eating fish and invertebrates.
- King snakes are more aggressive and they are reptile-eaters in the wild: they should be kept singly in a vivarium. Captive-bred individuals should have been brought up to eat dead mice but the feeding of wild-caught snakes can be a problem.
- Royal (or ball) pythons are the smallest of the larger snakes commonly available and can be very reluctant to feed in captivity if caught in the wild. Veterinary practices often see long-term anorexics and these require lengthy treatment to rehydrate and then force-feed—some never feed voluntarily in captivity.
- Indian (Burmese) pythons grow up to 4m or more; they are strong snakes and, though some remain easy to handle, others can be belligerent. Many of them become too much of a handful for their owners, who offer them to zoos that may be already overstocked. Yet they continue to be bred regularly in captivity and hatchlings are commonly available.
- Boa constrictors do not grow as large as Indian pythons: they have a slimmer build but they still tend to grow too large to be accommodated by the average household. They reproduce well in captivity and a snake that has been handled well when young usually remains amenable as it grows.
- Reticulated pythons grow as large and as strong as Indian pythons and are generally more aggressive.

Small lizards. Most lizards are territorial. There should be only one male of any species in a small vivarium, together with perhaps two or three females. The species generally recommended as a beginner's lizard is the leopard gecko, a nocturnal lizard that has been bred in captivity for many generations and is relatively easy to handle.

Large lizards. The large lizard most commonly kept is the green iguana, often imported as young animals at 30–45 cm long. Many purchasers fail to appreciate that the males can grow to up to 150 cm and that the species requires extensive heated accommodation: they are very demanding in time, space and money. In captivity they rarely reach their full potential size and offer suffer from fibrous osteodystrophy due to an inadequate or poorly balanced diet.

Handling

Snakes. It is assumed that the snakes brought to a veterinary practice are not venomous. Venomous snakes are kept by some herpetologists but usually only under the strict regulations of the Dangerous Wild Animals Act.

All snakes are susceptible to bruising: they should be handled carefully and never held more tightly than necessary. Those that are normally quiet and easy to handle will become upset in a new and possibly threatening environment or as a result of maltreatment during clinical examination, injection or blood-testing.

Small snakes, unless they threaten and strike at the handler, should be lifted gently by a hand under their widest part and then supported as they coil around the arm (Fig. 4.24). Aggressive small snakes can be caught with the aid of a towel or gloves and gently restrained behind the head.

To examine the head and mouth, support the snake just behind its head and then open its mouth (if required) by gently inserting a flat instrument in the labial notch at the front of the mouth. Wooden lolly-sticks and biro-tops have been found useful for this task; there are doubtless many other possibilities.

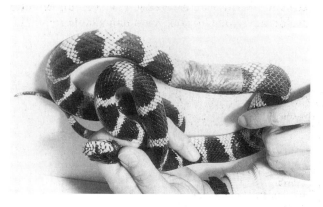

Fig. 4.24. Holding a king snake. This one has an adhesive dressing on a skin lesion, which needs careful nursing to avoid secondary infections.

Large snakes should be handled with care and never draped around the neck. Two or three competent people should be present to help with really large snakes. Those known to be aggressive should be sedated before handling.

Lizards. Small lizards should be picked up round the pectoral girdle. Very small and delicate lizards can be trapped against the side of the vivarium with a soft cloth. Never catch a lizard by its tail: the shedding of the tail is a defence mechanism in many species (but not all) and the tail breaks off cleanly a little way from the body.

Iguanas should be handled with care: they can inflict damage with their teeth, their short claws (particularly on the hind limbs) and their long, lashing tails. It is best to use a towel or gloves, unless they can be grasped briskly in two hands with one hand round the shoulders and one holding the thighs along the side of the tail.

Fish

The health and welfare of fish depend very much upon the quality of the water in which they live. Important features of water quality are:

- Temperature (less oxygen is present at higher temperatures).
- pH (6–8 is the usual range for freshwater species).
- Hardness/salinity (hard water is usually preferable).
- Metallic salts in solution.
- Ammonia and nitrate levels (deaths may occur if high—testing kits are available).
- Bacterial levels.

Aquaria

Aquaria are usually made entirely of glass but ones with frames are still in use. Setting up an aquarium needs planning and patience, and the following points are important:

- Choose a site away from direct sunlight.
- Ensure that the aquarium is properly supported—a tank full of water is heavy. Use pieces of polystyrene under all-glass tanks to minimise uneven pressures.
- Install gravel on floor. It must be several centimetres deep if there is undergravel filtration.
- Add rocks and ornamental structures as necessary.
- Add plants, ensuring that they come from a reputable dealer. Soak in 2ppm potassium permanganate for 48 hours before transfer.
- Let the aquarium settle for 2 weeks before stocking with fish. Some people then add 'cheap fish' to test the water before introducing other species.
- Tropical species need heating, either of the tank or of the whole room.

Feeding and maintenance

Proprietary foods should be the staple diet, supplemented with live food if necessary, but the latter can introduce disease. Various supplements are available and can be useful. Never overfeed: assess how much is being eaten and give slightly less than this, provided once or twice daily.

Maintenance includes:

- Regular observation of the fish and their environment.
- Weekly cleaning (removal) of gross dirt from the bottom of the aquarium plus 10–15% of the water. Dechlorinate tap water before it is added.
- Installing mechanical, biological or chemical filters for large tanks and the more sensitive species.
- Taking prompt action if fish appear unwell or die or if the water changes in appearance.
- Quarantining all incoming fish for at least 2 weeks.

Invertebrates

Invertebrates are increasingly being kept in captivity (Fig. 4.25). Their management differs according to their species, origin, age and other factors, and some examples are given in Fig. 4.26.

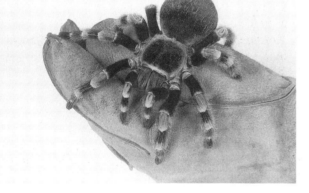

Fig. 4.25. A red-kneed tarantula on the hand. Gloves are not usually necessary but will reduce the risk of irritation from the spider's hairs (setae).

Wildlife

Space does not permit detailed discussion of the care of wildlife. Nevertheless, some basic information is important. Members of the public have traditionally brought wild mammals and birds that are in need of attention to veterinary practices and in recent years there has been an increased interest in work with such casualties.

Wild animals are likely to fall into one or more categories:

- Those that have an infectious or parasitic disease (e.g. tuberculosis, tick infestation).
- Those that have an injury (e.g. a broken wing).
- Those that have been poisoned, intentionally or accidentally.
- Those that have been electrocuted or burnt, e.g. on power-lines or following a fire.
- Those that are oiled or have other chemical damage (see Chapter 3, First Aid).
- Those that are, or appear to be, orphaned.
- Those that have been displaced for some reason, e.g. birds that fly off-course on migration.

There are several questions that should be asked when dealing with a wildlife casualty:

(1) When and where precisely was it found?
(2) What species is it? Some wild animals, particularly certain birds, are covered by special legislation (birds of prey in particular) and steps may need to be taken to register them or to keep appropriate records.
(3) Does the practice have the necessary facilities and staff to deal with the animal? Some species, such as badgers and herons, require a great deal of personal attention whereas others can be tended with a minimum of specialised accommodation or equipment. If the practice cannot cope, is there a wildlife centre that may better be able to assist?

From the outset it is necessary to ascertain whether it is in the animal's best interests to embark on care and treatment—and this can be a hard decision. Many factors have to be taken into consideration, of which the most important are:

MANAGEMENT AND FEEDING OF INVERTEBRATES		
Species	**Management**	**Main food**
Indian stick insect	Well-ventilated containers. Temperate.	Privet leaves.
Giant millipedes	Containers with ample substrate. Tropical.	Dead leaves, fruit, vegetables, waste organic material.
Giant snails	As above. Tropical. High humidity.	Fruit, vegetables. Calcium source.
Red-kneed tarantula	Spacious container with some substrate. Tropical. High humidity.	Insects, other invertebrates.

Fig. 4.26. Management and feeding of invertebrates.

- Is the animal so unwell or so badly injured that it is unlikely to survive and is probably in severe pain?
- Even if the animal is likely to survive, will it be possible to return it to the wild when recovered. (With all wildlife casualties this must be the aim, and is often a legal requirement.)
- If it cannot be rehabilitated in the wild, can it properly be retained in captivity? Will it have a reasonable quality of life?

Although the treatment of wildlife is challenging and stimulating, this must not be allowed to obscure the fact that the kindest approach to some casualties is euthanasia. Heroic surgery, expensive drug therapy and dedicated nursing have their place and will yield successful results in a proportion of cases but others, for a variety of reasons, fail to respond and are probably best humanely killed. Euthanasia is an option at each stage, as indicated in Fig. 4.27.

Assuming that the decision is made to attempt to keep the casualty, the following points are important:

- Keep proper records—species, date of arrival, diagnosis, treatment, outcome.
- Carry out all handling, examination and treatment with care—wild animals are easily stressed.
- Remember that nursing plays a very important part in the care of wild animals. Warmth, fluids and feeding, coupled with attention to wounds and discharges, will often go a long way towards keeping the patient alive and facilitating recovery.
- Getting the animal to eat voluntarily can prove difficult and needs a great deal of patience. Forced feeding may be necessary at first.
- Rehabilitation and release can prove time-consuming, difficult and sometimes impossible. Help can be obtained from people who specialise in wildlife care—for example, those who run the reputable rehabilitation centres.

The British Wildlife Rehabilitation Council publishes a Code of Practice and can give advice (contact through the RSPCA Wildlife Officers at Horsham).

Pain Assesment and Welfare Considerations

An important part of the veterinary nurse's responsibility is to promote the welfare of the animal and to minimise pain and distress. It is best to assume that all animals are capable of feeling pain (the majority, including invertebrates, are certainly capable of *responding* to it) and to give them the benefit of the nurse's skill in practice.

It is helpful to consider this aspect of welfare under three headings: pain, discomfort and distress.

- **Pain** is a physical phenomenon, with which all humans are familiar. We assume that exotic (and native wild) species can also experience pain of different degree (mild, moderate, substantial) and of different duration (acute or chronic).
- **Discomfort** is also a physical phenomenon but is milder than pain and may only be an inconvenience or irritation to the animal—for example, a piece of bandage that has become loose and makes it difficult for the animal to walk or to lie down comfortably.
- **Distress** is a psychological phenomenon and may be associated with pain or discomfort, or can be entirely distinct. It occurs, for example, when a mother is separated from her young, or a social animal is kept alone. These and other 'stressors' can cause 'stress' in the animal.

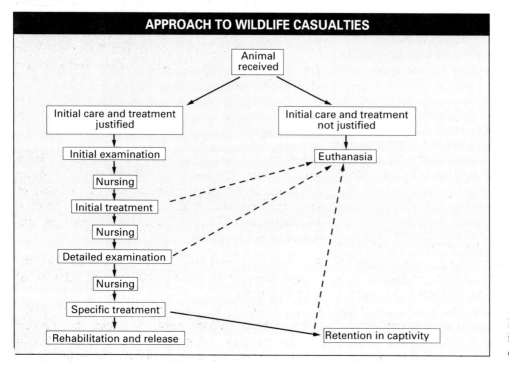

Fig. 4.27. Considerations in dealing with wildlife casualties.

There are many ways in which the nurse can contribute to the relief of pain, distress and discomfort in exotic species. For example:

- Ensure that the animal receives the best possible care in terms of good feeding, handling and general management.
- Provide an environment that is appropriate to both the species and the particular individual.
  - —Animals that like to burrow (such as gerbils) or to hide in a damp place (such as toads) should be permitted to do so.
  - —Social species should not be kept alone.
  - —Species that fight or strongly challenge one another should not be kept together in close confinement.
- Attend promptly to wounds, infections and other problems. Such attention must include supportive care (e.g. cleaning of ocular discharges, and hand-feeding) as well as specific therapy.
- Make appropriate changes to management—e.g. use rubber mats to reduce pain and to minimise further damage to a rabbit with 'sore hocks' or a guinea pig with pododermatitis.
- Administer analgesics to prevent or minimise pain. These can include local analgesics (e.g. lignocaine), systemic analgesics (e.g. buprenorphine) or general anaesthetics that have an analgesic effect (e.g. nitrous oxide).
- Administer other chemotherapeutic agents that, while not themselves analgesic, reduce the risk of further pain or distress (e.g. tranquillisers to prevent an animal from damaging itself in its cage).
- The question of necessary euthanasia must never be overlooked. As with other species, the exotic or wild animal that is in substantial pain which is likely to persist may need to be killed on humanitarian grounds.

The veterinary nurse is likely to ask: 'But how do I know when an unfamiliar species is in pain?' This is a valid question, to which there are three answers: subjectivity, clinical indications and responses.

Subjectivity. Subjectivity is probably a good guide. If under similar circumstances a human would be in pain, assume that the animal is also. Thus, if *any* species is anorexic and lethargic following surgery, consider post-operative pain as one of the likely causes.

Clinical indications. Certain clinical features are now considered to be indicative of pain in laboratory mammals and it is prudent to apply the same criteria to these same species in veterinary practice. Much has been written about pain assessment in laboratory animals in recent years (see Further Reading) and the veterinary nurse can gain from reading these publications and discussing the matter with experienced animal technicians. A scoring system is often used in laboratory animal work and this can be applicable to small mammals in practice.

Clinical features can be common to all species (e.g. anorexia, dehydration, lethargy, weight loss) or may be specific to the type of animal (e.g. failure of rats to groom or a tendency for rabbits to press their heads against the wall of the cage). An observant veterinary nurse will quickly develop the ability to recognise signs that indicate pain, discomfort and distress.

Responses. If in doubt, give the animal appropriate treatment (e.g. an analgesic) and see if there is a response. A ferret, for example, that looks dejected and is reluctant to move or feed following surgery on a broken leg may behave very differently after a subcutaneous injection of buprenorphine.

Common Problems and Diseases

Diseases of exotic species can be infectious or non-infectious. Often there is an overlap and many apparently infectious diseases (e.g. respiratory conditions of rabbits, foot infections of birds) are due to, or precipitated by, poor management or inadequate diet. When taking a history, or discussing a problem with an owner, the veterinary nurse should obtain as much information as possible about the housing, feeding and general management of the patient. Ideally the client's premises should be visited but in a busy practice this is not always practicable. Owners should therefore be encouraged to produce the animal in its own (uncleaned) cage together with samples of uneaten food. It can prove helpful if they also bring a photograph or drawing of the animal at home, in its own environment.

Common problems and diseases are summarised in Figs 4.28–4.30 and are looked at below for different groups of exotic pets. Much useful information on the diseases of small mammals can also be obtained by reference to the literature on laboratory animals.

Zoonoses

Veterinary nurses should be aware of the potential of some exotic animals to carry and/or transmit zoonoses. A zoonosis can be defined as a disease or infection that can be naturally transmitted from a vertebrate animal to a human. Each part of this definition is important:

- A zoonosis need not cause disease in its host: the organism may be present and transmitted without clinical signs.
- The disease or infection must be naturally transmitted. Many organisms can be spread experimentally—by injection, for example—but in that case they are not considered to be zoonoses.

SOME DISEASES OF SMALL MAMMALS

Species	Condition	Clinical signs	Treatment	Comment
All	Skin wounds and abscesses	Skin abrasions and lesions.	Clean with appropriate disinfectant or cleansing agent. Suture where appropriate. Irrigate abscesses.	Wounds may indicate fighting or other management problems. Rabbit abscesses may need to be excised in toto.
	Traumatic injuries	Incoordination, collapse, hyperpnoea, etc.	Warmth, fluids orally and/or by injection. Hand-feeding and nursing.	Some species, e.g. hamsters, are prone to fall off surfaces. Damage may also be caused by poor handling (especially by children), cats, etc.
	Fractures	Locomotor disturbances, swelling, pain, etc.	Euthanasia may be necessary. Limb fractures can be fixed (externally or internally) but in small rodents often heal spontaneously. Nursing.	Vetebral injuries are common in rabbits.
	Dental problems	Excessive salivation ('slobbers'), dysphagia.	Clipping of overgrown teeth. Removal of plaque, attention to inflamed gingivae.	Overgrowth of incisors and cheek teeth (malocclusions) is common in rodents and lagomorphs and may be associated with genetic factors, soft food, lack of wear, etc. Dental abscesses and periodontal disease are prevalent in ferrets.
	Ectoparasites (flea, mite, tick or louse infestation)	Vary from inapparent infection to marked pruritus and skin lesions.	Appropriate parasiticidal treatment of skin (and, in case of fleas, environment).	Skin lesions may also be due to environmental factors, nutritional deficiencies, or behavioural traits (barbering).
	Endoparasites (nematode, cestode, trematode, or protozoan infestation)	Vary from inapparent infection to diarrhoea. Rectal prolapse may be indicative of infestation with the pinworm Syphacia.	Anthelmmintic or antiprotozoal treatment. Various agents can be used orally including mebendazole (10mg/kg), praziquantel (5–10mg/kg) and, for protozoa, sulphonamides or dimetridazole (1mg/ml water).	Diagnosis of endoparasites will depend upon careful examination of faeces or (post mortem) body tissues.
	Respiratory disease	May range from mild respiratory signs, e.g. nasal discharge in rabbits, sneezing in rats, chattering in mice, to dyspnoea. Headtilt, due to labyrinthitis, may be seen.	Antimicrobial agents may be tried. Isolation of affected animals and attention to management (temperature and ventilation) are important.	Difficult, if not impossible, to eliminate from a group or colony of rodents. Many different microorganisms may be involved but the primary pathogen in rodents is usually a virus or Mycoplasma. Secondary bacterial infection is common and may respond to chemotherapy.
	Diarrhoea, enteritis (various types)	Loose faeces, fluid loss, electrolyte imbalance, etc.	Specific therapy plus fluids where appropriate.	Many different causes ranging from changes in diet to bacterial, viral, and parasitic infections. Specific therapy will depend on cause and laboratory investigation of faeces may be necessary. It is wise to check for Salmonella.
Mouse, rat, guinea pig and rabbit	Ringworm	Hair loss, occasionally erythema and pruritus.	Oral griseofulvin (25mg/kg) for 4 to 5 weeks.	Differential diagnosis in the rabbit includes plucking of hair for nest-building.
Mouse and rat	Mammary tumours	Swollen, usually hard, mammary glands.	Surgical removal.	Often malignant, especially in rats. May be confused with mastitis.
Mouse and rat	'Ringtail'	Raised, corrugated (usually hyperkeratinized) lesions on tail.	Raise relative humidity. Lesions which become infected can be treated topically.	'Ringtail' and certain other non-specific skin lesions are associated with a low relative humidity (<40%).
Mouse, rat, golden hamster, jird and guinea pig (occasionally rabbit)	Tyzzer's disease (Bacillus piliformis infection).	Diarrhoea, loss of condition, death.	Rarely successful. Tetracylines may be tried. Improve management.	Stressors may be responsible for onset of disease.

Fig. 4.28.—continued ♦

SOME DISEASES OF SMALL MAMMALS

Species	Condition	Clinical signs	Treatment	Comment
Golden hamster	Impacted cheek pouch.	Swollen side(s) to face.	Remove impaction manually or by irrigation with saline.	Often caused by artificial foods, e.g. sweets, pellets.
	'Wet tail' (proliferative ileitis)	Diarrhoea and perianal excoriation, especially in newly weaned animals.	Rarely successful. Fluids by mouth or injection. Oral neomycin, kaolin preparations, etc. Nursing.	Cause uncertain, possibly a form of colibacillosis. Often precipitated by stressors, e.g. change of diet or overcrowding. A similar condition may be seen in jirds but is probably not identical.
Jird	'Fits' (epileptiform seizures)	Convulsions, lasting for 10 to 90 s.	None necessary. Animal should be returned to cage and not disturbed.	Cause and significance are uncertain. Often precipitated by stressors, e.g. handling.
	Sebaceous gland disorders	Swollen gland on ventral surface of abdomen.	If inflamed and/or infected use topical antimicrobial agent and/or corticosteroid. If neoplastic—surgical removal.	
Guinea pig	Alopecia	Hair loss, usually without pruritus.	Change of environment. Improved diet (including addition of vitamin C and hay).	Cause often uncertain. Common in female animals during pregnancy.
	Scurvy (vitamin C deficiency)	Lethargy, swollen joints, weight loss, death. Often predisposes to infectious or parasitic disease.	Vitamin C orally (50 – 100mg/day per animal).	May occur even if diet contains vitamin C since deterioration of the latter can be rapid, especially at high temperatures.
	Pregnancy toxaemia	Depression and anorexia during last 1 to 2 weeks of pregnancy or immediately after parturition.	Corticosteroids by injection. Dextrose by mouth or injection. Avoidance of stress.	Probably associated with heavy and long pregnancy, and obesity. Often only diagnosed post mortem.
Guinea pig and rabbit	Pseudotuberculosis (*Yersinia* infection)	Diarrhoea, weight loss, enlarged mesenteric lymph nodes, death.	Rarely practicable or wise. Culling and disinfection are preferable.	Infection may be introduced by other animals (including wild birds and rodents) or contaminated greenfood.
Rabbit	Ear canker (*Psoroptes cuniculi* infestation)	Inflammation of external ear canal: pruritus and self-inflicted damage.	Soften exudate with liquid paraffin prior to cleaning and application of ear drops, for 5 days.	Regular inspection of rabbit's ears will enable early infestation to be detected. In severe cases light anaesthesia will facilitate cleaning.
	Sore hocks	Hair loss, swelling, ulceration and/or infection of hock(s).	Treat wounds. Provide soft bedding.	Often follows trauma or prolonged periods on hard floor.
	Hairball (gastric)	Anorexia, dehydration, sometimes diarrhoea. Hairball may be palpable.	Liquid paraffin by mouth coupled with manual massage to break up hairball. Surgery may be necessary.	Usually follows self-grooming and this may be due to boredom. Particularly prevalent in long haired breeds, e.g. Angora.
	Hepatic coccidiosis (*Eimeria stiedae* infestation)	Weight loss, anorexia, occasionally diarrhoea. Liver may be enlarged.	Oral sulphonamides (e.g. 0.2% sulphadimidine or 0.3% sulphaquinoxaline) in water for five days.	May be present in subclinical form—oocysts detectable in faeces. In severe clinical cases chronic hepatic damage may persist after treatment.
	Enteritis complex	Depression, diarrhoea, fluid intestinal contents, dehydration, mainly in recently weaned animals (5 to 10 weeks old).	Food with high fibre content, e.g. hay. Nursing and supportive care. Antimicrobial agents may be helpful.	Cause uncertain—probably multifactorial and associated with bacteria and change of diet. Differential diagnoses include coccidiosis and diarrhoea following a change in diet.
	Myxomatosis	Conjunctivitis, blepharitis, subcutaneous swellings. Anorexia, depression, death.	None specific. Nursing and supportive care, including hand-feeding.	Vaccination can be used prophylactically. Control of the vector – the rabbit flea (*Spilopsyllus cuniculi*) – is also important.

Fig. 4.28.—continued ▶

SOME DISEASES OF SMALL MAMMALS				
Species	**Condition**	**Clinical signs**	**Treatment**	**Comment**
Ferret	Persistent oestrus	Swollen, sometimes abraded, vulva. May be severe—depression, anorexia, pale mucous membranes, death.	Termination of oestrus by stimulation of vagina, mating (entire or vasectomised male) or hormonal therapy, e.g. proligestone 0.5ml sc. Ovariohysterectomy and/or blood transfusions in severe cases.	The mild syndrome is common but the more severe condition (oestrus-associated bone marrow depression) has only once been reported in Britain.
	Canine distemper	Respiratory signs, conjunctivitis, diarrhoea, neurological signs, death.	None specific. Nursing and symptomatic treatment.	Vaccination can be used prophylactically.

Fig. 4.28. Some diseases of small mammals.

- Only vertebrate animals can be sources of a zoonosis. An organism transmitted from an invertebrate, such as a mosquito or tick, with no involvement of another animal (mammal, bird, reptile, amphibian or fish) is not zoonotic.

Some zoonotic diseases are common to a wide range of species: bacteria of the genus *Salmonella*, for example, can be acquired from animals ranging from ferrets to frogs. Others are more specific: for example, the virus of lymphocytic choriomeningitis (LCM) is only likely to be contracted from rodents. Animals with zoonotic infections need not show clinical signs of disease, since they may either be incubating the disease or carrying the organisms asymptomatically, and therefore the veterinary nurse's approach to zoonoses must be based upon other factors:

- *Awareness* that such infections exist and that apparently healthy animals may transmit them.
- *Reducing unnecessary exposure* to animals that may be a source of zoonoses. This may involve not handling an animal unnecessarily; or ensuring that, when it is handled, it is unlikely to bite or scratch or to contaminate wounds.
- *Practising good hygiene* so that infections are less likely to spread. Hand-washing, protective clothing and other standard safeguards are usually adequate.
- *Taking prophylactic action* where this is available. For example, all veterinary nurses should be immunised against tetanus and those who come into contact with zoo animals or captive primates should consider rabies and hepatitis vaccinations.

Common Problems in Pet Mammals

Rabbits

- Overgrown claws.
- Malocclusion of front and cheek teeth—the teeth are not properly worn down, resulting in spikes and grossly overlong teeth that may require clipping or filing.

- External parasites—*Psoroptes cuniculi*, the rabbit ear mite, and *Cheyletiella parasitivorax*, the fur mite.
- Internal parasites—including roundworms (*Passalurus ambiguus.*)
- Coccidiosis—most commonly seen in litters reared in unhygienic conditions. Signs are diarrhoea, poor growth, weight loss. Hepatic coccidiosis may be seen in adults.
- Abscesses—usually round the head, sometimes associated with tooth-root infection.
- Gastrointestinal problems—anorexia; diarrhoea; faeces matted round the anus (possibly if rabbit fails to eat its 'night faeces' because it is too obese to reach its anus); furballs; gastric dilatation (an emergency). Rabbits that have been anorexic and had gastrointestinal upset can often be tempted to eat with fresh, coarse greenstuff such as long grass, raspberry or dandelion leaves.
- 'Snuffles'—purulent nasal discharge or pneumonia. Most pet rabbits develop some lung damage during their lives. The incidence of respiratory disease increases in poorly ventilated or too warm an environment.
- Myxomatosis—viral disease still widespread in the wild population, carried by the rabbit flea, which can reach pet rabbits via a cat or dog passing through the garden. Vaccination is recommended for all pet rabbits.
- Traumatic injuries—falls, attacks by dogs/cats. Rabbits have very powerful hindlegs and a sudden leap in fear can result in spinal injury.

Many rabbits bought as pets for young children end up unhandled and largely ignored because of the development of behavioural problems, usually related to the onset of sexual maturity. Males often become aggressive and may bite or urine-spray; females will bite and stamp in defence of their 'nest-burrow'. Neutering of both sexes is recommended: it will avoid these problems and will also reduce the incidence of uterine adenocarcinoma, a major cause of death in female rabbits.

Guinea pigs

In the case of any sick guinea pig, ascertain the likely vitamin C status—low dietary levels are likely to hamper recovery from skin and other diseases.

- Malocclusion—occurs but probably less commonly than in rabbits. Salivation may be a sign commonly called 'slobbers'.
- Skin disease—may be caused by sarcoptic mange mite (*Trixacarus caviae*) and less frequently by ringworm. Lice are also sometimes seen. Poor hutch hygiene may lead to pododermatitis (sore feet). Hair loss may be due to 'barbering' by other guinea pigs.
- Nutritional disease—guinea pigs may 'barber' (chew) each other's hair if there is insufficient roughage in the diet. Vitamin C deficiency shows in young animals as poor growth, reluctance to move, swollen joints; skin wounds take a long time to heal.
- Diarrhoea—a number of causes.
- Impaction of the anus—quite common, particularly in males. Faeces may be normal or softer than usual and accumulate just inside the anus.
- Cystic and urethral calculi—not uncommon in guinea pigs.
- Respiratory disease—common in guinea pigs.
- Pregnancy toxaemia—quite common in the last 2 weeks of pregnancy; more likely in obese or stressed animals. The disease tends to have a rapid course. Sometimes the animal is found dead by the owner.

Chinchilla

Common problems include malocclusion ('slobbers'), abdominal pain (often gastric dilatation), fur-chewing (where not enough hay is supplied) and, less commonly, ringworm.

Rats, mice, gerbils and hamsters

- Malocclusion may be occur in all the small pet mammals.
- Respiratory disease—all are susceptible and they may catch disease from owners with sore throats and colds.
- Parasitic diseases—including various mange mites (*Demodex* species in hamsters, commonly *Notoedres* in mice and rats).
- Nutritional disease—more likely to be subclinical than an obvious nutrient deficiency, but a great many clinical problems in small mammal pets can be helped by improving the diet. Animals allowed unlimited sunflower seeds may suffer from osteodystrophy.
- Impacted pouches—all species of hamster may suffer; the pouches may become impacted with either food or unsuitable bedding material (such as cotton wool).
- Traumatic injuries—not uncommon in the small pets (they may be dropped accidentally). The protruding eyes of Syrian hamsters are sometimes damaged and often require enucleation.
- 'Wet tail' disease in hamsters—seen in young, recently weaned animals which develop diarrhoea and quickly become dehydrated; often fatal. If the hamster was recently acquired, owners should not purchase a replacement from the same source.

Many small mammal pets develop behavioural problems, especially as a result of living in an inadequate unstimulating environment—often both too small and inadequately furnished. Gerbils without much to dig in will scrabble obsessively at one corner of the cage. Some will eat too much or drink too much or gnaw at the bars if there is nothing better to chew. Others exhibit stereotypic behaviour, performing a series of actions over and over again. Chipmunks kept in small cages indoors often repeatedly somersault in one corner of the cage.

Ferrets

The most common problems in ferrets are fleas, abscesses (which require veterinary attention) and endoparasites. They can also suffer from distemper (vaccination may be recommended if the disease is locally prevalent) and can catch colds or influenza from humans. Owners might also require advice about oestrus control, spaying, vasectomy and castration.

Common Problems in Birds

Nutrition and environment

General poor health in birds is often associated with the accomodation provided and poor nutrition. Only with experience can the distinction be made between a really healthy, fit and active bird with glossy plumage and one that is surviving but in suboptimal health. However, there are certain specific deficiencies:

- Iodine deficiency—common in budgerigars, often presents as respiratory distress caused by pressure of the enlarged thyroid gland on the trachea.
- Vitamin A deficiency—very common in all cage-birds, particularly those that have little fruit or vegetable in their diet. Clinical signs may be those of mild to moderate upper respiratory disease, with swellings around the eyes, nasal discharge and blocked nostrils. More severe cases have small abscesses on the palate.
- Calcium deficiency—may occur in any species but is a particular problem in African grey parrots. Initially inactivity, drooping wings and general

SOME DISEASES OF BIRDS

Condition	Clinical signs	Diagnosis	Treatment	Comment
Skin wounds	Skin abrasions and lesions, bleeding.	Observation and examination.	Clean with appropriate disinfectant. Control haemorrhage. Suture where appropriate.	Wounds may indicate poor cage design, pecking by other birds, or predation (e.g. by cats). See also Abscesses.
Traumatic injuries	Incoordination, collapse, hyperpnoea, etc.	Examination.	Warmth. Fluids. Hand-feeding and nursing. Attention to wounds.	As above.
Fractures	Lameness, drooping wing, swelling, pain etc.	Examination.	External (splints, taping, plaster) or internal (pinning, wiring, plating) fixation. Nursing.	Callus formation is rapid in small birds and fixation may not be necessary after 14–21 days.
Feather conditions (various)	Feather loss or damage. Irregular or abnormal moult.	Observation, examination of feathers.	Depends on cause. If parasites present parasiticidal treatment. If no parasites detected improve diet, change environment, provide company and/or a mate. Some cases are due to hormonal imbalance and may respond to thyroxine or testosterone.	A complex and often frustrating group of diseases.
'Scaly leg' and 'scaly face' (Cnemidocoptes infestation)	Raised keratinous lesions on feet and/or cere.	Observation. Examination of crusts for parasites.	Painting with liquid parafin to soften scabs, followed (if necessary) by weekly painting of affected areas with 10% benzyl benzoate or 5% piperonyl butoxide.	Deformity of the beak may be a sequel to 'scaly face'. Ivermectin may be effective against the mites.
'Bumblefoot' (usually S. aureus infection of foot)	Swollen, painful foot or digit.	Observation. Examination. Aspiration of pus and bacteriology.	Lancing, removal of pus and irrigation. Dressing of foot. Improved hygiene of perches.	Differential diagnosis can include visceral gout (see below), and traumatic injuries.
Articular gout	Swollen, painful joint(s).	Observation. Aspiration of urates.	None, other than removal of urate deposits. Improve renal function by ensuring adequate water intake.	Aetiology uncertain. May be associated with renal damage. Urates are deposited in joints and, in some cases (visceral gout), on the serosae of internal organs.
Skin tumours	External swellings.	Examination. Aspiration for cytology, or biopsy for histopathology.	Surgical removal.	May be lipomas, fibromas, adenomas, or malignant equivalents. Differential diagnosis includes haematomas, feather cysts (see below) and abscesses (see below).
Abscesses	External swellings.	Examination. Aspiration for bacteriology and cytology.	Surgical removal or lancing and irrigation.	Pus is usually caseous. Differential diagnosis includes haematomas, neoplasia (see above) and feather cysts (see below).
'Feather cysts' (hypopteronosis cystica)	External swellings, especially on wings.	Incision or excision to demonstrate whorls of keratin.	Surgical removal.	Particularly prevalent in certain strains of canary. May be a genetic predisposition.
Regurgitation	Food is regurgitated. In crop necrosis bird is unwell with fluid around beak and, sometimes, diarrhoea.	Eliminate 'normal' regurgitation (see Comment). Swab of crop for bacteriology and mycology (Candida).	Nursing. Fluids. Clavulanate-potentiated amoxycillin 12.5 mg/kg orally and/or nystatin orally. Vitamin B supplementation.	Male budgerigars regurgitate food as part of courtship and may do this in captivity, even when kept alone. Crop necrosis is an infectious condition, possibly secondary to a nutritional deficiency or overuse of antibiotics.
Sinusitis	Swollen periorbital region.	Observation and examination. Swabs for bacteriology.	Parenteral antibiotics. Change of environment. In severe or intractable cases surgical drainage and irrigation of sinuses.	Probably part of an upper respiratory disease sydrome, possibly precipitated or exacerbated by adverse temperature/relative humidity or prolonged exposure to smoke.

SOME DISEASES OF BIRDS

Condition	Clinical signs	Diagnosis	Treatment	Comment
Ectoparasites	May be none. Feather loss or damage, pruritus, anaemia.	Observation. Examination of birds and cage/aviary for evidence of parasites.	Pyrethrum-based powders or sprays. Dichlorvos strip in birdroom.	In cases of mite infestation treat environment as well as bird. *See also* 'Scaly leg' and 'Scaly face' and Feather conditions.
Endoparasites	May be none. Loss of weight or condition, lethargy, anorexia, diarrhoea.	Examination of bird and laboratory investigation of faeces and/or buccal/crop smears.	Depends on parasite. Nematodes treated with levamisole 10mg/kg orally or febendazole 100mg/kg orally. Do not use latter in pigeons.	Some parasites e.g. *Capillaria* may infest upper alimentary tract. High burdens of ascarids can block intestine.
Enteritis	Diarrhoea, loss of weight and condition.	Observation and examination. Investigation of faeces may or may not prove helpful.	Depends upon cause. Change of diet and/or oral antibiotics or sulphonamides (coupled with fluids and nursing) may be beneficial.	'Enteritis' is a general term and probably refers to many conditions. Normal droppings consist of two portions – white urates and brown/black/dark green faeces. Very green faeces are usually indicative of reduced food intake and excess bile production.
Repiratory disease	Noisy, difficult or exaggerated breathing. 'Clicking' or other sounds. Nasal or ocular discharge. Swollen sinuses.	Observation and examination. Laboratory investigation.	Depends upon cause. Antibiotics or sulphonamides – preferably by injection. Supportive care.	There is a whole range of respiratory diseases. Many are due to or associated with bacteria but fungi and mites may also be involved. Psittacosis (chlamydiosis) must always be considered: laboratory investigations (blood and faeces) will confirm. *See also* Sinusitis.
Poisoning	Usually found dead but may be collapse, diarrhoea, dyspnoea etc.	Examination of bird and surroundings. Laboratory investigations.	Depends upon cause. Generally similar to treatment in domesticated species. Supportive therapy of prime importance.	Important causes of poisoning in birds include carbon monoxide (car exhaust), polymer fumes (non-stick cooking utensils), pesticides and lead.
Egg binding	Abdominal distension, straining, collapse. Prolapse of oviduct or cloaca may follow.	Observation and examination.	Immediate warmth (30°–32°C), calcium borogluconate intramuscularly, manual removal. Surgery. Drainage of egg with syringe.	A relatively common condition. Many cases respond to warmth alone.
Dropsy	Swollen abdomen.	Observation and examination. Radiography, laparoscopy, laboratory examination of fluid aspirate.	Depends on cause. Internal tumours may be operable. Infectious conditions treatable with antimicrobial agents. Ascites can be treated temporarily by paracentesis. Constipation will respond to liquid paraffin.	A variety of causes. Differential diagnosis includes 'egg binding' (*see above*) and obesity.
'Going light'	Chronic loss of weight and condition, sometimes diarrhoea, often fatal.	Examination of bird and aviculturist's records.	Improved nutrition and supportive care may help.	A term used by aviculturists. The condition is recognised in several species of bird but the aetiologies may differ.

Fig. 4.29. Some diseases seen in birds.

discomfort, progressing in severe cases to fits. Also seen in birds that have been laying constantly over a period.
- 'Stuck in the moult'—a state of constant moulting. Birds normally moult in response to decreasing day length at the end of the summer but some indoor birds moult constantly under the influence of artificial lighting. There may be a nutritional factor as well; increasing the protein content of the diet has helped in some cases.

Infectious and parasitic disease

- Roundworm infestation—common in aviary birds, particularly ground-feeding grass parakeets. Birds should be wormed twice a year, before the breeding season starts in spring and after the moult in the autumn.
- Trichomoniasis—commonly transmitted to aviary birds (usually budgerigars) via the faeces of wild birds, especially pigeons. It is caused by a protozoon that infects the upper part of the digestive tract, particularly the oesophagus and crop, resulting in inappetence and regurgitation.
- Salmonellosis—not uncommonly diagnosed in birds showing gastrointestinal signs. The serotypes isolated may or may not be those that commonly cause disease in humans.

The two major infectious diseases in birds are psittacosis and PBFD. **Psittacosis** is caused by a chlamydia and may produce either respiratory or gastrointestinal signs. Suspect birds should be isolated. Remember also that there is a danger to human health: the disease is spread in dry faeces. Nurses caring for such birds should wear gloves and mask, and should dampen the paper at the bottom of the bird's cage before moving it (to minimise the spread of the spores). The disease can be treated but in many cases pet birds that are confirmed carriers are euthanased because of the risk to human health.

Psittacine beak and feather disease (dystrophy) (PBFD), a viral disease affecting the integument, is seen in many different species but most commonly in cockatoos. Birds often present as 'feather pluckers': in severe cases the birds have very few feathers and those that remain are broken and greasy-looking, while the horn of the beak is soft and crumbly. Affected birds eventually die of the effects of secondary bacterial and fungal infection of the damaged skin and feathers. This is a very infectious disease and could pose a serious threat in a breeding colony of rare or valuable parrots.

Reproductive disorders

Persistent egg-laying may occur in any species but is particularly common in cockatiels. In the wild, birds continue to lay until they have a full clutch. If an owner removes unfertilised eggs from a captive bird, it will persistantly lay more and will suffer severe depletion of stored calcium and protein. If a bird is 'broody' (wishing to lay eggs and then sit on them), it is far better that the owner should give her a nest-tray or box and allow her to sit, not removing the eggs until she has finished with them after a couple of weeks of fruitless incubation.

Egg-binding may occur with a first egg, or after a period of egg-laying. The bird may collapse and become anorexic: it will need supportive therapy as well as specific treatment to remove the egg.

Tumours and lumps

Tumours are common in pet budgerigars. Lipomas occur over the breast in obese pet birds and tumours may also affect internal organs, particularly the gonads. This can result in pressure on the sciatic nerve, causing difficulty in perching. Feather lumps, or feather cysts, are particularly common in canaries. They are caused by deformities of a feather follicle, which eventually forms a large mass.

Behavioural problems

Behavioural problems are particularly common in the larger pet birds. They include:

- Feather plucking.
- Nail chewing.
- Self-mutilation.
- Excessive screaming.

Stress-inducing factors that may contribute to such problems include:

- Poor diet.
- Boredom.
- Lack of companionship (bird or human).
- Lack of privacy.
- Sexual frustration (or wishing to breed).
- Lack of sleep (parrots need 8–10 hours of undisturbed sleep at night to remain healthy).
- Hot, dry atmosphere (often made worse by cigarette smoke or fumes). Rainforest species in particular prefer a high relative humidity.

Common Problems in Reptiles and Amphibians

Failure to feed (in an otherwise healthy animal) may be because of an inadequate environment (temperature too low, poor lighting) or unsuitable food (a wild-caught snake may not recognise a dead white mouse as food).

Failure to slough (shed the skin) may occur in any reptile but is most important in snakes. When a snake is ready to shed, the skin goes dull, the eyes appear milky and the animal will not feed. Sometimes the failure to shed is total but more often parts of the shed remain on the snake, including the eyelids or the tip of the tail. It is important that these are removed, and with great care, particularly the 'spectacles' over the eyes.

Other problems include:

- Stomatitis (mouth rot)—infection within the mouth. This is common in snakes and also in debilitated tortoises (particularly after hibernation).
- Scale rot—common in snakes. Predisposing factors may be too low a temperature, or too moist a vivarium so that the snake cannot dry out after being in water.

- Regurgitation of food—occurs for a number of reasons: the temperature in the vivarium may be too low for digestion; the snake may be suffering from endoparasites; and some snakes will regurgitate if they are handled too soon after feeding.

- Hypovitaminosis A—not uncommon in lizards and chelonia. The signs include swelling of the eyes, epiphora and unwillingness to feed. Hypervitaminosis A can also occur, usually as a result of over-supplementation, and causes skin lesions (commonly in chelonia a moist dermatitis).

SOME DISEASES OF LOWER VERTEBRATES

Species	Condition	Clinical signs	Treatment	Comment
All (Reptiles, amphibians and fish)	Skin wounds and abscesses	Skin abrasions and lesions.	Clean with suitable disinfectant. Suture where appropriate. Drain abscesses or remove surgically.	Abscesses are best removed *in toto*. Amphibians and many fish can be kept in a 0.6% salt solution to encourage healing. All lower vertebrates must be handled and transported with care to minimize risk of trauma.
	Traumatic injuries	Incoordination, collapse. External lesions, haemorrhage.	Optimum temperature. Fluids by sc, iv or ip injection. Hand-feeding and nursing.	
	External parasites	See individual groups.	See individual groups.	See individual groups.
	Hypothermia	Lethargy, anorexia. Colour changes.	Slowly raise temperature to PBT.	Species vary in requirements—see text.
	Bacterial septicaemia	Sudden death. Severe incoordination. Haemorrhage. Ascites. May be associated skin lesions.	Isolation. Antibiotics. Hygienic precautions to reduce spread.	Gram-negative bacteria usually involved—especially *Aeromonas* spp.
	Obesity	Increase in weight. Sometimes sudden death. Occasionally jaundice.	Reduction of food intake. Increased exercise.	Common in captive animals. Often diagnosed *postmortem*—fatty change in liver, kidneys etc.
Reptiles and amphibians	Fractures	Locomotory disturbances, swelling, pain etc.	External or internal fixation. Dietary changes; some fractures in small species will heal spontaneously.	Keeping an amphibian in shallow water will help to reduce pressure on limbs and facilitate healing. Fractures are often due to a nutritional deficiency (usually calcium).
	Endoparasites	Vary. Often diarrhoea. May be loss of condition and anorexia.	Depends on cause. Anthelmintics. Antiprotozoals. Fluids. Hygiene.	Laboratory examination of faeces necessary for diagnosis. Fresh wet preparations for demonstration of protozoa—e.g., ciliates, entamoebae.
	Inanition	Loss of weight and condition. Anorexia.	Control of parasites. Attention to other diseases. Correction of environment. Tube feeding.	A common problem in captive reptiles and amphibians but not so prevalent in fish (see 'Obesity'). Assess condition of tortoise by Jackson ratio
	Maladaptation syndrome	Loss of weight and condition. Anorexia. Difficulty in sloughing. Skin lesions etc.	As above. Attention to skin lesions and other secondary signs.	Common in captive animals. Cause often not clear, frequently multifactorial. Some species and some individuals particularly prone to maladaptation—possibly not suited to captivity.
	Dermatitis	Skin lesions. Various: often proliferative in reptiles, ulcerative in amphibians.	Depends on cause. Topical or systemic antibiotics. Antifungal agents. Excision may be advisable.	Biopsies and/or swabs can be helpful in diagnosis. Papillomatous lesions in certain lizards may be viral in actiology. Lesions in amphibians are often due to fungus.
	Dysecdysis	Difficulty in sloughing or abnormal frequency.	Attention to environment. Soaking of reptiles will facilitate sloughing.	Underlying hormonal disturbances may also be involved.
Amphibians and fish	'Fungus' (*Saprolegnia* infection)	Distinct fungal growth (like cotton wool) on body surface.	Treat underlying factors. Topical therapy with povidone iodine or malachite green	Usually secondary to other factors—e.g., skin lesions, poor water quality.
	Leech infestation	Leeches visible. Anaemia. Secondary infection.	Sodium chloride baths.	Often introduced with live food or vegetation.
	'White spot' (*Ichthyophthirius*) infection	Pinhead size white foci on skin.	Proprietary treatment—usually malachite green.	Parasites can complete lifecycles rapidly in warm water. Often fatal if untreated.

Fig. 4.30.—continued ◆

SOME DISEASES OF LOWER VERTEBRATES

Species	Condition	Clinical signs	Treatment	Comment
Fish	'Fin rot'	Damaged and necrotic fins and tail.	Depends on cause but attention to water quality essential. Antibiotics. Parasiticides.	Envoirmental factors often responsible. Saprolegnia may supervene (see above). Detection of gill parasites may prove difficult in life fish. Skin parasites can lead to ulceration and bacterial septicaemia (see earlier). Common causes are Mycobacterium marinum and M. fortuitum. Zoonotic. Often only confirmed after death but skin (and other) biopsies may permit ante morten diagnosis.
	External parasites: Protozoa, Monogenea, Crustacea	Various. Parasites may be visible on skin or gills. Hyperaemia and/or ulceration may occur.	Depends on cause. Large parasites (e.g. Argulus) may be removed manually. Others may require parasiticide baths.	
	Tuberculosis	Various. Weight loss, skin lesions, ascites.	Best to isolate/cull affected fish but treatment can be attempted. Hygiene.	

Fig. 4.30. Some diseases seen in lower vertebrates.

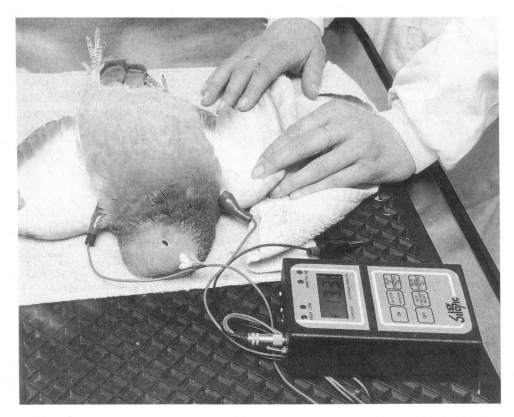

Fig. 4.31. Monitoring anaesthesia is important: a lightly anaesthetised pigeon being examined with a heart monitor.

Land tortoises may suffer from **post-hibernation anorexia (PHA)**, a blanket term to cover all those that do not start eating within a week or so of emerging from hibernation. They may have stomatitis, liver failure or kidney failure; or they may simply have exhausted their vitamin reserves or be dehydrated. The kidneys barely function during hibernation, so that waste products build up in the circulation and blood tests may reveal a very high blood urea. Some of those suffering from PHA respond well to basic fluid therapy and vitamin supplementation.

Other land tortoise problems include:

- Roundworms—particularly where a number of tortoises are kept, or where they have been on the same piece of ground for a number of years.

- Infectious rhinitis—a very infections and debilitating viral disease affecting the spur-thighed tortoise (Testudo graeca); it may take a year or more to clear. Young animals are much less susceptible and seem to develop a solid immunity once recovered.
- Osteodystrophy in young animals fed a diet low in calcium or with a poor calcium/phosphorus ratio.

Surgery and Anaesthesia

Animals that are to be anaesthetised (Figs 4.31 and 4.32) or referred for surgery may need to be hospitalised and nursed within the surgery. Sometimes there is merit in housing the patient in its own

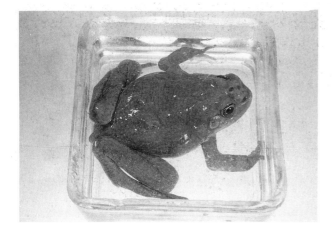

Fig. 4.32. Non-domesticated species may need special equipment or techniques for anaesthesia: this frog is being anaesthetised in water in a glass dish, using a water-soluble agent (benzocaine).

cage; at other times special accommodation may need to be constructed. The practice should ensure that it is always prepared for emergencies involving exotic pets by having one or more of each of the following:

- 'Hospital cages'—designed for birds but equally useful for small mammals and sometimes reptiles and amphibians.
- Glass or plastic aquaria—primarily used for fish but easily modified to accommodate other species.
- Other suitable containers, e.g. bird cages (preferably with solid sides), buckets.

Important aspects of nursing exotics include:

- Provision of warmth/maintenance of the patient at its preferred body temperature.
- Maintenance of fluid balance.
- Ensuring adequate nutrient intake.
- Minimising stress.

Further Reading

Alderton, D. (1992) *You and Your Pet Bird*. Dorling Kindersly, London.

Beynon, P. H. and Cooper, J. E. (1991), eds. *Manual of Exotic Pets*. BSAVA, Cheltenham.

Beynon, P. H., Lawton, M. P. C. and Cooper, J. E. (1992), eds. *Manual of Reptiles*. BSAVA, Cheltenham.

Butcher, R. L. (1992), ed. *Manual of Ornamental Fish*. BSAVA, Cheltenham.

Coles, B. H. (1985) *Avian Medicine and Surgery*. Blackwell, Oxford.

Cooper, J. E. (1976). 'Pets in hospitals', *British Medical Journal* I, 698–700.

Cooper, J. E. (1986a). 'Animals in schools', *Journal of Small Animal Practice* 27, 839–850.

Cooper, J. E. (1986b) 'Veterinary work with non-domesticated pets. II Mammals', *British Veterinary Journal* 142, 420–433.

Cooper, J. E. (1990) 'Feeding exotic and pocket pets', *Journal of Small Animal Practice* 31, 482–488.

Cooper, J. E. (1991) 'Caged and wild birds', in *Practical Animal Handling* (eds. R. G. Anderson and A. T. B. Edney). Pergamon, Oxford.

Cooper, M. E. (1987) *An Introduction to Animal Law*. Academic Press, London.

Crush, M. (1982) *Handy Homes for Creepy Crawlies*. Granada, London.

Flecknell, P. (1983) 'Restraint, anaesthesia and treatment of children's pets', *In Practice* 5, 85.

Flecknell, P. A. (1984) 'The relief of pain in laboratory animals', *Laboratory Animals* 18, 147–160.

Flecknell, P. A. (1987) *Laboratory Animal Anaesthesia*. Academic Press, London.

Forbes, N. (1993) 'Avian medical and surgical nursing', *Veterinary Practice Nurse* 5(2), 4–7.

Fox, J. G., Cohen, B. J. and Loew, F. M. (1984) *Laboratory Animal Medicine*. Academic Press, Orlando.

Hime, J. M. and O'Donoghue, P. N. (1979) (eds) *Handbook of Diseases of Laboratory Animals*. Heinemann, London.

Liles, J. H. and Flecknell, P. A. (1992) 'The use of non-steroidal anti-inflammatory drugs for the relief of pain in laboratory rodents and rabbits', *Laboratory Animals* 26, 241–255.

Murphy, F. (1980) *Keeping Spiders, Insects and other Land Invertebrates in Captivity*. Bartholomew, Edinburgh.

Poole, T. B. (1986) (ed.) *The UFAW Handbook on the Care and Management of Laboratory Animals*. Longman, Harlow.

Porter, V. (1993, revised edn) *The Complete Book of Ferrets*, D & M Publications, Bedford.

Price, C. J. (1988) (ed.) *Manual of Parrots, Budgerigars and other Psittacine Birds*. BSAVA, Cheltenham.

5
Management of Kennels and Catteries

C. A. VAN DER HEIDEN

It is essential that those who are responsible for animals should have a good basic knowledge of the needs, care and welfare of the normal healthy domestic animal, whether it is in a one-pet household or in a large kennel or cattery. This knowledge can then be built upon so that the many and varied requirements of the patients that are entrusted to the care of the veterinary nurse can be taken into account.

Although this chapter is relevant to accommodation for pets, and is therefore likely to assist the nurse in advising pet owners, it deals mainly with the care of groups of dogs and cats in kennels or catteries. Veterinary nurses are often responsible for running the hospital kennels and it is important to understand fully the construction and efficient management of such establishments and their effects on the health and well-being of the animals.

Basic Requirements for a Kennel or Cattery

The design and construction of a kennel or cattery will depend upon its main use. Kennels and catteries range from those owned by private individuals (for housing their pets, breeding and show animals or working dogs) to large boarding, quarantine or dog training establishments, as well as the specialist hospital animal accommodation provided within veterinary practices. The requirements for the housing of all dogs and cats are basically the same, with some variations for different use of accommodation.

Construction Requirements

Essential Requirements

Above all, kennels should be designed and managed to meet the needs of the animal to be housed in comfort. This first and most important consideration for the housing of any animal should not be prejudiced by other requirements such as ease of management, as this could result in housing to suit the human operators rather than the animals.

> The animals' basic needs are:
> - Warmth, comfort and security.
> - Companionship, mental stimulation and opportunities for expression of normal behaviour.
> - Protection from disease and injury.
> - Protection from fear and distress.
> - Exercise as appropriate to the animal.
> - Provision for appropriate feeding.
> - Opportunities for defecation and urination away from the sleeping area.

Warmth, comfort and security

For the normal healthy dog, a relatively cool environmental temperature is quite acceptable (though it should not drop below 7°C (44.6°F)) as long as the accommodation is dry and draught free and with suitable and sufficient bedding material. A higher temperature is required by very young, elderly or ill animals and some specialist breeds.

Dogs are generally more relaxed when they feel comfortable and secure. The design of the sleeping area will aid this: they tend to seek out darker areas where they can lie behind or underneath something or in a corner. All dogs should be given the opportunity to sleep in a conventional sleeping area, which they will usually prefer once settled into kennel life, but they often initially have the desire to create their own sleeping area by moving the bedding material. Some individuals pull the bedding out to the centre of the kennel or into the run if they can. This is a form of nesting behaviour and the dog will often be much more relaxed if it has been able to achieve this, though at times there seems to be quite a frantic period of activity before the dog finally settles.

Cats require a comfortable environmental temperature and a sleeping area in which they feel secure and comfortable. Many shy cats take to the 'igloo' style of bed, which has its own roof. Even a simple up-turned cardboard box might give a greater feeling of security in an unfamiliar environment.

Companionship, mental stimulation and opportunities for expression of normal behaviour

Dogs are pack animals and prefer companionship. Domesticated dogs need the attention and physical presence of humans as well as other dogs. Association with the latter can (or, in quarantine, must) be achieved without actual physical contact.

Kennelled dogs and cats need stimulation—by sight, sound, smell and touch, as found in their normal environment—to avoid boredom and, ultimately, the stereotyped behaviour patterns that boredom would produce. This can be a particular problem in long-stay establishments and in institutional or 'rescue' kennels.

Exercise

To understand the dog's natural exercise behaviour, it is necessary to look at the domestic animal's wild cousins. These dogs would exercise at a trot over many miles per day, with short bursts at full speed when hunting or at play, interspersed with rest periods (particularly after feeding). This behaviour is modified in the domestic dog, though it is still seen in some working dogs.

Age and health affect exercise requirements—for instance, young adult dogs require more than the middle-aged, elderly or very young. The breed of dog is also of enormous influence on the amount of exercise required. All dogs require daily exercise, though the requirement of gun dogs, herding dogs, sight hounds etc. is much higher than for toy breeds. Dogs are more contented and relaxed when exercised on a regular daily basis and so kennel design and practices must take the need for exercise into account.

Cats in a domestic environment exercise themselves by playing hunting games where stalking, pouncing and killing are practised on small inanimate objects. Cats at liberty act in contrast to dogs: they usually walk and then stalk, with jumping and running over short distances only. They jump much higher than dogs and they have the ability to climb. Cats that have outdoor access sometimes range a considerable distance when hunting. They are territorial and mark out their territory by scent, guarding the area against intruding cats. Intruders have the choice of standing and fighting or running away when challenged.

The normal exercise requirements for cats differ from those of dogs and this should be borne in mind when keeping cats indoors or in a cattery. The cat should be provided with suitable 'toys' to stalk and chase, some of which can be suspended to simulate airborne prey. Opportunity should be provided for cats to climb and jump by providing ledges or similar at different heights. In a cattery, windowsills or similar vantage points are provided within in the run.

Protection from disease and injury

This is one of the major contributions made by humans to the well-being of the domestic dog and cat. Many factors contribute to this and in a kennel or cattery environment they are as follows:

- Safe housing: no sharp edges; escape-proof accommodation and secure run fencing; no areas to get

caught or fall into; use of non-toxic and non-combustible materials; prevention of access to dangerous areas or materials.
- Hygiene and cleanliness of the environment: hygienically kept living areas; specialist kennels for sick dogs (e.g. hospital for non-infectious, isolation for infectious cases).
- Health care: vaccination and antiparasitic control programmes; grooming and checking for abnormalities; recognition of any ill health, presentation to veterinarian and application of prescribed treatments.

Protection from fear and distress

It is important to take into account that kennelled animals have been parted from their owners and are accustomed to living in a domestic situation, when put into kennels or a cattery for the first time may be distressed until they become accustomed to the new routine. They should be handled with consideration and care, taking into account their temperament and mental state (recognised by body posture and behaviour). Time should be taken to reassure distressed animals, particularly recent admissions.

Provision of appropriate feeding

Dogs and cats must receive adequate nutrition appropriate to their specific requirements and must have access to clean, fresh drinking-water at all times (unless contraindicated by a specific condition). Nutrition requirements are dealt with in Chapter 17 but automatic drinking-water systems can be incorporated into the design of the kennel.

Opportunities for defecation and urination

Dogs are instinctively reluctant to foul their sleeping area. During early training this instinct is extended to human living areas via house-training. It is therefore necessary to provide frequent opportunities for urination or defecation in designated areas to avoid the breakdown of this training.

Dogs prefer to relieve themselves on a similar surface to the area they used as puppies, which is often grass. This behaviour will probably have to be modified during a stay in the kennels, as it is not practical for kennel 'relief areas' for reasons of hygiene, but the preference should be borne in mind if a particular dog is very reluctant to relieve itself in the designated concrete area.

Exercise is the time used by many owners to give their dogs opportunities for urination and defecation, but elimination behaviour should be separated from free exercise where possible. Many local authorities are clamping down on the fouling of public areas by dogs and so owners are encouraged to 'relieve' their dogs on command in their own gardens before exercising. Alternatively they should clean up after their dogs have produced faeces and this is easier if the command is given just before exercise, so that the faeces are easily found and removed.

When dogs are in kennels, therefore, it is important that opportunities for urination and defecation are regular and are separate from exercise periods, so that training habits are not disrupted.

Cats are also instinctively reluctant to foul their sleeping area and they usually have the desire to bury their excreta. This assists greatly in normal domestic house-training as loose, readily dug materials considered suitable by the cat can be provided by the owner in a 'litter' tray. Sometimes cats deposit faeces that remain uncovered for marking their territory.

All cats which do not have free access to areas that they would naturally find suitable (e.g. loose soil) should be provided with sanitary trays containing material that is acceptable to the cat. The trays should be regularly cleaned and replenished.

Design Factors

Kennels and catteries should be built for the purpose for which the animals are housed (Fig. 5.1). They should meet all licensing, building and planning requirements and regulations and they should be designed with the factors set out in Fig. 5.2 in mind, as well as those essential requirements already discussed.

The sizes and construction materials also depend on the proposed use of the kennels. Many kennel owners refer to recommended boarding kennel sizes and construction details when building private kennelling, and this is increasingly made easier by the use of ready-made sectional kennelling (Fig. 5.3). Medium-sized to large establishments tend to build traditional permanent buildings, built to a specific design using suitable permanent materials—brick or breeze-block structures, walls with impervious

coverings, built on foundations and with internal concrete flooring laid with a fall towards built-in drains, or guttering and drains. The floor is then either painted or tiled, or covered with asphalt, vinyl or similar internal flooring material. Particularly useful are materials that can be moulded up at the edges and secured to create a watertight seal with the walls. Any material for kennel or cattery flooring must be impervious and capable of being regularly hosed and disinfected.

Sound-proofing

All kennels have a potential noise problem caused by the barking of the dogs and every effort should be made to prevent barking becoming a problem. The effective handling and control of the dogs is of great importance. All staff should be aware of dog behaviour, including why dogs bark and how to reduce the noise. Where a dog is barking from excitement, it should be handled calmly and firmly—and without shouting, as this can in itself contribute to further excitement and noise.

Staff cannot be in the kennel 24 hours a day and spontaneous barking will usually occur if the dogs are disturbed by external noises. Efficient sound-proofing will reduce the likelihood of such disturbance as well as assist in reducing the noise of barking reaching outside the kennels.

Soundproofing is achieved by either absorbing the sound—deadening it with suitable materials rather than reflecting it from hard surfaces—or preventing the free passage and escape of the sound from the buildings and perimeters (Fig. 5.4).

Purpose-built kennel blocks

Individual kennels designed and arranged together in a group under one roof are generally referred to as a kennel block. There are many different designs for differing requirements, each with certain advantages and disadvantages. The main features of the more common designs (run-access, corridor kennels, circular 'parasol' and H-block kennels) are given in Fig. 5.5 and illustrated in Fig. 5.6.

Contents of kennel accommodation

Whatever the design, each individual kennel should contain:

- A plinth for the bedding or a removable bed.
- Some form of heating, e.g. an infrared dull emitter (if not centrally heated).
- A bulkhead electric light or similar (unless corridor lighting is sufficient to light the kennel).
- A water bowl or automatic drinking-water system.
- Some form of ventilation, i.e. controllable vents, if there is no centralised active ventilation system.

EXAMPLES OF KENNELS AND USES

Private owner unlicensed
  pet dogs
  gun dogs/herding dogs
  small scale breeding (1–2 bitches)
  Show dogs
Private owner licensed breeding (2 breeding bitches +)**
Boarding kennels/cattery**
Training kennels
  Police, customs, security, Defence.
  Guide Dogs for the Blind, Hearing Dogs for the Deaf, Dogs for the Disabled, etc.
Charity rescue kennels
  e.g. Wood Green Animal Shelters, R.S.P.C.A., N.C.D.L. etc.
Quarantine kennels
Veterinary practices with hospital kennels

Those marked with a double asterisk require to be licenced. Requirements are available from the licensing body as regards building materials and accommodation sizes.

Fig. 5.1. Examples of kennels and uses.

The kennel block should contain:
- Electricity points.
- Water points or taps conveniently situated for hose connection.
- A sink and water-heating system.
- Work tops, shelves, cupboard.
- Dustbins and other waste disposal receptacles.
- Various items such as brushes, buckets, shovels, and other cleaning equipment; grooming equipment; feed and water bowls etc.

DOG KENNEL AND CATTERY DESIGN FACTORS	
Accessibility	Cleaning and disinfection. Safe handling of the animal (for animal and staff). Maintenance work. Rapid access in emergency situation.
Efficiency	Animal housing close to service area (food preparation areas, store rooms etc). Service fittings appropriately positioned, e.g. handles, switches and service controls within easy reach; work surfaces at the correct height and situation; storage space suitable for equipment and stocks. Construction materials should be easy to clean and dry with drains to remove water when cleaning (via a fall in the floor towards the drain); non-permeable surface materials should be used.
Adequate care facilities	Grooming and bathing areas for dogs. Food storage and preparation areas. (If both dogs and cats are kept, separate areas should be allocated for the foods.) Treatment room (surgery). Hospital and isolation facilities. Whelping or puppy facilities (where appropriate to the purpose of the kennels).
Health, safety and fire prevention	The accommodation should be designed to meet all the health and safety and fire regulations. Adequate fire precautions should be in operation with all staff aware of procedures. Safe construction materials should be used. Kennels and catteries should be designed to avoid hazards e.g. no deep drains or unsafe steps, no high shelves that may be difficult for the staff to reach. Safe working practices should be observed. Electric power-points should be covered with approved coverings when water is used near by.
Designed for the purpose	Designed to be appropriate for the purpose that the animals are housed for, e.g. quarantine kennels where high security from escape and contact between animals is of vital importance.
Licensing and planning regulations	Designed to meet all licensing, building and planning requirements and regulations.
Cost and maintenance	Construction materials and installations should be of a reasonable cost but able to withstand constant use. Balance between expensive and durable fittings and economy in construction. Materials used and basic design should contribute to maintenance required, being as low as possible; metal fitments may become corroded by urine and chemicals used for disinfection; wooden window frames should be avoided, due to the need for frequent painting.

Kennel construction and siting	It is usual to site a kennel/cattery in a reasonably isolated position but close to a large area of population, particularly if purpose is boarding animals.
	Factors taken into account when choosing a site for commercial kennelling include:
	  Site suitable for building e.g. not sloping excessively, not liable to subsidence etc.)
	  Sufficient space for the proposed kennels and ancillary buildings. (The space required depends upon the number of dogs to be housed and the type of kennel design to be built.)
	  Good road access for clients. Access for goods delivery etc.
	  Adequate space for parking of clients/delivery vehicles etc.
	  Whether a licence and planning permission is likely to be granted.
	  Noise control. If not totally isolated or there is any possiblity of future planning permission being granted for building within the area surrounding the kennel site, (this cannot be totally ruled out) then sufficient space must be available to erect noise control structures (earth banks) around the kennels.
	Availability of local services:
	  Sewage mains (mains or septic tank) where suitable for proposed use.
	  Availability of electricity, gas etc.

Fig. 5.2—continued

DOG KENNEL AND CATTERY DESIGN FACTORS

	Refuse collection or the possibilities of running an incinerator for kennel waste.
	Cattery siting
	As for dog kennels but noise control is not a major consideration. The Feline Advisory Bureau recommends that dogs are not housed in close proximity. It is also recommended that 1/3 to 1/2 of an acre is sufficient for building accommodation for 45–50 cats and that cat cabins are built with the run to face south or south-west. This is recommended for the following reasons:
	  It reduces the possibility of overheating the sleeping compartments in the summer.
	  It assists the drying out of runs after cleaning.
	  Cats can sit in the sun.
	It is also recommended that the runs are built giving the cats maximum visibility of the surrounding area, to provide mental stimulation. Dog kennels can also be built facing south or south-west for similar reasons, if they are designed with the runs all facing the same way. Other factors, such as allowing maximum visibility, may lead to excessive barking, therefore a balance must be made to ensure sufficient mental stimulation to combat boredom but a low noise level.

Fig. 5.2. Factors in kennel and cattery design.

SECTIONAL PREFABRICATED KENNELLING TYPES

Concrete kennel bases with drainage	Where any type of demounting kennelling such as sectional kennels (or catteries) are erected, first lay a concrete base and drainage system. This base usually forms the kennel floor (if a floor is not incorporated in the kennel design) and the kennel run. The base is laid on hard-core with a damp-proof membrane. The concrete is laid a minimum of 4 in thick with a fall towards drains and/or or drainage guttering. Precast concrete gutter units can be set into the concrete to assist water drainage towards the kennel and run drains. Drains are either connected to the mains effluent disposal system or other systems approved by the Water Authority.
Wooden kennelling	Generally wooden kennels are not recommended (unless covered by an impervious material) due to (a) the risk of escape by chewing out; (b) being impossible to disinfect properly. However many private owners do use wooden kennels, as cross-infection is not such a common problem when only the owner's own dogs are being accommodated. These kennels are relatively inexpensive and are easily erected and dismantled. Many designs are available.
Fibreglass and other modern materials	Twin insulated fibreglass and other easily cleaned modern materials are likely to phase out the use of wood; they are as convenient and have many advantages, such as the ease of cleaning and disinfection. Many new types of kennelling are appearing on the market aimed at all types of user, from the pet owner to the commercial kennel/cattery.

Fig. 5.3. Sectional prefabricated kennels.

SOUNDPROOFING ANIMAL ACCOMMODATION

Absorbing the sound	Use of acoustic tiles or materials with similar properties on upper walls and roof (hard surfaces are preferable for hygienic reasons lower down). Tiles must be out of dogs' reach (easily damaged if chewed or scratched). Some acoustic tiles cannot be cleaned/disinfected easily – carefully use spray disinfectants for those that should not be wetted. Washable tiles are now available but can still be damaged with rough use.
Preventing the free passage and escape of sound	Construct the building to prevent free passage of sound down corridors: use double doors offset to one another. Double glazing throughout the kennels. Perimeter structures such as earth mounds or 'buns' surrounding the kennels – require additional space and are expensive but can be very effective. To be fully effective: must be at least as high as the kennel roof; must be no near neighbours with buildings higher than the mounds. Other effective structures that take up less space: – 'Green' or 'willow' walls of woven willow fencing and earth. Shrubs that are planted in these 'walls' to stabilise and create attractive appearance. – Tree belts. Require large area for maximum effect with bushy non-deciduous trees/shrubs. Not effective until trees are well grown and even then not as effective as solid structures such as earth mounds.

Fig. 5.4. Soundproofing.

TYPES OF DOG KENNEL	
Run-access kennels	These are the type most commonly used by private owners and breeders as they are very convenient, relatively inexpensive and widely available as sectional units. Some of the more modern designs are used by small boarding establishments or as additional overflow/emergency kennelling. Any number of individual kennels can be erected side by side or back to back. The main drawback: this type is essentially basic outdoor kennelling – services are not usually installed such as active ventilation, central heating or internal kennel lighting. Therefore it is difficult to control the living environment of the dogs. Other drawbacks are: They are more time consuming for staff to run. They are not particularly suitable for dealing with aggressive dogs as staff cannot reduce contact with the dog by having access to the kennel without entering through the run and confronting the dog. The dogs when confined to the kennel cannot usually see out and cannot easily be seen by staff. With this type of kennel it is usual to allow the dog free access from kennel to run during the day. This can lead to noise problems of persistent barking occurring. Heating the kennels is also inefficient.
Corridor kennels	This design has been commonly used where a number of individual kennels are required to be incorporated into one compact block and as such is suitable for medium to large establishments. Large establishments may have a number of these blocks. These can be sectional buildings or traditionally built. Entry to the kennels is via a central corridor with individual kennels along the corridor at each side. The runs are connected to the individual kennels by either an external door which can be opened by staff walking through the kennel to let the dogs into the run or a hatch operated via a pulley system that can be operated without entry into the kennel. The dogs can be allowed either free access to the runs or limited access depending upon the weather, policy of the kennel or the control requirements for individual dogs. This kennelling usually has food preparation and grooming areas situated at the end of the corridor of kennels. This enables staff to work near the dogs and supervise them, which will help to reduce the noise and other problems. Any animals requiring close supervision should be kennelled near to the staff working area to assist staff having prompt access to deal with them. As the individual kennels face one another, all dogs can see another animal. This can help dogs to settle as it fills the need for companionship even if they have no physical contact. Where this design is used for large establishments many blocks require to be built. It is more time consuming for staff to run more than one block of kennels where they are separated this way. The dogs will also be supervised less if one staff member runs more than one block. However, where large numbers of dogs are housed the risk of spread of disease is higher. The construction of several separate blocks of kennels is therefore an advantage for disease control, providing the dogs have no external contact with others, and the kennel blocks are spaced to prevent contact via kennel runs. It is then possible to prevent infectious conditions such as kennel cough running through entire kennels. Drawbacks to this design, beside staff time etc. are that firstly the bed has to be along the side wall or in a corner. Therefore the type of bed that can be used is limited as the kennel shape is usually long but narrow. Secondly, if transparent external doors are used from the kennel to run, although it is light in the kennel and the dogs can see interesting things outside during the day time, during the night this is a disadvantage and can lead to restlessness, leading to noise problems when the kennels are unattended overnight.
Circular 'Parasol' kennelling	This more recent design is used for medium to large establishments. It has been notably successful when used for animals requiring a great deal of supervision and observation such as those housed in quarantine and animal rescue kennels. Although it has some advantages, it has been more expensive to build as it is circular. The individual kennels are built in a circle with a large circular central area instead of a corridor. The runs are attached to each kennel via an external door or hatch which can be operated in a similar method to the corridor kennel-run doors, i.e. staff opened or a pulley system.

Fig. 5.5—continued

	TYPES OF DOG KENNEL
	The main advantage of this design is an improved ability to supervise the dogs. A staff member in the central kennel area can see all the dogs in the block from one position.
Equally important the dogs can see both the staff member and more of the other resident dogs than with any other kennel design. This is particularly important for long-stay animals as it assists in fulfilling the need for companionship and mental stimulation: 'confinement without the solitude'. This also applies to the dog runs, as the dogs have a wide area of vision due to the area radiating outwards, ending with a relatively wide terminal fence.
As with the corridor kennels, a grooming area and food preparation area are usually incorporated in the design at the entrance to the block or in the central area that may otherwise be wasted space. For large establishments, rather than increase the size of the circular kennel it is usual to have either several individual units as with the corridor kennels with similar advantages regarding disease control) or two or three units joined. In the latter case, the normally separate auxiliary buildings can be incorporated resulting in the entire kennel buildings being under one roof and therefore more convenient and less time-consuming for staff. Some of the drawbacks to this design (apart from the cost of building by traditional methods) are:
The kennels use a larger amount of ground space per animal housed than in some more compact designs.
The size of each block is limited, as the larger the block becomes the larger the central space becomes, which unless utilised may be wasted floor space.
The kennels may be difficult to fit with some types of beds due to the shape of the individual kennels.
The size of the runs may be limited depending upon the number of kennels in the block and ground space available.
H-block kennels	The true H-block kennel has four main kennel blocks arranged together in the form of an H with the service areas forming the cross bar of the H. There is a corridor between the individual kennels and the runs therefore, allowing no free access option for running the dogs. This arrangement is used for training establishments such as those of the Guide Dogs for the Blind Association where a large number of dogs are to be housed with the best possible use of ground space.
All the normal auxiliary buildings and a hospital and other special need kennels (except the isolation block) are under one roof, and the space between the four wings of the H is fully utilised.
The major advantage to this design is that it is compact and therefore easy to manage. Staff time can be used very efficiently as all the major auxiliary service areas are close to hand, without having to leave the dogs unsupervised for long periods (thus aiding noise control). All four kennel blocks are quickly accessible from the central area.
Staff do not get cold and wet during the winter when moving from block to block, or to and from the main service areas. Another advantage is that centralised systems can be installed to control heating, air conditioning etc. in all areas under the one roof.
The drawback of this type of kennelling is that it is too large and therefore expensive for all but those establishments requiring to house a relatively large dog population of say 80 or more dogs.
Additionally, with a large number of dogs under one roof, a strict disease control regime is essential with an efficient active ventilation system being particularly important in the control of airborne diseases.
The presence of a corridor between the individual kennels and runs require staff to take each dog out of its kennel individually to the run. This is therefore not a suitable design where aggressive dogs are likely to be housed. The other disadvantage to the one-sided layout and corridor is that the dogs have restricted vision while in the kennel – they cannot see outside (but this is an advantage redarding noise control). They cannot see other dogs either and unless more than one dog is housed in one kennel the dog may lack companionship and mental stimulation.

Fig. 5.5. Main kennel types—advantages and disadvantages.

Cattery Design and Construction

The essential requirements in cattery design are similar to those for the housing of dogs but two further factors must be taken into account:

- The cat's agility in climbing to escape.
- The greater risk of infectious respiratory disease among cats, which means that segregation is more important.

The two common types of cattery (the 'outdoor' and the 'indoor') can both be built using traditional methods but modern sectional catteries are increasingly becoming available.

Outdoor catteries

These are similar to the run-access kennels for dogs, with entrance to the cat accommodation through the outdoor run. Major differences are that the run is totally roofed and that the run access is via a safety passage to prevent any likelihood of escape. The cat accommodation units are side by side, with full height 'sneeze barriers' and/or gaps of 0.6–1.2 m (2–4 ft) minimum between the runs (Fig. 5.7).

(a)

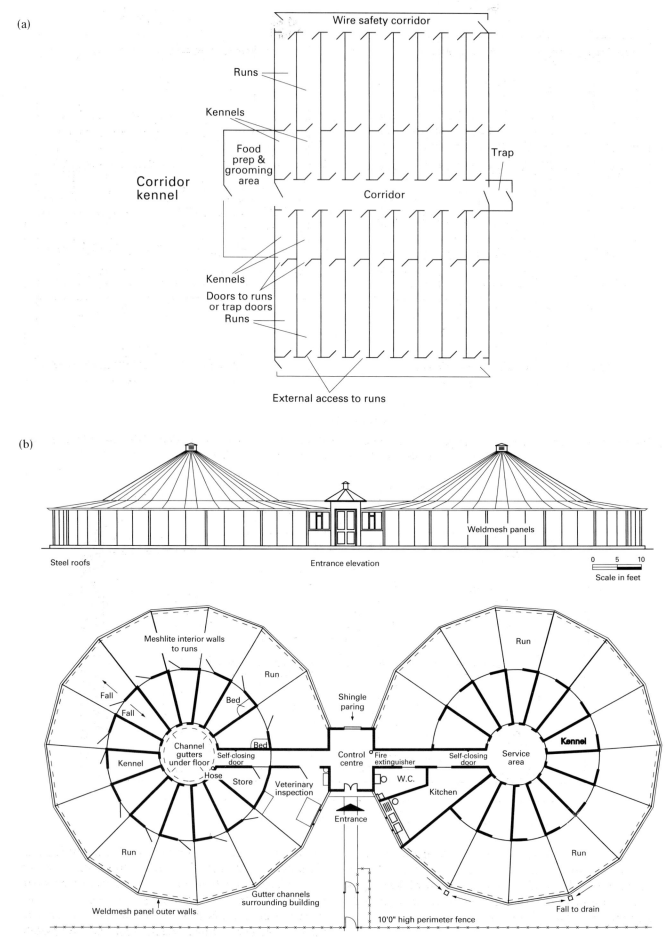

Corridor kennel

Wire safety corridor

Runs

Kennels

Food prep & grooming area

Trap

Corridor

Kennels

Doors to runs or trap doors

Runs

External access to runs

(b)

Steel roofs   Entrance elevation

Weldmesh panels

0   5   10

Scale in feet

Meshlite interior walls to runs

Fall

Fall

Run

Bed

Bed

Shingle paring

Run

Channel gutters under floor

Self-closing door

Kennel

Control centre

Fire extinguisher

Self-closing door

Kennel

Service area

Hose

Store

Veterinary inspection

W.C.

Run

Entrance

Kitchen

Run

Run

Gutter channels surrounding building

Weldmesh panel outer walls

10'0" high perimeter fence

Fall to drain

Circular 'parasol' kennel

(c)

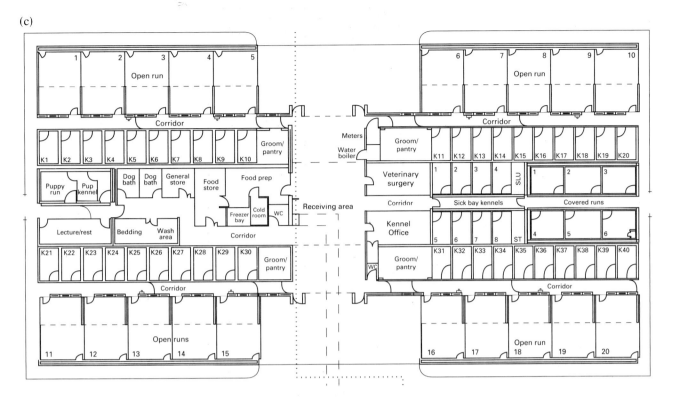

H-block kennel

Fig. 5.6. Main kennel types. (The design of the 'H' block kennel is credited to The Association of the Guide Dogs for the Blind. The kennel plan is courtesy of the Animal Inn in Kent.)

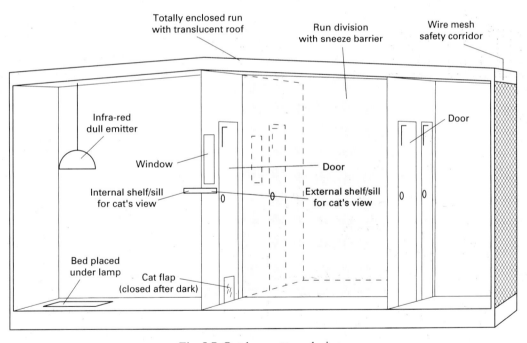

Fig. 5.7. Outdoor cattery design.

Correctly positioned and managed, outdoor catteries provide the least risk for cross-infection between cats. This advantage can be lost if two of the blocks are positioned with their runs facing into the same safety passage from opposite sides.

Indoor catteries

Indoor catteries are similar in layout to corridor kennels for dogs, with access to each cat housing unit via a central passage. The major disadvantage is the risk of cross-infection due to air exchange between the units via the central passage. The exterior doors from the units on both sides of the block open into totally enclosed runs. Each unit is completely enclosed, to prevent escape. Within the cattery building, the doors and internal walls should be solidly constructed to prevent air circulation between the units.

Contents of cat accommodation

Each cat accommodation unit should contain:

- A cat bed, possibly on a shelf or plinth.
- Heating, such as an infrared dull emitter or a heated bed.
- Lighting and ventilation systems.
- Dustpan and brush (for exclusive use in a single unit).
- Two each of water bowls, feed bowls and litter trays (for exclusive use of one cat).
- Scratching post.
- Toys (possibly suspended) to encourage play.
- A shelf or window-sill in the run to allow the cat a view.

The cattery block should contain:

- Electricity points (for heating and lighting).
- Water points, external stand pipes/taps (one over a sink), with a drain for litter trays and one tap for a hose connection.

Auxiliary Buildings and Facilities

Kennels and catteries require some auxiliary facilities, the size, contents and type of which depend upon the type of kennels. Three facilities are essential to all establishments:

- Reception office (attached to the block, or separate).
- Small kitchen (Fig. 5.8).
- Isolation unit (described in depth later in this chapter).

Other facilities (Fig. 5.8) might include:

- Stores for equipment, cleaning materials, bedding etc.
- Grooming and bathing room.
- Surgery or veterinary examination room.

Specialised Animal Housing

Specialised housing is used for animals that have specific needs regarding their environment and care. Specialised housing includes:

- Hospital kennelling.
- Whelping kennelling.
- Puppy kennelling.
- Isolation kennelling.

The same type of kennelling can be used for veterinary practice kennels or private kennelling, as the principles are the same. The precise requirements depend upon the category of animal.

KENNEL SERVICE AREAS	
Kitchen with food stores	It is advisable to have the kitchen separate from the kennel blocks, particularly if it is to service more than one block. Where it is separate each kennel block should have a small utility area with worktops and sink, for final mixing of feeds, washing of dishes etc. The main dog and cat kitchen should be easy to clean and disinfect and be equipped as follows: At least one sink with hot and cold water. At least one refrigerator. A deep freeze (size dependent on the kennel use of frozen foods). A small cooker and/or microwave oven. Work surfaces, shelves and cupboards. Vermin-proof bins for in-use sacks of food. A cool, dry and vermin-proof store room where sacks of food can be stored, raised off the floor. Various cutlery scoops, tin openers, etc. Scales for accurate weighing of feeds.
Stores for equipment, disinfectancts, cat litter, bedding, etc.	The size of the stores will depend upon the size of the kennels and the types of materials used. Relatively large storage areas may be required if it is possible to bulk-buy items.
Grooming and bathing room	The size of the grooming area, type of bath and equipment held depend on the use. Some kennels run animal grooming services where owners bring the animals in for the day; they therefore require a large fully kitted grooming and bathing room with small holding kennels. Where the grooming facilities are for boarding/hospitalised animals a small area in each kennel block may be used for grooming individuals. A small central bath room/area can then be used if bathing of animals is fairly infrequent.
Surgery or veterinary consulting room	This room, built as a separate facility for non-veterinary practice kennels, is usually only necessary for large establishments. Separate facilities are particularly useful where the animals are long-stay and the population is relatively static. It is more usual for the animal to be examined and treated either in its own housing or in a hospital ward where suitable examination facilities are made available.

Fig. 5.8. Other facilities in a kennel or cattery.

Hospital kennelling

Hospital kennels or cages are designed and constructed for animals that are undergoing treatment or for post-operative convalescence. These short-stay animals require a high degree of supervision and the kennelling is deliberately restrictive in size (Fig. 5.9). In many cases strict rest is required, particularly for post-operative animals that may dislodge sutures etc.

It should be remembered that these units are designed for a short stay. Where animals do not specifically require confinement and their stay is likely to be medium to long-term, they should be housed in a larger kennel.

Hospital kennelling can be either of the 'walk in' type or the more restricting 'locker' type. It is usual to have a choice of both types in a hospital ward to allow selection of the most suitable housing for each animal, depending upon the animal's size and temperament and the degree of confinement required.

Metabolic kennels. Metabolic monitoring kennels, available in some veterinary hospitals, are usually smaller and therefore even more confining than standard hospital kennels. Animals are only housed in them for the short duration of any tests before being rehoused in standard hospital kennelling.

Intensive care kennels. Some form of intensive care kennelling is available in many hospitals. It is usually in the form of an airtight kennel with a supply of oxygen to the interior. The front of the kennel is transparent to allow constant observation of critically ill animals.

Whelping kennelling

A whelping kennel and its run should be large enough to accommodate a whelping bitch and her litter up to at least 6 weeks of age. The whelping box should be designed to allow the use of an additional heating unit (such as an infra-red dull emitter) and to give the bitch privacy, with an observation panel that enables staff to observe her unnoticed. It should be borne in mind that the bitch will be housed solely in the kennel as long as the pups are in the whelping kennel. Her kennelling must be escape-proof; she should never leave the confines of the whelping area, because of the high risk of introducing disease to her pups from her contact with other dogs. The whelping kennels should be situated away from other dog housing and be managed in a similar manner to the isolation unit to achieve 'protective isolation' for the vulnerable pups.

In a hospital, it is highly unlikely that the bitch and pups will be housed longer than the duration of the whelping itself. It is therefore only necessary to have a kennel large enough to hold the whelping bed but it should be the quietest site available. The bitch and pups should still be subject to protective isolation procedures within the hospital environment.

Puppy kennelling

Breeding kennels and others that commonly house very young animals for a short time usually require safe housing for these vulnerable animals. Puppy kennels should be situated away from adult dogs and managed so as to reduce the risk of unvaccinated youngsters coming into contact with disease. A puppy kennel should be able to house an additional heating unit, with any possible animal contact with electric wiring totally eliminated.

There must be no gaps between the dividing partitions and the floor for kennelling and runs—puppies can squeeze through very small spaces, including those used for drainage in the kennels of adult dogs.

Where litters of puppies are to be housed, a divided 'stable door' is invaluable: when its top half is opened, attending staff can step over the closed bottom half which confines the pups. (When a standard kennel door is opened, it is very difficult to stop a number of pups escaping or, worse, getting trapped by the door.)

Kennel Services

Lighting

It is necessary for the kennels to be well lit so that all procedures can be carried out effectively and safely, from cleaning the kennels to safe handling and observation of the boarders.

Lighting and its effects on dogs

Dogs require mental stimulation for their general well-being, and in this the use of sight plays its part. It is therefore important for the welfare of the dog that adequate lighting is provided during the active hours of daylight. This may seem obvious but, in kennels that have no natural light through windows, the dogs can be left in total darkness when staff switch off the lights. The dog should be able to observe other dogs and staff, creating an interesting environment preventing boredom.

HOSPITAL KENNEL SIZES			
Size of dog	Width	Depth	Height
Large (Locker)	130 cm	100 cm	60 cm
Medium (Locker)	85 cm	75 cm	55 cm
Small dog/cat (Locker)	60 cm	65 cm	45 cm
Minimum size (Walk-in)	140 cm	100 cm	1.8 m

Fig. 5.9. Hospital kennel dimensions.

It is preferable to allow as much natural light as possible but to bear in mind the likelihood of overheating the kennels in mid-summer.

Lighting and restfulness

While it is necessary to have good lighting to create a interesting environment during the active daylight hours, it is also necessary to have reduced lighting in sleeping areas to encourage rest.

During daylight periods of inactivity, dogs take short periods of rest. To sleep, they often seek out darker areas. This should be taken into account when designing kennel sleeping areas—for example a 'skylight' over the sleeping bench should be avoided. Where a great deal of natural light is provided (via windows and glass doors) it is useful to be able to reduce this overnight so that the dogs are more restful and less likely to bark. In winter, the long hours of darkness achieve this naturally but in summer months the dogs become restless at dawn and start to bark, which can cause problems with neighbours.

Artificial lighting

It is usually necessary to supplement natural light with some form of artificial lighting in a kennel block. The most prevalent is fluorescent strip lighting with a diffuser, which provides few shadows and is therefore helpful when cleaning.

The lighting is usually situated in the corridor, or in the central area of circular kennel blocks. If this does not provide sufficient visibility for cleaning, bulkhead lights can be positioned in the kennels. These are securely attached, to either the ceiling or the upper wall, and are completely covered. Hanging light-bulbs are not recommended: some dogs may try to grab them if they dangle low, and there is also a danger of kennel staff knocking the bulbs while scrubbing out the kennels.

All wiring and switches should be inaccessible to the dogs and all electrical fittings should be protected from contact with water. One method is to use waterproof switch units and screw-on covers for power points when not in use.

Ventilation

Ventilation must be provided in kennels and catteries to:

- provide transmission of clean air for the animals and staff by removing any foul air containing fumes, obnoxious gases and smells—for example stale air (CO_2 from exhalation), ammonia, methane and unpleasant odours from animal soiling;
- reduce to a minimum the concentration of possible airborne infective agents that may cause disease.

The two types of ventilation commonly used in kennels are known as active and passive.

Active ventilation

Active ventilation mechanically pulls air into or out of the kennels, usually by means of extractor fans or an air-conditioning system. In the case of air-conditioning, a heat exchange system to prevent loss of heat from the unit can be incorporated with a heating system, providing a dual-purpose ventilation and heating system.

In some specialised kennels much thought is given to the ventilation system and attempts are made to reduce the potential transmission of airborne infection. The aim is to introduce clean air into each kennel, and extract the 'used' air from the kennel, in such a way as to reduce the likelihood that the air exhaled by one animal is inhaled by another. There are two common systems: either air-conditioning with induction vent, or extractor fan with vent.

Air-conditioning system with induction vent. In this system there is an induction vent in each kennel unit, actively pushing air into the kennel from an external 'clean' source such as the central area of the kennel roof. The air is actively extracted by another vent immediately outside the individual kennel in the corridor (Fig. 5.10).

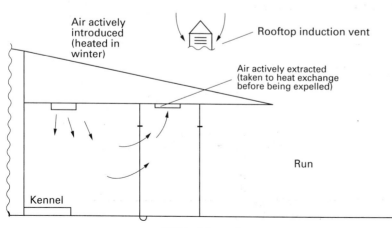

Fig. 5.10. Active ventilation: air-conditioning system with vents.

Air-conditioning units are usually installed to suit the conditions within the unit when closed, which means that leaving doors and windows open can effect their efficiency. Always seek advice from the manufacturers or installation engineers to ensure effective management and operation .

Active ventilation enables control over the number of air changes per hour, usually set at 6 for kennels, with the ability to increase up to 12 changes (or to decrease the rate in some circumstances), depending on weather conditions, number of kennel occupants etc.

Extractor fan and vent. Vents to introduce air are placed in the kennels and are themselves passive, the air being drawn through them by the activity of the extractor fan. The success of the system depends upon the correct placing of the vents in relation to the extractor fan. Figure 5.11 demonstrates the system in use in a circular 'parasol' kennel. The system is also suitable for the smaller indoor cattery and small-scale hospital accommodation.

This system can be used in reverse, with air drawn in through the central fan rather than being extracted by it. This creates positive pressure so that the air is forced out through the passive vents.

Even though a ventilation system is designed to reduce airborne infection in a working kennel, it should be remembered that it is not infallible. There is a strong possibility of the transmission of airborne infection if the dogs are passing along the corridor to grooming or relief areas or for exercise, or if they are allowed to exercise in adjoining runs with free airflow between them. For disease control, in addition to a scientific ventilation system:

- The kennels should be managed in such a way as to reduce likely contact, particularly at high risk times (e.g. when kennel cough is known to be affecting dogs in the area, or the kennels are full). All staff should be aware of the risk of airborne disease and quickly identify suspect cases.
- Animals infected or suspected of being infected should be placed in an isolation unit immediately.

Passive ventilation

Passive ventilation is achieved by opening and closing vents, windows and doors. Although widely used in many kennels and found to be satisfactory for situations where only a few animals are kept, there are some disadvantages:

- No control over air changes.
- Draughts may be caused.
- Loss of heat may be a problem.

Insulation and Heating

Insulation and heating are provided for several reasons:

- For the warmth and comfort of the dogs.
- To enable rapid drying of kennels and service areas after cleaning and disinfection (heating combined with through airflow provides the most rapid drying).
- For the maintenance of buildings and contents (without heating, some deterioration or damage may occur—such as the freezing and fracturing of insufficiently insulated water pipes). A good heating system, combined with proper ventilation, also controls condensation, the dampness of which leads to mould and other problems.
- To a lesser extent, for the comfort and health of staff working in the kennel area: they benefit from dry, well ventilated and warm environments.

Temperature control

It is advisable to check the temperature at different sites within the kennel building, particularly within the kennels themselves. The use of a maximum/minimum thermometer can be helpful in assessing the variations in temperature throughout the day and night. The range may be significant enough to warrant changes to the system. During the day the general opening and closing of doors associated with the normal running of kennels may have a noticeable effect. During the night, when there is no movement,

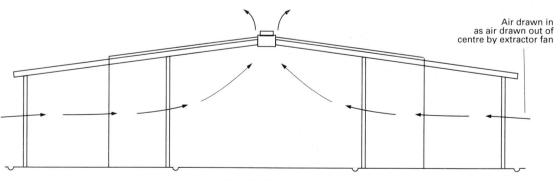

Extractor fan actively draws air out

Air drawn in as air drawn out of centre by extractor fan

Circular kennels

Fig. 5.11. Active ventilation: extraction fan and vents.

the temperature range and air quality may be significantly different from that in the daytime. Figure 5.12 gives recommended environmental temperatures for housing dogs.

Types of heating

Heating for kennelling and catteries should be:

- economical to install and run;
- easy to control, operate and maintain;
- safe, e.g. not easily knocked over, with no naked flames, and free from fumes.

Various options are available for heating kennels but they generally fall into two groups: environmental or 'central' heating of the whole kennel space, and local heating for individual animals.

Central heating is controlled by thermostat. Local heating is more economical to run: it provides additional heat for individuals with special needs, enabling the overall environmental temperature of the block to be lower so that it is more comfortable for individuals not requiring such a high degree of warmth, thus allowing animals with different needs to be housed in the same block. Figure 5.13 sets out the advantages and disadvantages of typical systems used for both central and local heating.

Insulation and draught-proofing

Whatever type of heating is installed, it will not be efficient or economical if heat can easily escape through a lack of insulation or if draughts cause chilling.

Automatic door closures may be found helpful, as if doors and windows are unnecessarily left open when the heating is operating, this will also reduce the effectiveness of the heating systems.

Beds and Bedding

Beds are used to contain the animal while resting or sleeping. They should provide a sanctuary where the animal may retire to feel safe and secure. The bed will represent its own territory in the kennels.

For these reasons all dogs and cats, whether housed in human accommodation or in any type of kennelling, should have a bed. The basic requirements for most types of bed are that they should:

- be raised to some extent from the floor;
- give easy access for the animal (particularly the old and very young);
- have sides and back (and front where used) high enough to prevent draughts, to promote the animal's feeling of security and to contain the bedding material.

Types of bed

Many types of bed are available for purchase (Fig. 5.14). The majority are designed with the domestic pet owner in mind, rather than for kennel use, though some are suitable for both. Most require the addition of bedding material but some have this incorporated in the bed.

Bedding

Bedding is used:

- to provide warmth by insulation of the animal's body heat;
- to provide comfort, by allowing padding between the animal and hard surfaces;
- to avoid injury from constant contact between skin over bony areas and hard surfaces that cause pressure or 'bed' sores.

Good bedding material has certain properties:

- It is a good insulator.
- It is soft and, depending upon its use:
  - —it can be arranged by the animal when curling up to sleep; or
  - —it is flat, with some give, and large enough to accommodate a stretched-out animal (it is important that older animals should not be forced to sleep curled up).
- It permits drainage of body fluids in case of 'accidents' when used for normal healthy animals. (This is essential in keeping ill or incontinent animals dry.)
- It does not contain anything that is harmful if ingested or that is irritant to skin, eyes etc.
- It is easy to manage.
- It is easily cleaned, disinfected or disposed of.
- It is easy to store.
- It does not soil or damage the animal's coat.

ENVIRONMENTAL TEMPERATURE FOR HOUSING DOGS	
Adult average healthy dogs	Should not drop below 7°C (44°F) in a kennel environment.
Whelping kennels and puppy accommodation	10–21°C (65–70°F), with the temperature in the whelping bed for pups in the nest at 26–29°C (80–85°F) during their first week, 21–26°C (70–80°F) in their second week, then 20°C (68°F) thereafter until weaning. The pups require a higher temperature than the bitch. The bitch can leave the bed if she becomes too hot without the pups becoming chilled.
Hospital and isolation kennels	Should be 18–21°C (65–70°F).

There are differing views regarding the correct ambient temperature for the housing of dogs

Fig. 5.12. Environmental temperatures for housing dogs.

- It is economical to use—inexpensive if disposable—durable, long-lasting and not easily chewed or destroyed if reusable.

The materials that are commonly used for bedding are either disposable or non-disposable (Fig. 5.15).

Non-disposable bedding. Non-disposable materials are laundered, disinfected and reused; they are used mainly in longer-stay kennels. They can be expensive to purchase and require suitable facilities for laundering and disinfection. The size of storage area for this type of bedding is far less than for the

TYPES OF HEATING		
Type	**Advantages**	**Disadvantages**
Central heating Gas, oil or electricity powered boilers. These heat water-filled radiators, usually placed outside individual kennels in the corridor.	Easy to operate and maintain, commonly available.	The corridor is often warmer than the kennels (thermostat or thermometer should be used to ensure individual kennels are at the corect temperature, not only the corridor). Requires suitable wall space for fitting. Likely to be difficult to keep clean and disinfect as many pipes/corners in the apparatus.
Electrical underfloor heating. Usually situated under the individual kennel flooring.	Floors dry very quickly, dogs have local heating when in closer contact with the floor when resting.	If insulation is poor the floors can become uncomfortably hot as the system attempts to increase the air temperature. Animal faeces dry hard to the floor, making removal difficult. System faults may be difficult and expensive to repair if the fault is under the floor. Electrical 'leaks' may eventually require the excavation of the whole floor.
Electric fan-assisted warm air heating. This form of heating is more often used to provide supplementary heating but can be installed in some cases as a central heating system.	The main advantage of this form of heating is its ability to provide rapid heat by circulating heated air.	As the air is very hot when it leaves the heater, great care should be taken not to place a heater too close to a patient's kennel as overheating of the patient could occur. This type of heating is fairly noisy and relatively expensive to run if used for more than as a supplementary heating option.
Total air conditioning/heating system. This system is usually installed when the building is purpose-built and is centrally operated. It is only suitable for large establishments where many kennels or kennel blocks are under one roof.	Heat and clean air can be fed directly into individual kennels and extracted in the corridor, ensuring the kennels themselves are at the correct temperature and air is pushed/pulled out of the kennels. This reduces the air flow from kennel to kennel, which is advantageous in reducing the distribution of air-borne infection. As the heating is introduced through the kennel ceiling, the dogs have no potential contact with the heating unit and finding suitable wall space is not an issue, as for radiators.	Expensive to install and not suitable for many types of kennel design with low roofs. Running costs may be high in winter.
Local heating Infra-red dull emitter. Widely used in all types of kennels, the unit is suspended from the roof by a chain or other strong adjustable material over the sleeping area. This is assessed before the animal is housed by placing a thermometer on an object such as a box,	Easy to install. Correct heat can be directed into the animals sleeping area. Produces heat without light thus aiding restfulness. The height of the unit can be adjusted to regulate the heat reaching the animal.	Requires a power point either in each kennel or the means to direct an electric lead safely into the kennel. Unless correctly positioned the animal may be either too hot or cold. (The F.A.B. recommend the use of individually thermostatically controlled infra-red dull emiters in cat accommodation to reduce the risk of over- or under-heating.) Some animals may be able to tamper with it with disastrous

Fig. 5.13.—continued

TYPES OF HEATING		
Type	**Advantages**	**Disadvantages**
at the height of the sleeping animal's back. Once the optimum temperature has been reached by raising and lowering the unit and leaving for a few minutes each time, the unit can then be fixed in position and a mark or strip of tape can be permanently put on the wall indicating the height and temperature expected.		results if hung too low and not firmly fixed to the ceiling (by a chain or similar). Fires can occur if: – the animal pulls it down and it is in contact with bedding. – It is hung too low scorching the bedding. – Water is splashed onto the bulb which then bursts.
Heated bed/pad. This type of supplementary heating is widely used and enjoyed by many animals, healthy or ailing in kennel or hospital situations. It is essential that this type of heating is only used to supplement the environmental heating system as only the bed is warmed.	The animal can be directly heated by contact with a low constant heat being emitted from directly below.	Frequently damaged by chewing (even when metal casing used for wires) leading to a risk of electrocution of animal. These should be used with a circuit breaker to minimise the risk. Increased risk of contamination as directly in contact with the animal and may prove difficult to disinfect thoroughly. Some users feel that continual contact with a heated surface can lead to hair loss.
Hot water-bottles. Hot water-bottles are often used as temporary heaters for very young puppies (with the water at normal body temperature).	Cheaply available for providing rapid direct warmth to the animal. They are suitable for sending home with tiny puppies or kittens after a Caesarean operation.	There is a danger of using water too hot and burning the animal. There is also a risk of bursting and wetting and/or scalding the animal particularly as the animal may bite or claw the hot water-bottle. The water cools rapidly and therefore hot water-bottles are only used for short-term emergency use where an animal can be supervised.
Portable radiant heaters.	Widely available and provide rapid heat. Good for emergency use, heaters can be hired.	They should never be used when they cannot be supervised as if in contact with any combustible material can cause fires. They should never be used in a busy ward where they can be knocked over or have anything dropped on them, as fires can start very rapidly.
Electric fan heaters	Can be used to boost the heat rapidly in cold weather or act as a temporary rapid emergency heating in the case of the main heating system malfunctioning.	As for electric fan-assisted warm air heating.
Electrically heated oil-filled radiators. Widely available and provide heat without light.	Mobile and relatively safe as there is no single concentrated heat source.	Can take much longer to heat an area than some of the other forms of supplementary heating. They therefore may not benefit the animals for a long time after switching on.

Fig. 5.13. Types of heating: advantages and disadvantages.

disposable type as less stock is required. Non-disposable bedding includes blankets, acrylic bedding and covered foam pads.

Disposable bedding. Disposable materials are relatively inexpensive and are discarded once soiled. A large stock of material will be required and needs a suitable storage area situated as near to the kennel accommodation as possible. Provision must also be made for disposal according to current regulations.

TYPES OF BEDS FOR DOMESTIC ANIMALS			
Type of bed	**Use**	**Qualities**	**Additional bedding type**
Wicker basket	Domestic	Popular with owners, flexible, attractive, traditional. Liable to chewing by some dogs, difficult to clean/disinfect, can harbour flea eggs.	Blanket or similar
Bean bag	Domestic	Liked by many dogs and can be "arranged" by dog. Warm polystyrene beads insulate. Beads mould to body shape assisting comfort. Outer cover is washed/disinfected, remainder difficult to wash. Not suitable for incontinent animals. Not suitable for chewers as small holes allow the polystyrene beads to escape.	None
Foam and fabric (traditionally shaped)	Domestic	Are popular with more designs becoming available. Are available for cats and small dogs with a "roof", igloo style. Flexible, small beds are machine washable.	Foam pad. (Additional blankets can be used)
Metal frame	Domestic	Collapsible dog bed raised animal well off floor, liked by many dogs. Removable covers or blankets used to allow washing. Some elderly animals may have difficulty in getting in.	Blankets or similar for some types.
Radiator cat beds	Domestic	Radiator fixed cat beds, a fixed radiator is required. The bed hooks over the top of the radiator. A removable washable cover is used. Popular with some owners and many cats. The bed protrudes and can not always be conveniently placed. Elderly/very young or infirm cats may not be able to get in and out. Cats will seek warmth while radiator is on, but will be less comfortable when the heating is off e.g. at night.	
Plastic moulded	Domestic/kennels	Widely available in many sizes. Used with removable bedding. They can be washed and adequately chemically disinfected. Can be chewed by some dogs resulting in quite sharp edges being formed. Occasionally animals have been found to have allergic reactions to prolonged contact with some types of plastic, especially if the dog's nose rests on the plastic.	Covered foam pad, blankets etc.
Sleeping benches	Kennels	A. Fixed (built in plinth) This is an area of kennel that is raised. It is either a low, slightly raised floor in one area, or a structure projecting from a wall with supports at each end. Bedding material must be used. It may have difficult corners to clean/disinfect dependent on design. B. Removable Slide/lift out. Fold down. Wood laminated (aluminium reinforced edges). These have the advantage over the fixed plinth in that they are removable, and have some degree of "give" or flexibility and usually are slightly better at insulating body heat. Bedding material used should be either of the disposable or non-disposable type. It may be chewed by some dogs if any unreinforced edges are accessible to the dog.	Blankets or similar, or disposable bedding such as shredded paper can be used, if retaining board used. Bedding as above.

Fig. 5.14. Types of bed.

Commonly used disposable materials include newspaper, shredded paper and woodwool. Less frequently used (and not advised for regular use) are straw, straw bags, peat, woodshavings and sawdust.

General Principles of Kennel and Cattery Management

Kennel and cattery management consists of ensuring a planned and methodical approach, by designing and executing efficient routines and procedures for the care and welfare of the animals. Such management will ensure that:

- All tasks are carried out in a logical order, with the needs of the animals high in priority.
- The best possible use is made of labour and materials.

- Health and safety requirements are met.
- All staff are fully instructed about how to carry out their tasks.
- All staff are aware of set standards and can recognise when they have been achieved.
- Consistency of standards is maintained by supervision and by checking procedures.
- Morale of staff is kept high as they are fully aware of what is expected and the reasons for carrying out their tasks.
- Confidence generated by the staff and management conveys to clients that their animals are being well cared for.

Daily Work Routine Within the Kennel Block

The daily work routine is an amalgamation of tasks that must be carried out to a strict timetable (e.g.

| TYPES OF BEDDING USED ||
Non-disposable	Disposable
Blankets Unless donated or old blankets are used they can be an expensive form of bedding, particularly as they may be chewed and torn up by some destructive dogs. Dogs with allergies to dust mites may not be suited to this type of bedding if it is not laundered regularly using very hot washing water. Blankets are however a traditional warm bedding and are often used in domestic circumstances, and owners like to see them used in kennels. They are not suitable for hospital kennels or housing infectious disorders as they are difficult to sterilise. **Acrylic bedding** This type of bedding is widely used both domestically and in kennels. It is very expensive to purchase but more resistant to chewing than blankets. This type of bedding is easier to launder than blankets as it is resistant to organic material, even dried on debris can usually be removed by soaking. The properties that makes it particularly suitable for hospital use are that it allows body fluids through thus keeping an animal relatively comfortable and dry and it is sufficiently supportive as to reduce the occurrence of pressure sores in elderly and recumbent animals. **Covered foam pads** These are generally used in conjunction with a traditionally shaped foam-and-fabric or plastic-moulded bed. They can also be chewed and once damaged should be repaired or removed as soon as possible as chunks of foam can be more easily torn off by a dog once the pad has been initially damaged. This bedding is fairly easily laundered and warm and comfortable. It is sufficiently supportive as to reduce the occurrence of pressure sores. In some cases thick foam pads covered with waterproof material are found useful in a hospital situation where very large breeds are recumbent. The additional thickness assists in the support of these very heavy animals. Due to the thickness and size of these pads they are very difficult to launder. The waterproof covering can however be cleaned/disinfected by using chemical disinfectant and a cloth to wipe over.	**Newspaper** Newspaper is widely used by kennels and hospitals as it is freely available and absorbent. Many kennels line the bed area with newspaper and place a blanket or similar on top. It is rarely used on its own as a bedding as it is not warm or comfortable enough for the animal. A disadvantage of newspaper is that the newsprint will stain, particularly when wet. Dogs with light coloured coats and light coloured kennelling are likely to stain. **Shredded paper** This has the advantage over newspaper in that it is bulky and therefore warmer. If shredded newspaper is used the staining previously mentioned can be a problem. It can be messy to deal with in kennels as are all materials with similar properties unless retained in the sleeping area by some method. It will stick to an animal's coat if damp and is not suitable for use with animals that have discharging wounds as it is liable to attach itself to such areas. Healthy dogs in a kennel situation find this form of bedding very comfortable and appear to enjoy arranging it and burying their toys in it. Some animals may eat it and small amounts usually cause little harm. **Woodwool** Woodwool is used in some kennels as it is warm and liked by the dogs though it is more recently being replaced by the use of shredded paper. Woodwool is expensive and can on occasion cause allergic reactions. Small pieces may occasionally get into an animal's eyes. It is less absorbent than paper but this can be an advantage if body fluids are required to drain through a bedding rather than being absorbed. (It is thought that pine oil may repel ectoparasites where wood-origin materials are used.)

Fig. 5.15. Types of bedding.

animals receiving medications at specific times of day) and other tasks that are more flexible and which experienced staff will fit into the routine as appropriate. All new and inexperienced staff, however, should carry out tasks as instructed by their supervisor.

The five main factors to consider when planning daily work are as follows.

External influences. These can be almost anything that will affect the working day, from the weather (e.g. ice and snow hampering the cleaning of external exercise runs and requiring more time to complete the task) to several owners being due to collect their dogs on a particular day, or an unusual number of long telephone calls.

Weekly or non-routine tasks. The relevant documentation (usually a diary) should be checked for weekly or non-routine tasks due to be carried out on a particular day.

Time allowed for completion of tasks. Because many and varied tasks have to be included, it is important that all work is started promptly and that the time taken for each task is assessed appropriately.

Adaptability. Adaptability is essential when working with animals, as sudden changes will require the rescheduling of tasks. Animals may become ill or there may be unexpected requests to collect animals, for example when an elderly owner has been admitted into hospital as an emergency.

Communication. As in any business where more than one person is working, it is important to communicate effectively with all other personnel likely to be affected by any decision or actions. In addition to verbal communication, it is advisable to use some form of written instructions. Typical systems are kennel diaries, check-lists that can be ticked, and clearly written lists of the routine daily tasks. Figure 5.16 gives practical examples of daily kennel and cattery routines.

Kennel Management Procedures

The kennel manager should design and introduce set procedures within the kennels to ensure smooth running and minimise error. These should be supported by some form of documentation for

---

DAILY KENNEL AND CATTERY ROUTINES

Example of a daily kennel routine

7am start. Open kennels: check all dogs (walk through kennel block).
Gather equipment.
When initial excitement subsides, take dogs quietly to the runs.
Clean kennels and replace or change bedding.
Check that each dog has urinated and defecated (record) and return dogs to the kennel.
Remove faeces from runs and rinse away urine patches.
Check water supply, water bowls and buckets.
Carry out any early morning treatments or medications.
Breakfast. Break for staff.
Make up feeds; feed dogs; wash dishes (if water bowls/buckets are used, wash and renew water supply)
Take dogs quietly to the runs and see to any soiled kennels.
Record any urination and defecation; return dogs to kennels.
Remove faeces from runs and hose-clean entire run area.
Carry out kennel tasks (e.g. washing blankets/cleaning dog kitchen, checking feed/disinfectant/bedding supplies)
Exercise dogs according to type, age, condition, etc.
Remove any faeces from exercise runs.
Commence grooming and checking long haired dogs (if time).
Lunch. Break for staff.
Take dogs to runs etc.
Continue checking and grooming all dogs (long haired dogs first)
Bath/groom any dogs being discharged and prepare belongings for return to owners.
Feed any dogs receiving p.m. feeds; wash dishes.
Take dogs to runs etc.
Disinfect and thoroughly rinse and dry all runs.
Reception/discharge of dogs (there may be two reception/discharge times during the day, one in the morning, one in afternoon).
Settle in new dogs, feed, take to runs, etc.
Supper. Break for staff.
Any uncompleted documentation, paperwork; discussions, planning.
Break for staff; then in late evening:
Take all dogs to runs etc, opportunities for urination and defecation.
Check all dogs.
Lock up kennels. Set any security devices.

Example of a daily cattery routine

Starting 7–8am. Check all cats.
Remove feed and water bowls.
Adjust heating if necessary.
Wash water bowls.
Feed cats and supply water (with milk as appropriate.)
Clean kennels (cat units). Sweep cat housing unit and tidy bed (using the units individual dustpan and brush).
Wash down any soiled surface (with disinfectant/detergent solution).
Litter trays emptied, disinfected, cleaned and refilled (records of urination/defaecation kept).
Thoroughly sweep clean.
Sweep safety passage. Soiled litter/waste bags removed and prepared for disposal. Clean and disinfect any vacated units.
Treatments carried out. Grooming carried out.
Feed list for afternoon feeds made up and dated as necessary. Second feed given (8 hours after a.m. feed).
Attend to litter trays (check at intervals and attend to trays as necessary during the day).
Prepare any documentation for any admissions or discharges the following day.
Dusk
Secure cats in housing units.
Late evening
Check each cat, adjust heating if necessary.
Lock up all buildings. Set fire and other security alarm systems.

Fig. 5.16. Daily routines in kennels and catteries.

record and checking purposes. Set procedures should include admission (intake of animals), discharge (animals leaving the kennels) and others as appropriate to the type of kennels.

Documentation

All documentation must be:

- legible and accurate;
- up-to-date and relevant;
- able to record action taken;
- in the correct terminology.

All documentation must be easy to read and accurate in order to avoid mistakes being made (e.g. special feeding requirements or medication) and to ensure that all legal requirements are covered. Information should be recorded promptly (to ensure that records and instructions are up to date) and should be concise and brief. When instructions have been followed, the action taken must be recorded (this can be simply a tick column, or initials and date where two or more members of staff are responsible for the duties). The correct terminology should be used, and any abbreviations must be those that are understood and commonly used by all staff.

EXAMPLES OF ADMISSION AND DISCHARGE PROCEDURES	
Admission On arrival	The date/time of admission should have been previously written in the diary/day book. A kennel should be available/prepared for the animal. *Vaccination certificates must be checked BEFORE the animal is admitted to ensure animal is properly vaccinated and up to date.* Record details of admission – card or forms are usually designed to fulfil the individual kennel needs. However generally the information is: Owner details; Owners name, address and telephone number (plus a contact address/number if the owner is working or on holiday); Animal details: name, species, breed, age, sex (and if neutered) ; Animal's normal behaviour, characteristics or peculiarities; Details of food/normal feeding time/normal relief pattern and surface used (urination and defecation)/normal amount exercise given. List items admitted with the animal and label them: collar, lead, toys, carrying box, etc. (Try to avoid admitting many personal items as even if labelled they can still be lost causing embarrassment to the kennels or veterinary practice). Details of stay: arrival time and date; Reason for stay e.g. boarding, hospitalisation. Time and date of the animal's discharge: Other details/policies. Consent forms may be required to be filled in, or if the kennels are not attached to a veterinary practice details of the client's veterinary surgeon will require to be recorded. It MAY also be policy in some kennels to: a) Ask the owner how they will be paying b) Inform the owner if they are expected to settle all debts upon collection c) State the cost of the service. This is usually done in a pre-determined way as part of the normal administration procedure so as it does not offend or embarrass the owner. It does however save embarrassment or misunderstanding when the account is to be settled on collection as the owner knows what to expect. Any other kennel policy may need to be stated and the owner may be asked to sign a form in some cases agreeing to abide by the policy. If it is possible check the animal over in the presence of the owner and identify to the owner any abnormalities found. It is sometimes possible that they are aware of, say, a small swelling for example, but have forgotten to inform you of it which later may develop into a large hernia. It is helpful to carry out this check with the owner present to avoid any disagreement regarding whether an animal sustained an injury while in your care or was injured prior to admission. Check at this stage for signs of parasites and if present deal with them with the consent and knowledge of the owner.
Weigh the animal	If the animal is likely to stay in kennels for a prolonged period it should be weighed on entry and thereafter at weekly intervals. This should be part of the condition monitoring of all long stay animals.
Admit the animal	Firmly but pleasantly take the animal from the owner. Always remember that the separation may in some cases be distressing for both animal and owner. Make sure the animal cannot escape from you if it should struggle. It is best to use a kennel slip lead for dogs but with cats due to their agility when determined to escape strict precautions should be imposed to prevent possible escape. The cat should be presented in an escape proof container (basket, carrying box, cage) and the owner accompany the member of staff to the kennel.
Kennel the animal securely	All animals should be transferred to their housing using an escape proof technique, as when first admitting an animal is the time when the risk of potential escape is very high. The animal should be offered water and food if appropriate. The animal should be closely observed and reassured as it settles into the kennel routine.

Fig. 5.17—continued

EXAMPLES OF ADMISSION AND DISCHARGE PROCEDURES	
Discharge	The date and time of the animal's discharge should be written in the diary or day book. The day prior to departure, any preparations that are required for the animal's departure should be carried out. These may be, the preparation of any written materials such as reports/special care instructions for the owner to continue, or the preparation of any prescription. The account should be prepared and checked.
Feeding	Animals travelling a distance or not used to car journeys should not normally be fed less than four hours before their departure. This will help to reduce the likelihood of the animal vomiting, and if it does vomit there will be less solid vomit for the animal to soil itself or the owner's car.
Grooming	The animal should be checked and groomed before departure. This may fit in with the animal's normal daily grooming depending on the departure time. If not the grooming will require to be rescheduled to be carried out earlier in the day to ensure that the animal is groomed before collection.
Items admitted with the animal	Check that all the items admitted with the animal are ready for collection and are clean and undamaged.
Report on the animal's stay	If the animal has been hospitalised a written or verbal report may be required. Where an animal has been boarding a verbal report will be required by the owner. This should never come as a surprise and efforts should be made to report as fully as possible on the animal. This inspires confidence in the establishment as the owner is satisfied that the staff have taken an interest in the animal that is naturally regarded as special to them. This should ensure future custom from them and enhance the reputation of the kennels when they relay to others the high standard of care and attention that they feel was given to their pet. The account or method of payment must be resolved. If it is policy for the account to be settled on collection of the animal, the itemised bill should be ready. The owner, having been previously made aware of the kennel policy, will be expecting it to be ready for payment.

Fig. 5.17. Admission and discharge procedures.

Figure 5.17 gives examples of admission and discharge procedures.

Kennel Cleaning and Disinfection

All animals require a hygienic environment in order to remain healthy. Where animals are housed in large numbers or the population is constantly changing, as in most kennels and catteries, an effective cleaning and disinfection routine should be in place and strictly followed. When setting up such a routine it is important to set a balance: constant washing creates damp kennels and a humid atmosphere in which micro-organisms thrive and, in any case, dogs and cats are more comfortable in dry accommodation.

Daily cleaning

Whilst animals are resident one thorough cleansing and disinfection daily (using the method described below) should be sufficient and is better than, say, three half-hearted floor wipes with a cloth or mop and bucket. When animals accidentally soil their accommodation, this is dealt with on a local area basis and must be attended to at once.

Tidying kennels

For removal of dust and hair from the kennel during the day, consider the use of a vacuum cleaner. It is more effective and less time-consuming than a broom or dustpan and brush and it reduces the amount of water used in the kennels. (Take care to use a quiet machine and be aware that some animals may object to the noise.) At this point the bedding is usually tidied and shaken out.

Cleaning and disinfection on departure

On an animal's departure from the kennels, its accommodation can be thoroughly cleaned and disinfected, and preferably left empty for a few days. All bedding is removed and either disposed of or disinfected. All toys belonging to the kennels (rather than to the individual) should be disinfected, or discarded if this is not possible.

Post-operative kennelling

The highest possible standards of disinfection are essential in veterinary hospital kennels, especially where a risk of infection is likely, as in post-operative kennelling.

Principles and methods of cleaning and disinfecting kennels

The cleaning and disinfection of kennels is achieved by physical and chemical actions. The action of all chemical disinfectants is dependent upon being in direct contact with the target micro-organism, which means that all traces of organic material such as dirt, grease, faeces, urine, blood and vomit must be physically removed from the surface prior to disinfection, as it will prevent such contact. Begin by removing the bulk of the material with a shovel and scraper (or similar). Tackle the remainder by hosing out the kennel liberally with water; then use a detergent and energetically scrub with a suitable brush.

Precautions and use of chemical disinfectants

When using any chemicals, including disinfectants and cleaning materials, care should be taken to ensure their correct handling:

- Store in the original containers with the lids fully secured.
- Keep away from animals and children.
- Wear protective clothing when recommended and take care to avoid contact with skin.
- Wash hands thoroughly after use, particularly before eating and drinking.
- Only use disinfectants for the purpose recommended by the manufacturer.
- Use the correct concentration.

Manufacturers of disinfectants give recommended dilution rates. There is usually more than one rate, depending upon where the chemical will be used and the type of organisms to be killed or inactivated. To simplify use, most manufacturers do not provide a list of micro-organisms and a recommended strength for each, but they give a recommended strength for routine or general use and (usually) a stronger solution for certain specific disease-causing organisms.

In some kennels the recommended 'routine' strength is used for the normal daily cleaning and disinfection of kennels where no specific problems exist. A recommended higher concentration is often used in disinfecting a kennel after its occupant has been discharged and before admitting another animal into it. Some general rules can be applied to the use of disinfectants:

- Too weak a solution will be ineffective, whereas a solution that is stronger than the recommendation is not only wasteful but also may, with some types of disinfectant, lead to problems with the animal's feet, eyes etc. Inadequate rinsing may lead to similar problems.
- A disinfectant should have no substances other than water added to it. It is potentially dangerous to mix disinfectants together, unless recommended by the manufacturer, as combinations of chemicals can produce noxious gases or corrosive action. This problem can occur accidentally if adequate safeguards are not in place—always be aware of the chemicals and always use and store as recommended.
- Use at the chemical's optimum temperature for action. Many disinfectants are more effective when used with hot water than with cold, though with others there is no advantage. It is advisable to check this feature.
- Using very hot water can be hazardous. If it spills on the operator or the animal, injury will occur. Safety should be of paramount importance with all actions in kennels.

- The contact time should be taken into account when planning a disinfection routine. All disinfectants require time to kill or inactivate micro-organisms and are ineffective if rinsed off immediately after application. The required contact time varies considerably, depending on the type of disinfectant and the organism to be killed. Take note of the manufacturer's recommended contact times when selecting a disinfectant: it may be able to kill certain organisms but may take up to 24 hours contact time to do its work.
- Use freshly made up solutions. Some disinfectants begin to deteriorate when made into solution with water. To ensure effectiveness, use only freshly made up solutions.
- Equipment and receptacles used with disinfectants should be thoroughly clean and rinsed before use. Any organic material present on them may reduce the effectiveness of the disinfectant.

It should also be noted that the efficiency of some disinfectants may be hindered by 'hard' water, some plastics and certain other materials. Read all the literature relating to the chemicals before use.

- All disinfectants should be thoroughly rinsed off once the contact time is completed, unless otherwise recommended.
- Always adhere to recommendations on product COSHH sheets. Specific use and precautions to be taken when using chemical disinfectants are stated on the COSHH sheet provided by the manufacturer.

It is essential that veterinary nurses understand the COSHH (Control of Substances Hazardous to Health) regulations introduced in 1989 and adhere to standard procedures (Chapter 11: Occupational Hazards).

Summary of routine procedure for cleaning and disinfection of kennels
  (1) Remove animal from kennel into a run or other secure holding area (not another dog's kennel).
  (2) Remove bed, bedding, toys etc.
  (3) Remove any gross soiling with shovel and scraper or similar equipment.
  (4) Hose out hair and any debris.
  (5) Scrub out with detergent.
  (6) Rinse with water.
  (7) Apply disinfectant.
  (8) Time contact.
  (9) Rinse thoroughly.
 (10) Dry (remove excess water with a 'squeegee' drier).
 (11) Leave to air dry.
 (12) Return/replace bedding as necessary.
 (13) Return animal to kennel.

ANTISEPTICS AND DISINFECTANTS

Product name	Active ingredients	Presentation and recommended use
Antiseptics: some examples in common use		
Hibiscrub Vet	Chlorhexidine gluconate.	Rapid bactericidal skin cleanser/surgical scrub. Solution.
Nolvasan Surgical Scrub	Chlorhexidine acetate.	Skin and wound cleanser. Solution.
Povidine Antiseptic Solution	Povidone-iodine.	Topical application, burns/wounds etc.
Savlon Vet Concentrate	Chlorhexidine gluconate Cetrimide.	Solution. Wounds (dilute), pre-op.
Disinfectants: some examples in common use		
Anprolene	Ethylene oxide.	Gas (in ampoules). Equipment sterilisation (in enclosed fume cupboard).
Cetavlon	Cetrimide (quaternary ammonium compounds).	Liquid concentrate. Environmental use and skin disinfectant.
Cidex	Glutaraldehyde.	Liquid concentrate. Environmental use.
Clearsol	Phenol compounds (clear soluble).	Liquid concentrate. Environmental use.
Chloros	Hypochlorites (bleaches).	Liquid concentrate. Environmental use and skin disinfectant.
Dettol	Chloroxylenol (chlorinated phenol).	Liquid concentrate. Environmental use and skin disinfectant.
Dinex Foam	Chlorhexidine gluconate 1%.	Foam. Pre-op. skin disinfection.
Dinex Scrub	Chlorexidine gluconate 4%.	Liquid concentrate. Pre-op. skin disinfection.
Domestos	Hypochlorites (bleaches).	Environmental use.
Formula H routine spray	Formaldehyde.	Spray. Environmental use.
Formula H Conc. Disinfectant	Formaldehyde.	Liquid concentrate. Environmental use.
Halamid	Sodium tosychloramide.	Skin and pre injection, hands, udder. Powder (concentrate). Environmental use.
Ibcol	Chloroxylenol. (Chlorinated phenol).	Liquid concentrate. Environmental use and skin disinfectant.
Izal	Phenol compound (white fluids).	Liquid concentrate. Environmental use.
Jeyes fluid	Phenol compound (black fluids).	Liquid concentrate. Environmental use.
Marinol Blue	sodiochloramide trithydrate Benzalkonium chloride	10% or 50% solution. Pre-op. instruments. Topical (diluted).
Parvocide	Glutaraldehyde Q.A.C.	Liquid concentrate. Environmental use.
Resiguard	Benzalkonium chloride plus picloxydine.	Liquid concentrate. Environmental use.
Roccal	Benzalkonium chloride.	Liquid concentrate. Environmental use and skin disinfectant.
Tego	Ampholytic surfactants.	Liquid concentrate. Environmental use.
Vet-cide	Tri-n-butyltinbenzoate, Formaldehyde, Isopropyl alcohol.	Liquid. Environmental use.
Virkon	Peroxides.	Powder (concentrate). Environmental use.

Fig. 5.18 Common disinfectants.

Detergent-type disinfectants are available which are designed to clean and disinfect in one application (with the help of physical scrubbing). They are often used in kennels for daily application where no disease problems exist, as they shorten the time of the whole process.

Cleaning and disinfection of kennel equipment

Equipment such as shovels, buckets, mops, dustpans and brushes, kitchen utensils, feed bowls, beds and bedding must all be cleaned and disinfected regularly.

Wash them first in detergent and water to remove any organic material. To disinfect, soak the equipment in a solution of disinfectant appropriate to the material (some items can be corroded by certain chemicals) at the manufacturer's recommended strength and for the recommended contact time. Then thoroughly rinse and dry the equipment before storing it. Bedding can be laundered in the normal way after disinfection.

Antiseptics and Disinfectants

The terms 'antiseptic' and 'disinfectant' are often used loosely when referring to chemical agents but they actually describe the chemical's action against micro-organisms.

DEFINITIONS
- **Disinfectant** This term describes a process that causes the removal or destruction of pathogenic organisms (not usually including bacterial spores) on inanimate objects. The result is **disinfection**. Methods of achieving disinfection include the use of chemicals and some physical processes such as boiling.
- **Antiseptics** are chemicals that cause the destruction or inhibition of micro-organisms, preventing their growth or multiplication, without damaging an animal's cells. Antiseptics applied topically have many uses, such as the treatment of wounds or the cleansing of the skin. Many applications contain antiseptic components and some are described in Fig. 5.18.
- **Skin disinfectants** are antiseptic preparations designed either for pre-operative skin cleansing or for use with inanimate objects.
- **Environmental disinfectants** are designed for use on inanimate objects only; many of them require the user to wear protective clothing and they should *never* be used on the skin.
- **Sterilisation** is the term applied when an inanimate object is rendered free from all micro-organisms, including bacterial spores, by their removal or destruction. This procedure must be used when the efficient destruction of all micro-organisms is vital, such as in the preparation of instruments for surgery. When selecting methods for destroying micro-organisms on inanimate objects, it is important to remember that a method producing sterilisation is far more satisfactory than one that produces disinfection.

Suffixes:
- **-cide** indicates that a chemical kills a particular type of micro-organism. For example, a bactericide kills bacteria; a fungicide kills fungi.
- **-stat** describes the action of a chemical that prevents or inhibits the growth of a particular type of micro-organism—a characteristic of some antiseptics. It is preferable to select a disinfectant with the ability to kill the micro-organism rather than one that merely prevents or inhibits its growth.

Selecting disinfectants and antiseptics

Figure 5.18 lists commonly used disinfectants, their main active ingredients and recommended uses (for detailed information regarding each product's suitability in veterinary practice, the manufacturer's data sheets should be read). The choice of product depends upon many factors but some of the main considerations are:

- The intended use of the product.
  —environmental (kennels, runs, equipment);
  —on living tissue (skin, wounds, body cavities etc.).
- The product's activity against specific micro-organisms.
- The contact time required.
- Known local conditions (e.g. water hardness).
- Safety of staff and animals (the product should be non-irritant, non-toxic and non-corrosive—check manufacturer's COSHH sheets for details of any hazards and for recommended suitable protective clothing for the user).
- Stability of the product in storage.
- Odours and smell (most products should be either odourless or with a pleasant aroma that is agreeable to staff and animals).
- Ease of use (it should disperse easily in water if dilution is required).
- Economy of use (assessed by cost per litre of ready-to-use solution).

It should be noted, for example, that:

- some products which are very effective for kennel disinfection will stain bedding and other porous materials;
- the presence of even relatively small amounts of organic material in water may affect some products;
- some animal species are sensitive to some types of disinfectant (e.g. cats are sensitive to phenol; and formalin vapour irritates many animals' eyes);
- strong odours or perfumes are offensive to some animals, promoting sneezing and irritation to the ocular mucous membranes.

Effectiveness. The action of the product against specific organisms should have been tested and the results should be available so that the user knows whether it is effective against organisms such as parvovirus, and at what dilution strength and contact time. Early tests, such as the Rideal–Walker and Chick–Martin, only give accurate results for phenolic disinfectants; more modern techniques such as the Kelsey–Sykes test are suitable for the assessment of most disinfectants.

The bacteria-killing capability of a disinfectant varies as some forms of bacteria are more resistant than others. The Gram-positive group are the most easily destroyed; the Gram-negative group, acid-fast group and bacterial spores are progressively more difficult to destroy. Disinfectants that have been found most effective against bacterial spores are the aldehydes, ethylene oxide and the halogens (to a lesser extent).

The literature for many disinfectants now available for use in kennels and catteries states that they are effective against certain important viral diseases of the dog and cat. Disinfectants known to destroy viruses include the hypochlorites. Glutaraldehyde is also effective but can be relatively slow-acting. Ampholytic surfactants will destroy some types of virus.

Many disinfectants are able to destroy fungal spores. The notable exceptions are pine oil fluid and quaternary ammonium compounds.

Disposal of Waste

All establishments, whether domestic or industrial, have to dispose of waste materials. Veterinary practices and commercial kennels are classed as industrial users for this purpose.

Since April 1992 the Environmental Protection Act 1990 imposed a 'duty of care' on the disposal of waste classed as Controlled Waste, of which there are three types: household, industrial and commercial. Of particular importance to the veterinary practice is the fact that some of the items in the Industrial class are further classified as Clinical Waste and it is essential that the veterinary nurse should be aware of items in

this category, with particular regard to methods of disposal and how they should be handled and stored prior to disposal. Figure 5.19 identifies items classed as clinical waste and their ultimate disposal.

Handling clinical waste

For the health and safety of staff and to comply with the regulations, clinical waste must be handled, segregated and disposed of with great care. It must be placed in yellow polythene bags marked 'For Incineration Only', with the name and origin of the waste. The specification is in 'The Safe Disposal of Clinical Waste' published by HMSO.

Disposal of clinical waste

All items classed as clinical waste must be disposed of by incineration in a licensed high-temperature incinerator. These incinerators must conform to the regulations regarding clean discharge into the atmosphere.

As clinical waste is classed as Industrial Waste, the duty to arrange for it to be collected and correctly disposed of is with the person who controls it—the veterinary practice is responsible, not the local authority. Some local authorities do offer a service for the disposal of clinical waste but licensed contractors must be used where this service does not exist. The collection and disposal of clinical waste incurs a charge if collected by either the local authority or licensed contractors.

In the veterinary context, clinical waste includes carcasses. The veterinary profession has the 'duty of care' for the disposal of dead dogs and cats. The advice of the Department of Environment is that pets which die on veterinary premises remain the property of the owner and may then be disposed of by the owner within the 'curtilage' of their own dwelling in their capacity of a private individual without breach of the veterinarian's 'duty of care'. Bereaved owners may wish to take bodies home with them for disposal (see Chapter 8).

CHART OF THE SUBSTANCES THAT COMPRISE CLINICAL WASTE AND WHAT IS DONE WITH IT		
Sharps. Needles, syringes, broken glass, scalpel blades, etc.	Waste containing blood, body fluids, excretions, drugs. Swabs and dressings, blood/body fluids.	Non-agricultural animal carcasses and animal tissue. Non-domestic kennel excreta and bedding.
Unless rendered safe is Clinical waste.		
Pre disposal handling		
Sharps. Approved sharps container (sealed).	Swabs and soiled disposable bedding. Kennel excrement. Approved yellow containers or bags identifiable (with name and source of waste) prior to collection.	Cadavers. May be deep frozen for storage prior to collection.
Collection by local authority or licenced contractors. All clinical waste is destroyed by high temperature incinerator, licenced for this use.		

Fig. 5.19. Clinical waste and its disposal.

If an animal has suffered from an infectious disease, however, or for any other reason may be significantly hazardous, then it should be dealt with by the veterinarian as clinical waste and disposed of by licensed incineration.

Non-clinical practice waste

Non-clinical waste is classed as domestic waste. This includes empty food cans, outer packaging and office waste. (All confidential records should be shredded prior to disposal.) Domestic waste continues to be collected regularly by the local authority. Normal 'day-to-day' deposits of pet owners' dog faeces are also classed as refuse rather than clinical waste. Black plastic bags are commonly used for the refuse that is not classified as clinical waste.

Animal Care

Daily Care of Hospitalised Animals

The specific requirements in the care of hospitalised animals depend to some degree on the conditions under treatment. Figure 5.20 suggests a care routine.

Defecation and urination

Dogs. The opportunity to defecate and urinate is sometimes referred to as 'relief' and sometimes as 'exercise'. Most hospitalised dogs require restricted exercise but frequent opportunities to relieve themselves. It is therefore less confusing to refer to 'opportunity for relief' rather than 'exercise' in this context.

All dogs should be taken to a run and given frequent opportunities for relief, unless they are not mobile or movement is contraindicated by their condition. It is important not to leave a dog so long that it is forced to urinate or defecate in its kennel, which would cause considerable distress to normally clean house-trained dogs.

When the dog is taken to a run, its gait and general body stance should be noted. When it passes urine and faeces, any difficulty should be noted along with the appearance and the amount passed.

Reluctance to urinate or defecate in kennel runs. A reluctant dog should not be returned to its kennel until every effort has been made to encourage it to urinate and defecate. This is particularly important if the dog has been confined for a long period (such as overnight) and has not soiled its kennel.

Some dogs are reluctant to relieve themselves with the handler in close proximity. If so, retire a suitable distance to observe. If the dog is still reluctant, it may be unused to defecating on a hard surface such as concrete or slabs (as described in the discussion on kennel design earlier in this chapter). These dogs may be used to relieving on grass or soil surfaces, and it may need a little ingenuity to encourage them. Initial effort will ensure less stress to the dog and will save time for the handler on future occasions as the dog should relieve itself without delay once it understands the routine:

• Put some sawdust or peat on a small area at the end of a run and then praise the dog when it urinates or defecates there, so that it understands that this is the right place. The sawdust or peat can be lifted along with any urine or faeces and the run cleaned as normal.

CARE ROUTINE FOR HOSPITALISED ANIMALS	
Check	**Care routine**
General check	All animals are inspected briefly by touring the kennels/cages. This is to establish that there are no urgent problems that require immediate attention.
Individual checks	Each individual should be looked at for some time, noting the behaviour of the animal compared with its normal e.g. whether it is lively, aggressive, unresponsive.
	Its posture should be noted – whether it is standing, lying down or in an abnormal position.
Observe respiration	This should be done before the animal is disturbed.
Pulse and temperature	The animal's pulse and temperature may be taken (before exercise).
Soiling etc.	Check for soiling of kennel, and record details of quantity and type of eliminations. If the animal has urinated or defecated note if it is normal. If the animal has vomited note the appearance or amount, assess what has been eaten and record the observation before removing it.
	It is not usual practice to leave food with dogs overnight except in the case of difficult or shy feeders. It is more frequently necessary to leave food in with cats, as overnight is often the only time that some hospitalised cats will eat.
Check the water bowl	Note how much has been taken and if any spilling has occurred (if there is spilling the assessment of intake will be inaccurate.)
Physical check on patient	Any abnormalities should be noted and recorded. Wounds may be inspected.
	Any discharges should be gently removed.

Fig. 5.20. Care routine for hospitalised animals.

If this ploy fails, it may be necessary to walk the dog for some distance and then 'leash relieve' it on grass. However, this is not generally recommended as it is unhygienic: grass cannot be disinfected. (Dogs with suspected infectious disease should never be relieved on an area that cannot be adequately _isinfected.)

Cats. All hospitalised cats should be provided with a litter tray unless their condition contraindicates. Clean the tray regularly and record the presence and characteristics of the faeces and urine produced. If the tray is not cleaned frequently enough, some cats are so fastidious that they will not reuse the tray but will soil elsewhere in the kennel.

Some cats prefer privacy, which can be provided by covering the litter tray with an upturned box with an entrance hole cut into it.

Feeding

All animals should be observed when feeding to check that they are eating normally and without difficulty.

Each animal should have the same feed and water bowls throughout its stay to reduce the possibility of cross-infection. The bowls can be labelled or numbered to identify them with the kennel or animal.

Medication

Adhere strictly to any specific medication times, as instructed by the veterinary surgeon. Keep up-to-date records of all medication given.

Where medication has been given with food, check that the food has been consumed.

Weighing

All dogs should be weighed on entry to the hospital and weekly thereafter. This is important with long-stay animals to ensure that the feeding and exercise regime maintains the dog's condition and that any loss of weight due to illness is monitored and reported.

Grooming of hospitalised animals

Every effort should be made to keep hospitalised animals in a hygienic and comfortable condition. The grooming of hospitalised dogs should be carried out as part of their general nursing care, unless their condition contraindicates it (e.g. an animal admitted for warfarin poisoning should not be handled vigorously—see Chapter 3, First Aid).

Grooming as Part of Normal Animal Care

There are various reasons why grooming is beneficial and all of them can be placed broadly under five headings:

- **C**leanliness.
- **H**ealth.
- **A**ppearance.
- **I**nspection.
- **R**elationship.

The initial letters of these headings form a useful memory aid: CHAIR.

Cleanliness

Keeping the animal clean by the removal of dirt and discharge and assisting in the casting of hair contributes towards the animal's health and well-being. At home, the regular grooming of dogs and cats reduces the amount of hair deposited on furniture and carpets.

It is important that animals with dense or long coats are groomed regularly, as their coats rapidly become tangled, matted and soiled.

Health

By keeping the animal's coat clean, grooming assists the condition of the skin and hair and thus contributes to the animal's health:

- Grooming stimulates anagen (the hair growth stage) by the removal of dead, shedding hairs.
- The removal of discharge and prevention of matting prevents skin irritation.
- The close inspection of the animal during grooming assists in early problem recognition.
- During grooming, daily care and attention to any bony prominences, skin folds, feet and claws, eyes and ears, mouth and teeth, anus, vulva and prepuce contribute to the health of the animal.

Appearance

Owners usually give this as the first reason for grooming, though it is the least important for the animal itself. Many owners take a pride in the appearance of their animals—and this becomes very apparent when a post-operative animal with large areas of denuded skin is returned to an owner who was not forewarned. Owners of pedigree dogs often want their pets to look like the breed as seen at championship dog shows and this means that many dogs are trimmed and clipped by professional groomers, a practice that also assists the owner's daily grooming of the dog. The appearance of the true show dog is of major concern to its owner and show preparation often involves hours of careful grooming and trimming or clipping.

The veterinary nurse needs to appreciate this emphasis on appearance: many owners, rightly or wrongly, judge the standard of care at the practice or kennels by the appearance of the animal when it is returned to them.

Inspection

The daily inspection of an animal during the grooming routine contributes to its health by giving an opportunity for early recognition of problems. For example, flea excreta will only be discovered on close examination of the coat. It is recommended that inspection is carried out in a logical daily sequence so that any problems found can be attended to before further damage or discomfort is caused to the animal during the actual grooming.

Relationship and contact

This may seem a strange reason for grooming, but for the dog in the wild state grooming is part of pack socialisation activities. Dogs lower in the pack order submit to grooming by a more dominant member, while dominant dogs make it clear whether or not they consent to being groomed by other members of the pack. When dogs are groomed by their handlers, the activity strengthens the bond between them and confirms to the dog its place in the hierachy: the handler is the 'pack leader'. The act of grooming, therefore, should assist in the handling and training of the dog.

Grooming can also assist in teaching a dog to sit or stand still whilst the procedure is carried out, which will be of great assistance for veterinary examinations. If a dog resents grooming for no physical reason, it is likely to prove generally difficult to handle.

Introducing an animal to grooming

Ideally the process of grooming should be introduced (to all domesticated species) at a very young age as part of socialisation and habituation. Even short-haired puppies and kittens should be handled each day and introduced gently to brushes and combs. The experience should be made pleasant for the animal, with praise given for good behaviour but a firm tone if the animal struggles.

As with all training, grooming should be carried out for a few minutes at a time at first and gradually built up as the animal becomes accustomed to it. Each session should end on a successful note with the animal being praised for compliance.

Owners of long-haired animals should in particular be advised that time spent in the early stages of ownership will ensure that the animal is easier to groom in later years and is less likely to be presented at the practice for de-matting when an owner is unable to groom the pet because it objects, struggles or even attempts to bite.

Routine grooming

Routine grooming is part of the daily care of a normal healthy animal but the veterinary nurse can be faced with quite a problem as there are so many different types of coat. In addition, various factors have a direct effect on the coat and it is necessary to have a broad understanding of them so that the coat can be correctly maintained while the animal is in the nurse's care and so that owners' queries regarding grooming at home can be answered. It can be seen from Fig. 5.21 that the major factors affecting hair growth include:

- Environmental temperature and time of year
- Health
- Endocrine and reproductive status
- Feeding and nutrition.

The type of coat is governed by combinations of individual hair types that make up the coat. These are the rigid primary or 'guard' hairs and the soft, thinner secondary or 'lanugo' hairs. The various proportions, lengths and weights of these hair types account for the many and varied types of coat seen in dogs and cats (Fig. 5.22).

Grooming equipment and methods

A fairly wide range of attention and equipment is required to deal with the various types of coat. For the routine maintenance grooming of patients and boarders, it is advisable to stock a range of basic grooming equipment (Figs 5.23 and 5.24).

Although different coats require different attention, a logical general sequence can be adopted for all common breeds to ensure that nothing is missed out during the grooming session:

(1) Assess the animal's temperament.
(2) Carry out a physical inspection of the animal (Fig. 5.25).
(3) Loosen dead hair.
(4) Comb, brush and finish (Fig. 5.26).

De-matting

Sometimes the coat of a long-haired animal has been so grossly neglected and become so matted that it would be unkind to try to de-mat it while the animal is conscious. The neglect may have arisen because the animal has been so difficult to groom when conscious anyway.

In such cases the veterinary surgeon might sedate or anaesthetise the animal and request the veterinary nurse to 'de-mat' it. This should be carried out with great care: it is very easy to cut the skin and scissors should not be used by unskilled nurses. Cats are especially at risk when hair lumps are cut away .

Clipping and trimming

Under normal circumstances a nurse is unlikely to be involved in the long-term maintenance of a coat that

HAIR GROWTH	
Factors	The average rate of hair growth in the dog is 0.5mm per day. An average smooth-coat type takes about 6 months to regrow completely. Fine, silky long-haired coats taking up to 18 months; a similar growth rate can be expected in cats.

Environmental temperature and time of year	Dogs kept in housing with constantly high environmental temperatures, (usually centrally heated) will often shed hair almost continuously throughout the year but with noticeable increases in spring and autumn. Shedding in dogs kennelled out of doors or with less environmental heating tends to be more obviously seasonal – shedding is very noticeable in spring and autumn. This seasonal coat change is a natural process triggered by increasing day length in spring and decreasing day length in autumn.
	Spring = increasing day length
	      Production of summer coat triggered
	      Increased hair shedding (shedding winter coat)
	      Coarser coat with reduced density
	plus
	      Increased sebaceous gland activity
	        = Summer coat
	      Allowing increased air circulation through coat
	Autumn = decreasing day length
	      Production of winter coat triggered
	      Increased hair shedding (of summer coat)
	plus
	      New coat growth and reduced sebaceous gland activity
	        = Winter coat
	Increased coat density = Insulating against the cold.

Health and reproductive status	Condition can often be assessed by observing the coat and noting any unseasonal loss or thinning of hair. Thinning during periods of ill health is due to interruption of the growth cycle: fewer individual hairs are in the growth stage. An animal suffering from ill health may also have a dull and harsh coat. The reproductive status of an animal can have an effect on the coat growth and this can be quite obvious during pregnancy and lactation and occasionally after neutering. These and other so-called hormonal alopecias usually involve thinning of hair on certain areas of the body.
Feeding and nutrition	Diet affects hair growth, as it does all other functions. Nutrients essential for good health of skin and hair include amino acids, essential fatty acids, zine, iodine etc. (Chapter 17: Nutrition).

Fig. 5.21. Factors affecting hair growth and type.

COAT TYPES		
Coat	**Type**	**Example**
Most coat types can be divided into five broad groups for the purpose of grooming:		
1. Smooth coat	Short fine Intermediate or Coarse dense	Boxer, Dachsund, Chihuahua German shepherd dog, Pembroke corgi. Wild dogs and wolves have this coat type and it is therefore sometimes referred to as a normal coat.
2. Wire coat		Wire haired terriers.
3. Double coat		Rough collie, long haired German shepherd dog.
4. Silky coat	medium long fine	Most spaniels, setters and some retrievers. Afghan hounds, Bearded collies.
5. Woolly coat		Poodle, Bedlington terrier, Curly-coated retriever, Irish water spaniel.
There are some more unusual or specialised coat types, such as corded coats. Where animals with such coats are under the nurse's care, a professional groomer or the individual breed society should be contacted for specific advice if the owner is unable to provide details on coat maintenance.		

Fig. 5.22. Coat types.

requires clipping or trimming. However, it is essential that all those who care for hospitalised animals should know how to look after a variety of coat types.

The routine clipping or trimming of some areas in long-haired dogs will assist in maintaining cleanliness but care should be taken not to take the scissors to an animal without its owner's consent—it may be a pedigree show dog, which needs experienced clipping and trimming.

The clipping, hand stripping and trimming of specific breeds is generally within the realms of the professional dog groomer and showing kennel. Interested veterinary nurses can attend special courses on this art but in general practice it is more usual for a nurse to clip or trim a pet dog at its

GROOMING EQUPMENT FOR DOGS AND CATS		
	Types	**Features and use**
Brushes	Pin brush	Metal pins with rounded ends, mounted on a rubber back cushion. If used correctly, cannot break or pull out hair. The straight pins are able to be used more effectively than bristle with silky coats. Used for general grooming-out of silky and double coats and on feathering. Used to separate hairs and smooth and lay the coat. The action assists in promoting a smooth shine by distributing natural oils. Not so useful for tangled coats (a comb should be used first).
	Bristle brush	Often wooden or plastic with natural or synthetic bristles, with or without a handle. Denser than pin brushes and less able to brush through thick coats to achieve hair separation. Used for removal of dirt and debris. As the bristles are flexible, can be used with more pressure: flicks dirt deep in the coat on to the surface and then removes it with the following brush action. To remove dirt and debris from most types of coat, is most commonly used for routine grooming of short-coated breeds. For short coats it can be used fairly vigorously on the animal's back, sides, hindquarters and shoulders.
	Slicker brush	One-way hooked pins on a rubber pad. Stiff and softer pinned varieties are available. The hooks assist in pulling out dead hair. The action can be quite fierce and care should be taken with its use. Pressure should not be used as the hooks easily damage the dog's skin. Usually designed for one-way use only, towards the handle; the operator pulls the brush through the coat. Very useful for removing dead hair clogging coats and can be used to break up some coat tangles. Commonly used in the grooming of dogs with silky coats (especially feathering), wire, woolly and double coats.
	Hound glove	Designed to fit over the hand; flexible, with either short wire or plastic bristles, small plastic projections or a velvet surface or similar type of material. Often double sided with short bristles one side and velvet on the opposite side. As the glove is flexible it allows palm pressure and vigorous use (heavy pressure and vigorous use should be avoided with wire bristle types). Can be used to assist moulting by removing dead hair, with the smooth velvet side being used to promote a shine. Commonly used for the routine grooming of short-coated breeds.
Combs	Metal combs	Two types of comb commonly used for dog grooming: handle and non-handle comb. Both are ridged combs with metal roundend teeth, available in various tooth widths depending on density of coats being groomed. Handle comb has one size of teeth at one end and handle at the other. Easier to use for a longer period than a non-handle comb. Advantage of a non-handle comb is that it usually has two widths of teeth on the one comb. The combs are used only with the lay of the hair, at approximately 45° angle. Used for removing dead hair and the selective grooming of longer hair behind ears in silky coats etc. Also used for de-tangling and breaking up small matts.
	Rake	Ridged metal teeth with rounded ends set perpendicular to the handle. Designed to achieve a greater pull through dense coats. Great care should be used with the rake as damage can easily be inflicted on the dog's skin. Commonly used with dense coats for removal of dead undercoat and breaking up and removal of some small matts (with great care).
	De-matting comb	Specialised teeth, rounded and blunt on one side with sharp blades on the opposite side of each tooth. Substantial handle and thumb grip. Only used to cut out mats; it is a much safer way to remove mats than by the use of scissors. Used by placing blunt side towards the animal's skin and drawing the sharp edge against the mat, thus cutting and breaking up the mat for removal. Allows the maximum amount of coat to be preserved once the mat is removed.
Scissors	Trimming scissors	Long very sharp blades tapering to a point. Different sizes available. Used to trim neatly around the edges of ears, etc.
	Toe scissors	Short blades with blunt ends. Used to trim delicate areas between toes, etc.
	Thinning scissors	Specialised blades cut small amounts of hair and leave an equal amount uncut at intervals with easy use. The hair is thinned by this action without leaving 'steps' in the coat. Used anywhere the coat requires thinning to enhance features, e.g. the shoulders, sides of chest.

Fig. 5.23. Grooming and trimming equipment.

owner's request because the animal is difficult or impossible to groom. This may be due to the animal's temperament, or because the dog is elderly or infirm with perhaps an elderly owner. In the latter case, trimming or clipping may be carried out as part of a geriatric care policy (for the dog, that is). Where temperament is the problem, it is usually necessary to sedate the dog or, in extreme cases, to anaesthetise it as already discussed for de-matting.

In general practice, then, the veterinary nurse needs to know how to use common equipment for trimming or clipping a dog neatly and tidily. The regular trimming of some types of coat assists grooming and general hygiene, while clipping can assist in grooming by keeping the coat short enough to be managed easily.

Trimming is carried out with special scissors (Fig. 5.23). Areas that are commonly trimmed to assist in

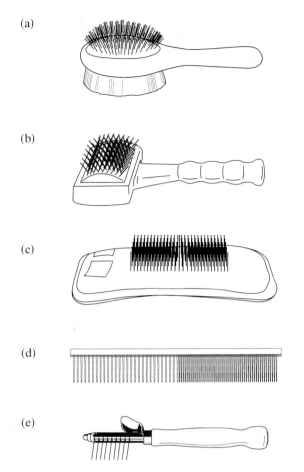

(a)

(b)

(c)

(d)

(e)

Fig. 5.24 Grooming equipment: (a) double-sided grooming brush (pins and bristles); (b) slicker brush; (c) hound glove; (d) metal grooming comb; (e) dematting comb.

grooming are those prone to matting or collection of soiling in breeds such as some spaniels and setters. This includes the ears, to avoid the collection of food when eating, and the matting of the long silky hair just behind the ears. Feet are trimmed particularly between the toes, where mud can collect and dry on the hair so that it causes discomfort by rubbing and by pushing the toes apart. In bitches, it may be necessary to trim soiled areas post-whelping if soiling and staining from whelping fluid cannot be removed easily any other way.

If a dog soils itself or mats easily, grooming will be simplified if hair is judiciously trimmed from the anal area and hindleg feathering—but do not be scissor-happy. Strike a balance between the need to keep the dog hygienic and the owner's need for the dog's appearance to be acceptable.

Clipping is by means of special clippers. There are set styles of clip designed to enhance breed features; for example, some of the hair of terrier breeds is removed or thinned out by professional hand-stripping. Non-showing owners of breeds with long, heavy coats such as the Old English sheep dog will have their animals clipped out for the summer. Dogs such as poodles do not moult normally and it is essential to clip the coat regularly, otherwise it would become unmanageable for the owner and would cause discomfort and distress to the dog.

Clippers should only be used according to the manufacturer's instructions as they are easily damaged by misuse. For example, the hair must be completely dry, as wet hair quickly blunts the blades. The blades should not be forced through a thick coat or matting as they may be clogged by the hair and stop the machine, possibly causing damage to the equipment. If the clippers become hot during use, they should be allowed to cool down before continuing.

Clipping machines should be regularly serviced and maintained. They need to be thoroughly cleaned and oiled after each use and then stored in a dry environment. A variety of blades should be available, with spares of those used most commonly to enable a rotation for regular sharpening.

Bathing

Bathing is carried out for three main reasons:

- To eradicate and control ectoparasites.
- To treat skin conditions and apply topical medication.
- To cleanse and condition the coat.

Cleansing may be required for various reasons, such as:

- The coat is soiled with a substance that cannot be removed by normal grooming.
- To remove odours (e.g. when a dog has rolled in excreta).
- To assist in the removal and masking of the scent from a bitch just out of season who is still receiving the attention of male dogs.
- To improve the appearance of the coat before a show.

Shampoo

There are many products for shampooing dogs. Some are generally available; others (for specialised medical or antiparasitic use) are only available by prescription. The preparations fall into three categories:

- Insecticidal (to eradicate and control parasites, most commonly fleas, lice and ticks).
- Medicated (containing some form of antiseptic or other active ingredient and prescribed for dogs with minor skin problems).
- Cleansing (general purpose, or also for conditioning).

The latter category includes those most widely used—shampoos for general coat cleansing. A conditioning agent is often added to improve the hair texture by lubrication, so that the coat is more manageable for brushing out when dry.

PHYSICAL INSPECTION OF THE ANIMAL BEFORE GROOMING	
Aims	Method
Assess the state of the animal's coat and therefore the need for the use of non-routine equipment such as the de-matting comb. Assess the state of the animal's health. This is very important as it ensures close observation of the animal so that lesions normally obscured by the coat are found prior to the use of any equipment that may cause injury to the animal. (It is too late to find a wart once you have stuck the comb in it causing it to bleed!)	The inspection should be carried out in a logical sequence, checking the dog from head to tail, checking closely both visually and by running the hands carefully over the animal. Areas requiring special attention, particularly with elderly or hospitalised animals, include: Mouth, teeth, gums and lip folds. Eyes and ears – discharges wiped away with clean damp cotton wool. In some breeds the long hair on the ears (and face) may gather food whilst the animal is eating. This should be removed by washing. Either trim the hair carefully to prevent recurrence; or, for a pedigree breed where this long hair is a feature, make a note to use a 'snood' when feeding the dog (these hold the long hair and ears back during feeding and are often used for Afghan hounds) or a narrow but deep feeding bowl that allows the long hair and ears to fall on each side of the bowl and not in the food. Hocks and elbows – any pressure sores noted and attended to (improve bedding and apply white petroleum jelly if there is hard skin but no sign of breaks in the skin). Foot pads – may be cracking, or in dogs that pace about continually in hard surfaced runs they may be reddened and thin due to the abrasive action. Claws – these should be checked for injury and condition (e.g. they may be overgrown when a dog has restricted exercise or is walked on grass). Some dogs that have a long-term abnormal gait may wear their claws unevenly, resulting in the need to trim some of the claws on a regular basis. Body orifices – Anus, vulva and prepuce may require the regular removal of discharges/soiling. With long-haired animals it may be necessary to trim or clip away some of the surrounding hair to allow easier cleaning of these areas. Any treatment or attention to any abnormalities found should be dealt with at this stage.

Fig. 5.25. Physical inspection routine before grooming.

Specialised shampoos are available from the pet trade for different types of coat. The two most notable are the 'mild' shampoo for puppies and dogs with sensitive skins, and 'colour enhancing' shampoos for particular coats, such as products containing optical whiteners for white coats.

Note that if the shampoo is in a glass bottle the amount required should be decanted into a plastic cup or a similar small, unbreakable receptacle before bathing commences. A small amount of water may be added to the shampoo at this stage so that it is easier to distribute when applied to the dog's coat.

Dog baths

The ideal dog bath should:

- allow the handler to get the dog in and out of the bath easily but also to contain the dog safely, deterring escape;
- allow access to all parts of the dog being bathed without the handler having to bend or reach excessively;
- have a non-slip area for the animal to stand on, with the surrounding area also non-slip for the safety of the handler;
- have a flexible shower hose with a spray head;
- have easily adjustable water and heat controls;
- have an easily cleaned surface allowing access for cleaning all parts of the bath.

Many specially designed dog baths are available from the pet trade but in some small establishments, where the bathing of dogs is not carried out

regularly, it is possible to modify other installations—for example non-slip mats can be added to a shower cubicle in which the floor has been raised and the shower-hose and controls lowered, or the mats can be added to a bath designed for a disabled person and fitted with a shower-hose.

The domestic bath. Clients who bath their dogs in a domestic bath should always be advised to use a non-slip mat and that they should not put the plug in the bath. An inexpensive mixer shower-hose can be fitted to the bath taps. Clients should be warned that some modern domestic baths scratch easily and can be damaged by the claws of a scrambling dog.

Drying the dog. Several towels are needed to dry a dog after it has been bathed. It is always advisable to put out at least two extra ones, to save having to search for more towels while a half-dry dog shakes itself and distributes water all around the bathing area.

The number of towels needed can be reduced by first using a synthetic chamois cloth to remove excess water. This can be wrung out several times and reused before towels finish the drying off.

Dogs that are bathed regularly may be familiar with hair-driers but these can frighten a dog that is new to the experience. Never blow the drier towards the dog's face. Instead, blow towards the hind end from the front, moving towards the rear and directing the hot air along the hair shaft, not directly at the skin. Continuously test the heat by keeping a hand in

GROOMING PROCEDURES	
Procedure	**Aim**
Loosening the dead hair	Most coats will benefit from the groomer pulling the fingertips along the skin through the coat against the lay of the hair. This will help to loosen the dead hair and therefore stimulate normal hair growth. Dogs tend to find this procedure pleasant and some will get excited and see it as a game, so firm but friendly handling is required to insist that the dog stays fairly still.
Combing	Using a traditional comb, any tangles can be eased out gently and any loose hair removed from the coat at this stage. The comb is used with the lay of the hair at an angle usually about 45°. Particular attention should be paid to areas on the longer haired breeds that have a tendency to tangle and mat such as behind the ears and feathering between and on the backs of the hindlegs. As the comb is more accurate than a brush and is usually smaller it can be used with care on areas that are difficult to assess, ensuring that no areas are missed or tangles remain underneath a superficially groomed coat. If mats are found during combing and they are not able to be removed or teased out gently during a traditional comb, then a specialised de-matting comb can be used where appropriate to remove the mat, followed by a combing out of the remaining hair gently with the traditional comb. Where a mat has been removed it is important to check the skin underneath it for damage as the area may be reddened or even suppurating. If the mat has caused irritation to the skin, this should be dealt with, depending on the severity.
Brushing	This is carried out with a brush type depending upon the coat, the action of brushing depends on the brush. Exercise great care when grooming with pin or slicker brushes, as it is possible to damage the skin with some types if used too vigorously. It is not generally advisable to use this type of brush against the lay of the hair. For a smooth coat of the intermediate type the following brushing technique could be adopted: Once the combing is complete a bristly brush can be used. Firstly it is used on the hair covering the trunk. The brush is used against the lay of the hair in short straight strokes. This is begun at the base of the tail and thighs and moves gradually forward as each area is brushed. The brushing against the lay stops at the back of the head and at the base of the skull, leaving the head untouched at this stage. The brush is then used gently on the head with the lay of the hair and thereafter working downwards and backwards with short straight strokes, until the entire body and legs has been brushed. Taking hold of the tail, gently but firmly brush carefully from base to tip. Care is required when grooming tails as many dogs are quite sensitive about their tails being groomed and some may react sharply to all but the most gentle brushing. During the brushing phase the brush should be periodically cleaned to remove any build up of hair. This can be done by drawing a traditional comb through the bristles.
Finishing	After combing and brushing a smooth or silky medium type of coat can be finished off by using a damp cloth or smooth hound glove (or a piece of velvet of damp synthetic chamois cloth). The face is gently wiped over followed by the remainder of the body, working from front to back. This action smooths down the coat and removes stray hair and dust from the coat surface. Giving a sleek shine to a healthy coat. This is not done generally with coats that are of the woolly or wire coat type, as these are usually required to stand up and are brushed into shape and left.

Fig. 5.26. Grooming procedures.

front of the air jet at the approximate distance of the dog's skin. The same hand can assist the drying process by lifting the dog's hair, running the fingers through to ruffle the coat.

The dog should be sitting comfortably. Panting or shivering would indicate distress or discomfort.

Protective clothing

It should be standard practice for the handler to wear protective clothing when bathing a dog. It not only keeps the handler's clothes dry but may also be required for safety. The usual clothing is:

- Waterproof overall or apron.
- Water-resistant boots or shoes with non-slip soles.
- Protective gloves where suggested by a shampoo manufacturer. (Those who have sensitive skin may prefer to wear protective gloves anyway.)

Handling and restraint for bathing

All dogs must be adequately restrained during bathing. A large wet dog leaping out of a bath can injure both itself and handler, and back injuries are not uncommon. A collar and lead, or nylon slip-lead, should be looped over the handler's arm so that it is readily accessible if restraint is required. With a large or boisterous dog, it is advisable to have a second person to steady or restrain it.

> WARNINGS
> - A dog should never be encouraged or allowed to jump in or out of the bath at any time, as it may easily slip on a wet surface and injure itself.
> - A dog should never be left unattended in a bath, as it may try to jump out, injuring itself if it slips.
> - A dog should never be tied up in the bath as it could leap over the side and strangle itself in a few seconds while the handler reaches away.

Where there are no steps for the dog to be encouraged to walk into the bath, it will require to be lifted. With large dogs, this should be carried out by two people for safety.

Bathing procedure

The procedure for bathing dogs depends to some extent on the reason for the bath. The following is a general procedure for coat cleansing:

(1) Know why the dog is being bathed.
(2) Assess the dog's temperament and arrange assistance if necessary.
(3) Assemble all the equipment and prepare the bathing area.
(4) Put on protective clothing.
(5) Bring the dog into the bathing area and encourage it up steps into the bath, or lift it in (with help if needed).
(6) Reassure the dog and start water flow away from the dog, running the water over a hand until a constant acceptable temperature is maintained.
(7) Carefully apply the water, soaking the dog well but taking care not to alarm it. Protect the dog's eyes with a hand and do not spray water directly on to its face.
(8) Apply shampoo sparingly to the entire coat but avoid sensitive areas such as the face, or into the vulva or sheath. (If the head requires particular attention due to a medical condition, protect the eyes by applying a bland eye ointment or smearing the lids with petroleum jelly.)
(9) Massage shampoo into the coat, or use as directed (e.g. leave it on for the recommended time before rinsing).
(10) Rinse thoroughly, starting at the upper front and moving in a downwards and backwards sequence so that every part is thoroughly rinsed.
(11) Squeeze out excess water; then remove as much water as possible with a synthetic chamois leather cloth, squeezing it out as necessary and reapplying.
(12) Remove the dog from the bath, either by encouraging it to step out or by lifting it carefully.
(13) Towel-dry.
(14) Use hair-drier if it is safe to do so (keep electric driers away from risk of contact with water) and if the dog's temperament permits.
(15) Return the dog to a warm kennel to avoid chilling.
(16) Record that the bath has been carried out, stating what shampoo has been used.

Dental Care (Oral Maintenance)

Dental disease is one of the most common problems seen in veterinary practice and the veterinary nurse is increasingly involved with client education in this respect. Many owners of show animals have been carrying out some form of teeth-cleaning for cosmetic reasons for some years but the routine brushing of pets' teeth as part of the daily grooming procedure has been overlooked by most pet owners until quite recently. Changes in the consistency of petfood have led to a greater need for routine teeth-cleaning, which is now recognised as necessary for dental health and therefore referred to correctly as 'oral maintenance'. For optimum results, all teeth should be cleaned daily.

Introducing a animal to the oral maintenance procedure

Advice regarding the method of cleaning teeth and the introduction of an animal to the procedure is offered by the manufacturers of the various products that are now widely available. Some general considerations are as follows:

- Before attempting oral maintenance, always assess the temperament of the animal and handle accordingly but always proceed with caution.
- As with all training it is better (where possible) to begin by simulating the procedure while the animal is still very young, so that it becomes accustomed to being handled in this way.
- The experience should be as pleasant as possible for the animal.
- Always reward good behaviour but be firm if the animal struggles or misbehaves.
- Exercise patience and do not try to proceed too quickly. Initially, do not expect the animal to tolerate the brushing for more than a few minutes at a time.
- Incorporate short rest breaks into the routine to avoid the animal becoming uncomfortable and restless.

Practical application. Begin by gently handling the animal's mouth daily and praising good behaviour. Increase the handling time to 5 minutes or so after a few days.

Once the animal tolerates the handling, hold its mouth closed with one hand, opening the mouth on one side, and gently rub the teeth with a finger of the other hand. When this stage is tolerated, use a toothbrush on a few teeth and increase the number brushed as the animal becomes accustomed to the experience.

When the animal has accepted brushing of the outside of its teeth, gently pull its top jaw upwards to open its mouth. Gently introduce the brush into the mouth to clean the inner surfaces of the teeth, again increasing the number brushed as the animal becomes accustomed to the procedure. Finger-stall toothbrushes are useful for cleaning the inside of dogs' teeth.

Clipping Claws

The average healthy animal does not usually require attention to its claws which, under normal circumstances, wear naturally with everyday use—with the notable exception of the 'dew claw' (though this claw tends to be slow growing). Dogs that have dew claws should be checked regularly for signs of abnormal length or the claw curling into the skin.

Where disease, injury or any type of immobility occurs, the claws may overgrow. This can lead to further immobility if the claws have grown to such an extent that they prevent or restrict the animal's normal gait. In extreme cases the claws may be so long that they curl around and begin to grow in towards the foot pad, causing the animal discomfort or even pain if the skin is penetrated.

Where animals do require some attention, the problem usually arises in one of the following categories:

- Animals that are only exercised on soft ground. (Dogs exercised on grass only, particularly very lightweight ones, are more likely to require claw-clipping than those that do a lot of road work or use concrete or similar runs daily.)
- Animals whose normal behaviour or exercise is restricted by their housing and management. (This includes most small mammals kept as pets—the problems of rabbits and budgerigars, for example, are discussed in Chapter 4.)
- Elderly animals that are unable to exercise normally. (Dogs that are stiff or generally less active due to old age are more likely to require regular attention to their claws.)
- Dogs with immobilised fractured limbs. (The nails will not wear on the injured limb and therefore need to be trimmed while the leg is immobile.)
- Animals with injury or disease conditions of the foot or nail. (The claws of a foot affected by disease, such as fungal infection of the nail bed, may need to be trimmed. A nail that is partly broken off will need to be trimmed.)

- Previous injury to the foot or leg causing abnormal gait. (Previous injuries such as fractures or damaged tendons may cause a change in the normal gait, leading to uneven wearing of some of the claws.)
- Puppies in the nest. (The claws of nursing pups are very sharp and grow rapidly, and the bitch's glands can become very sore from their scratches. To prevent or reduce damage to the lactating bitch, clip the puppies' claws weekly.)
- Animals causing damage to owners' property. (Cat owners often request claw-clipping when a pet damages their furniture. Waterbeds are especially at risk. However, clipping of cat claws is a controversial issue and only of very short-term usefulness in this situation. Instead, owners should be encouraged to provide scratching-posts.)

Equipment

Essential equipment for claws includes clippers suitable for the size and thickness of the claw. There are various types available. They should be kept sharp and in good working order and should always be used as recommended by the manufacturer.

In case bleeding occurs due to inadvertent cutting of the quick, have cotton wool to hand and a silver nitrate pencil (to be applied with care).

Procedure for claw-clipping

(1) The animal should be suitably restrained and reassured throughout the procedure.
(2) Take the foot firmly, using thumb or fingers to push up each toe in turn and fully expose the nail.
(3) Inspect each nail in turn for damage and length of quick (if it can be seen—if the nail is black the quick will not be seen). A very bright light is helpful.
(4) If the quick is visible, place the clippers below the quick and cut the nail at an angle (Fig. 5.27). Do this with a rapid action before the animal detects pressure and attempts to withdraw its foot.
(5) Take great care not to cut into the quick—it causes pain. An animal that has been caused pain during claw-clipping is likely to be very uncooperative and distressed on all future occasions.
(6) If the quick is *not* visible, estimate where it should be. Apply slight pressure with the clippers and note the animal's reaction. If necessary, revise the estimated position and cut well below it. Err on the side of caution: it is better to make one or two safe small trial cuts than to make one large cut that causes pain and bleeding.

(a)

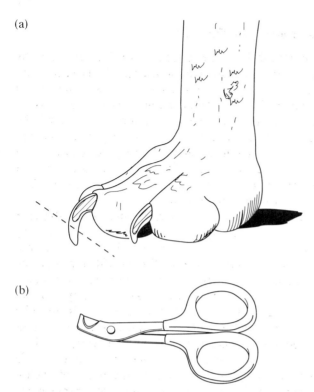

(b)

Fig. 5.27 Nail-cutting: (a) where to cut; (b) special cat claw scissors for precise timming.

(7) If the animal reacts strongly, watch for bleeding. If bleeding does occur it may be stemmed by pressure from a pad of cotton wool. If bleeding persists, traditional styptics such as friars balsam can be applied with a cotton bud but a silver nitrate pencil, applied with great care, is more effective.

(8) Once each foot is completed, move to the next. Check each time for the presence of a dew claw, which can easily be hidden in long-haired dogs.

(9) Once the procedure is over, always praise the animal for compliance. A food reward may be offered at the end.

Quarantine and Isolation

The terms 'quarantine' and 'isolation' both refer to the separation and segregation of animals to protect and prevent the transfer of infectious disease. This usually means that an animal which is infected, or is suspected of being infected, is housed in such a way as to prevent other animals coming into contact with the disease-causing organisms.

In the UK, 'quarantine' usually refers to a period of detention of animals entering the country from overseas to avoid introducing infections, especially the virus disease, rabies. 'Isolation' is a situation of reduced contact with infectious disease, e.g. in an isolation kennel at a veterinary hospital or boarding kennels. In the case of 'protective isolation', an uninfected but susceptible animal—a very young one,

perhaps, or an animal with an lowered resistance (for example, a post-surgical case)—is itself housed in such a way as to prevent its contact with disease-causing organisms.

Methods of Isolation

The methods used for isolation or quarantine depend upon the mode of transmission of the disease and the species of animal involved. Four factors are essential to the transmission of infectious disease from one animal to another:

- A micro-organism capable of causing disease and capable of transmission.
- An environment favourable to the growth of a particular micro-organism.
- A mechanism by which the micro-organism can be transferred.
- A susceptible host.

Micro-organisms capable of causing disease are always present under normal conditions in most environments where animals are housed. A favourable environment for the spread of many micro-organisms usually exists where several animals are housed together, such as in kennels or hospitals. Animals that are likely to be more susceptible as hosts to disease are generally more common in a hospital situation (for example, post-operative cases are more susceptible than the average healthy adult animal) and hospital accommodation is therefore designed and managed to reduce this risk by means of high standards of hygiene. Unfortunately, even with the best standards of kennel design and hygiene, risks can never be totally removed, particularly where there is a potential mechanism by which micro-organisms can be transferred.

Thus it becomes apparent that three out of the four factors in the above list can never be wholly removed. It is therefore important to concentrate on the other factor—the essential link of the transfer mechanism by which a micro-organism is transferred from one animal to another. The prevention of this mechanism is achieved by 'barrier nursing' or 'isolation nursing' of the infected animal.

To achieve effective isolation of a infected animal, the particular transfer mechanism of the specific disease must first be understood (Chapter 23, Medical Disorders and their Nursing).

Admission of infected animals

As general kennel or practice policy, ideally no animal should be admitted that has (or is suspected of having) an infectious disease which poses a potential risk to other animals housed. An infected animal should *never* be admitted into a hospital or kennels where no separate, specific isolation facilities exist.

The usual reason for providing isolation facilities in kennels and catteries is to enable the isolation of animals that have developed suspicious symptoms *after* they have been admitted. By then, this will be the only course of action to protect the other animals housed. Where this occurs, the correct care and housing depends upon the nature of the disease and the type of infection risk.

Isolation kennelling

When isolation kennelling is being designed, all possible disease transmission factors should be taken into account. The kennelling should comprise a totally self-contained unit so that all procedures can be carried out within the unit itself. All equipment should be kept and used in the isolation unit only, and the unit should be equipped to enable the intensive care of acutely ill patients.

Isolation and Infectious Disease

Certain disease management methods are used routinely when managing a case in isolation.

- If possible, one or two staff members should be allocated to deal only with the infected animal and they should not handle any other animals. If this is not practical, they should be restricted to handling animals that have a low risk of contracting the disease. On no account should they also care for high-risk animals such as the very young.
- A foot-bath should be used at the entrance of the isolation unit and should contain a freshly prepared disinfectant solution. The disinfectant type depends upon the disease.
- All hygiene procedures should be carried out using disinfectants known to be effective against the disease concerned.
- A change of protective clothing should be available in a suitable area at the entrance to the isolation unit. The type of clothing depends upon the disease but may be:
  —a boiler suit or other coverall;
  —wellington boots;
  —disposable gloves and apron;
  —surgical mask;
  —hat (particularly for staff with long hair).
- There should be facilities for washing and disinfection and for safely discarding disposable items at the exit from the isolation unit.
- The infected animal should be nursed and treated as is appropriate to the disease.

Where purpose-built isolation facilities are not available, a measure of isolation can be achieved in less than ideal situations by strict nursing techniques (Chapter 20).

Quarantine in the UK

The British Isles are fortunate in being separated by sea from the continent of Europe. This separation has provided a natural barrier to diseases that spread through wild or domestic animals where free passage across borders is otherwise difficult to prevent. Pet animals require human assistance to cross that sea and it is therefore relatively easy to control and restrict the entry of animals, despite the constant movement of humans and even when a tunnel link with Europe is now available.

Britain has been free from the disease of rabies for many years and the continued prevention of its entry is of major concern. The principal control measure has been the quarantine of all dogs, cats etc. entering the country but in recent years there has been much debate with the other European Community member states regarding the freer movement of animals. The argument put forward is that vaccination is thought to reduce the likelihood of rabies entering the UK. Although the use of quarantine still stands as the principal method of preventing the entry of rabies, Britain has now agreed to certain new arrangements regarding the movement of animals. The Ministry of Agriculture, Fisheries and Food (MAFF) announced that changes relating solely to breeding animals came into force in July 1994 and will be due for further review by 1997:

(1) Under tightly controlled conditions, commercial traders in dogs and cats for breeding may use an alternative to quarantine. Movements between registered premises will depend on residency, vaccination, blood test, identification and certification requirements involving checks at origin, notification of a consignment, controlled movement and checks at destination. These arrangements take into account the most recent scientific advice and the need for arrangements to be fully enforceable. Any trader who fails to observe the rules will lose this possibility and their animals would be subject to quarantine, as will dogs and cats which do not meet these very strict conditions.

(2) The second change reflects the fact that some categories of animal present no real risk of bringing rabies into the British Isles—for example rabbits, rats and guinea pigs. From 1 January 1994 there is no requirement for quarantine for such animals, provided that they have been born and bred in the holding of origin. (Domestic farm livestock and horses have never been included in the rabies quarantine arrangements as they are not considered a risk on import.)

MAFF agreed to these changes providing that the British quarantine arrangements for pet animals can only be changed if measures with at least the same level of protection can be found.

Animals still subject to quarantine are:

- Primates
- Carnivores
- Wild mammals not born and kept in captivity.

In case there are any further changes to the rules, it is strongly recommended that those who wish to import or export dogs and cats into or from the UK should contact the MAFF for the most recent information regarding relevant regulations and the specific requirements for each country of destination. At present the quarantine period for dogs and cats entering the UK is 6 calendar months, the only exceptions being as previously mentioned.

The requirements of quarantine kennelling

The principles of quarantine kennelling for the prevention of rabies entering Britain are that the animal should be confined humanely for a period of 6 months in a secure establishment. The animal must have no possibility of contact with other animals (either internally or external to the kennels) that may risk being infected by rabies. To meet these principles:

- No physical contact of any kind is allowed between animals.
- No animal may have contact with the body fluids of another animal. (For example, urine must not seep through or be directed from one run to

another through fences; and screens must protect cats from spitting at one another.)

- No animal may have contact with any item used by another animal prior to disinfection (e.g. dog beds and non-disposable bedding materials).
- There must be no possibility of escape from the kennel or compound.

The only exception to the above is where animals from the same household share a kennel, in which case both animals are isolated from others as if they were one animal.

The standard sizes and other factors regarding quarantine accommodation for dogs and cats are set out in Fig. 5.28.

Licensing of quarantine kennels

Kennels and catteries used for the quarantine of animals in the UK are licensed and controlled by MAFF. The primary concern is that the kennels should be secure and meet the requirements necessary to achieve all the principles previously mentioned.

Licences are granted only to veterinary surgeons but the kennels may be owned by either a veterinary surgeon or a lay person.

If a lay person owns the kennels they must employ a veterinary surgeon who is available to visit the kennels every week day.

QUARANTINE FACILITIES			
	Sleeping area (not less than)	Adjoining exercise area (Run) (not less than)	Other comments
Small dogs (less than 12kg (26lb))	1.1m² (12 sq ft) Width and length: 0.9m (3ft)	3.7m² (40 sq ft) Width: 0.9m (3ft)	*Height of dog compartments*: not to be less than 1.8m (6ft). Walls of sleeping area must be floor to roof or with all walls measuring at least 1.8m (6ft) and any gap above partitioned with escape-proof weld mesh. Wire diameter must be not less than 2mm (14swg), with mesh size not exceeding 50mm (2in). Runs should be constructed to allow dogs to see beyond the confines of the unit wherever possible.
Medium sized dogs (12kg (26lb) to 30kg (66lb))	1.4m² (16 sq ft) Width and length: 1.2m (4ft)	5.5m² (60 sq ft) Width: 1.2m (4ft)	They must be constructed to allow no nose or paw contact and no passage of urine from one run to another. *Dividing partitions between runs*: At least 1.8m (6ft) high. An impervious material with a smooth hard finish is used for the first part of the dividing partition, to a height of 0.4m (18in) for small to medium sized dogs, and 0.6m (2ft) for large dogs.
Large dogs (more than 30kg (66lb)	1.4m² (16 sq ft) Width and length: 1.2m (4ft)	7.4m² (80 sq ft) Width: 1.2m (4ft)	The upper part of the dividing partition must be constructed of a see-through material that is nose and paw proof. *Run fencing*: Minimum height of 3m (10ft) with a weld mesh guard of 0.6m (2ft) set at an inward 45° angle; or Runs roofed over completely.
Cats	Total floor area (sleeping compartment and run) not less than 1.4m² (15 sq ft). Width and length: 0.9m (3ft). Height not less than 1.8m (6ft).		Quarantine accommodation for cats should be of the 'walk in' type. It must be securely roofed with all partitions solid to prevent cats spitting at one another.

Fig. 5.28. Quarantine facilities.

General safety procedures in quarantine establishments

- All staff must be instructed on the dangers of rabies.
- Quarantine kennels must be run separately from all other units on the same site.
- Security and fire precautions and procedures must comply with current regulations.
- All animals must be transported to the kennels by an authorised carrying agent from the airport or ship's dock, and in a special vehicle and container.
- A high-security area must be used for the transfer of animals from the transporting vehicle to the kennel accommodation units.
- Rabies vaccination should be carried out on arrival or within 24 hours (regardless of current vaccination status).
- An animal must be kept in one accommodation unit for the duration of its stay.
- Animals housed in each accommodation unit should be clearly identified.
- Strict hygiene procedures should be observed at all times, using approved disinfectants.
- Animals in quarantine have restricted access by owners or any other person. Special authorisation is required if owners visit before 14 days of the arrival in quarantine.
- Strict recording procedures must be carried out regarding any movements of the animal, visits by the owner and all health records.

Procedure if a Rabies Case is Suspected

Where the suspected case is held in quarantine

If an animal in quarantine displays unexplained nervous signs, it should immediately be confined and the MAFF should be informed that a case of rabies is suspected.

If the suspect case dies or is euthanased, the animal is removed by a Ministry veterinary officer. Its head will be removed and taken to the MAFF diagnostic laboratory where the brain is removed under very strict conditions for tests to determine if the animal was infected by rabies.

Where a suspected case occurs in general practice

> The veterinary nurse should always have emergency plans prepared for various events, including natural disasters such as fire and flood. Rabies is a real 'disaster' and requires a plan of action by the head nurse to keep the veterinary practice prepared.

It is possible that an animal brought into the practice for consultation with a veterinary surgeon displays clinical signs and a case history which raise the suspicion that it may be a case of rabies. Even a sick bat brought in might have to be viewed with suspicion. The veterinary surgeon will take into account all the symptoms and the history in making a decision to report the case as suspected rabies.

Where an animal is a suspected case but with insufficient grounds to report. In these circumstances a second opinion may be requested.

The MAFF Divisional Veterinary Officer (DVO) should be contacted to arrange for a veterinary officer to visit and examine the animal in consultation with the veterinary surgeon. The animal will be isolated and the veterinary surgeon will remain with the suspect animal until the veterinary officer arrives.

Where the veterinary surgeon makes a decision to report a suspected case. There is a statutory requirement that any suspicion of a case of rabies must be reported to:

- a MAFF inspector (Veterinary Officer); or
- the local authority animal health inspector; or
- a police constable.

Where a case is suspected in general practice, it is likely that the first contact will be with the DVO, by telephone.

The owner or person in charge of the animal should be advised by the veterinary surgeon:

- that rabies is suspected;
- that the animal must be detained and isolated;
- that it will be necessary for an official enquiry to be carried out by the Ministry veterinary officer who is being called to attend the case.

Isolation of the suspected case. The suspect animal must be isolated in escape-proof accommodation in order to prevent any further contact with animals or humans. It must remain on the premises on which it has been examined by the veterinary surgeon until the Ministry veterinary officer's enquiries are completed.

Identification of all contact animals. The names and addresses of the owners or person in charge of all animals that may have come into direct contact with the suspect case, along with descriptions of those animals, should be recorded. Reception records for the day will be needed for verification.

Any animal that has been bitten, scratched or come into contact with the saliva of the suspect animal should be detained at the premises until the Ministry veterinary officer's enquiries are completed.

The officer will advise if any further action is necessary with regard to contact animals.

Human contacts. Once the animal has been detained and isolated, all persons who have handled it should carry out a thorough personal disinfection:

- Hands should first be washed with soap or detergent and hot water.

- Clothing or overalls, if contaminated with discharges from the suspected animal, should be removed and sterilised before reuse.
- Equipment used on the animal should be removed and sterilised before reuse.

> WARNING
>
> **It is of paramount importance that anyone bitten or scratched by the suspected animal should have the wound treated immediately.**
>
> (1) Wash and flush the wound with soap or detergent and water.
> (2) Flush repeatedly with running water alone— **this is imperative**.
> (3) Apply either:
>   —40–70% alcohol; or
>   —tincture of aqueous solutions of iodine; or
>   —0.1% quaternary ammonium compounds (NB: soap neutralises quaternary ammonium compounds, therefore all traces of soap must be removed before application).

All cases of human contact with the suspected animal will be referred to the Medical Officer or the Environmental Health Office for further action and advice.

General Routine of Admission of Dogs and Cats into the UK

The routine of admission at the time of writing is as follows. For up-to-date information, contact MAFF.

Import licence

No dog or cat may be imported unless an import licence has been granted by or on behalf of MAFF (or the Secretary of State for Scotland, Northern Ireland or Jersey or the Welsh Office Agriculture Department if appropriate).

A condition of the licence is that the animal will be held in quarantine for 6 calendar months from the date of its landing in the UK.

Application for import licences must be made in good time. As it is essential that the licence is issued on time, it is necessary for applications to be made at least 8 weeks in advance of the proposed date of importation.

Licences will not be granted unless the Ministry or relevant Department of Agriculture is satisfied that the necessary arrangements have been made, i.e. that the quarantine kennels and carrying agent have given notice of the booking.

Quarantine kennels. Accommodation must be reserved at approved quarantine premises well in advance of the proposed date of importation. A list of approved premises is available from MAFF or the relevant Department of Agriculture.

Authorised carrying agent. The services of an authorised carrying agent must be reserved to meet the animal at the port or airport and be responsible for its safe custody to the quarantine premises (some quarantine premises are also authorised carrying agents).

The port of entry. Animals may only be landed at certain ports and airports. A list is available from the Ministry or relevant Department of Agriculture.

Granting of the licence. The Ministry or relevant Department of Agriculture will confirm the booking with the quarantine premises and carrying agent. They will then:

- Send the import licence to the carrying agent. (The carrying agent is responsible for clearing the animal through customs.)
- Send a boarding document to the applicant (usually owner of the animal) or a named representative. (The boarding document will confirm the licence number and act as written evidence that a licence has been granted. This document will be shown to the shipper or airline before the animal will be allowed to leave for the UK.)
- Send a red label to the applicant or named representative if the animal is to be transported by air. The red label is to be completed and affixed to the crate prior to embarkation.

Container or crate. If the animal is to travel by air, the container or crate must conform to IATA standards; i.e. it must be large enough for the animal to stand and lie in a natural position and turn around.

The animal will travel to the UK as manifest cargo in the freight compartment.

Procedure for Exporting Dogs and Cats from the UK

The factors governing the requirements for the export of dogs and cats from the UK are determined by the country to which the animal is being exported. No British laws are in force which govern the export of animals—the only laws presently in force govern imports.

The regulations relating to the export of dogs and cats to other countries vary considerably and may change depending upon the circumstances within the individual country at the time.

It is recommended that the export section of MAFF be contacted for the up-to-date requirements for each country.

Breeds. The Recognised Groups of Dogs and Cats

Pedigree Dog Breeds

In the UK, all dogs exhibited at official shows must be of a breed recognised by the Kennel Club and must be registered through a system by which each has a registered name, usually combined with its breeder's registered prefix. Any change of ownership is also registered with the Kennel Club. The breeds recognised by the Kennel Club are broadly classified as 'sporting' and 'non-sporting', subdivided into 'groups' as follows:

- *Sporting*
  Hound group
  Gundog group
  Terrier group

- *Non-sporting*
  Utility group
  Working group
  Toy group

Names are not necessarily a guide to the breed's group. For example, not all dogs with the word 'terrier' in their name are classed as terriers. The Australian silky terrier, English toy terrier and Yorkshire terrier are in the Toy group, while the Boston and Tibetan terriers are in the Utility group. Most but not all spaniels are in the Gundog group but the Tibetan spaniel is in the Utility group and the King Charles and Cavalier King Charles spaniels are in the Toy group.

The following information gives maximum/minimum or ideal height and weight where stated in the breed standard.

SPORTING BREEDS		
Breed name	**Height at Withers (Top of shoulder) Ranges**	**Weight**
Hound group		
Afghan Hound	Dogs 68-74 cm (27-29 in) Bitches 63-69 cm (25-27 in)	
Basenji	Dogs 43 cm (17 in) Bitches 40 cm (16 in)	11 kg (24 lb) 9.5 kg (21 lb)
Basset Hound	33-38 cm (13-15 in)	
Basset Fauve De Bretagne	32-38 cm (12.8-15.2 in)	
Beagle	33-40 cm (13-16 in)	
Bloodhound	Dogs 63-69 cm (25-27 in) Bitches 58-63 cm (23-25 in)	41-50 kg (90-110 lb) 36-45 kg (80-100 lb)
Borzoi	Dogs 74 cm (29 in) Bitches 68 cm (27 in)	
Dachshunds	Standards Miniatures	9-12 kg (20-26 lb) 4.5-5 kg (10-11 lb)
Deerhound	Dogs 76 cm (30 in) Bitches 71 cm (28 in)	45.5 kg (100 lb) 36.5 kg (80 lb)
Elkhound	Dogs 52 cm (20.5 in) Bitches 49 cm (19.5 in)	23 kg (50 lb) 20 kg (43 lb)
Finnish Spitz	Dogs 43-50 cm (17-20 in) Bitches 39-45 cm (15.5-18 in)	14-16 kg (31-35 lb)
Grand Bleu De Gascoigne	Dogs 63.5-70 cm (25-27 in) Bitches 60-65 cm (23.3-25.5 in)	
Greyhound	Dogs 71-76 cm (28-30 in) Bitches 68-71 cm (27-28 in)	
Hamiltonstovare	Dogs 50-60 cm (19.5-23.5 in) Bitches 46-57 cm (18-22.5 in)	
Ibizan Hound	56-74 cm (22-29 in)	
Irish Wolfhound	Dogs 79-86 cm (31-34 in) Bitches 71 cm min.(28 in)	54.5 kg (120 lb) Min 40.9 kg (90 lb) Min
Norwegian Lundehund	Dogs 35-38 cm (14-15 in) Bitches 32-35 cm (12.5-14 in)	7 kg (15.5 lb) 6 kg (13 lb)

Fig. 5.29—continued   ◆

SPORTING BREEDS		
Breed name	**Height at Withers (Top of shoulder) Ranges**	**Weight**
Otterhound	Dogs 67 cm (27 in) Bitches 60 cm (24 in)	
Petit Basset Griffon Vendeen	34-38 cm (13.4-15 in)	
Pharaoh Hound	Dogs 56 cm (Ideal). (22-25 in) Bitches 53 cm (Ideal). (21-24 in)	
Rhodesian Ridgeback	Dogs 63-67 cm (25-27 in) Bitches 61-66 cm (24-26 in)	
Saluki	Dogs 58.4-71.1 cm (23-28 in) Bitches proportionately smaller	
Sloughi	Dogs 60-70 cm (23.5-27.5 in)	
Whippet	Dogs 47-51 cm (18.5-20 in) Bitches 44-47 cm (17.5-18.5 in)	
Gundog Group		
Brittany	Dogs 65-68 cm (25.5-27 in) Bitches 61-65 cm (24-25.5 in)	15 kg (33 lb) 13 kg (28.5 lb)
English Setter	Dogs 65-68 cm (25.5-27 in) Bitches 61-65 cm (24-25.5 in)	
German Shorthaired Pointer	Dogs 58-64 cm (23-25 in) Bitches 56-62 cm (24-25.5 in)	
German Wirehaired Pointer	Dogs 60-67 cm (24-26 in) Bitches 56-62 cm (22-24 in)	25-34 kg (55-75 lb) 20.5-29 kg (45-64 lb)
Gordon Setter	Dogs 66 cm (26 in) Bitches 62 cm (24.5 in)	29.5 kg (65 lb) 25.5 kg (56 lb)
Hungarian Vizla	Dogs 57-64 cm (22.5-25 in) Bitches 53-60 cm (21-23.5 in)	20-30 kg (48.5-66 lb) 20-30 kg (48.5-66 lb)
Irish Red and White Setter		
Irish Setter		
Italian Spinone	Dogs 56-69 cm (23.5-27.5 in) Bitches 58-64 cm (23-25.5 in)	34-39 kg (70-82 lb) 29-34 kg (62-71 lb)
Large Munsterlander	Dogs 61 cm (24 in) Bitches - 59 cm (23 in)	25-29 kg (55-65 lb) 25 kg (55 lb)
Pointer	Dogs 63-69 cm (25-27 in) Bitches 61-66 cm (24-26 in)	
Retrievers		
- Chesapeake Bay	Dogs 58.4-66 cm (23-26 in) Bitches 53.3-60.9 cm (21-24 in)	
- Curly Coated	Dogs 68.5 cm (27 in) Bitches 63.5 cm (25 in)	
- Flat Coated	Dogs 58-61 cm (23-24 in) Bitches 56-59 cm (22-23 in)	25-35 kg (60-80 lb) 25-34 kg (55-70 lb)
- Golden	Dogs 56-61 cm (22-24 in) Bitches 51-56 cm (20-22 in)	
- Labrador	Dogs 56-57 cm (22-22.5 in) Bitches 54-56 cm (21.5 in)	
Spaniels		
- American Cocker	Dogs 36.25-38.75 cm (14.5-15.5 in) Bitches 33.75-36.25 cm (13.4-14.5 in)	
- Clumber	Dogs Bitches	36 kg (80 lb) 29.5 kg (65 lb)

Fig. 5.29—continued

SPORTING BREEDS		
Breed name	**Height at Withers (Top of shoulder) Ranges**	**Weight**
– Cocker	Dogs 39-41 cm (15.5-16 in) Bitches 38-39 cm (15-15.5 in)	28-32 lb) (28-32 lb)
– English Springer	51 cm (20 in)	
– Field	45.7 cm (18 in)	18-25 kg (40-55 lb)
– Irish Water	Dogs 53-58 cm (21-23 in) Bitches 51-56 cm (20-22 in)	
– Sussex	38-41 cm (15-16 in)	(50 lb)
– Welsh Springer	Dogs 48 cm (19 in) Bitches 46 cm (18 in)	
Weimaraner	Dogs 61-69 cm (24-27 in) Bitches 56-64 cm (22-25 in)	
Terrier Group		
Airedale Terrier	Dogs 58-61 cm (23-24 in) Bitches 56-59 cm (22-23 in)	
Australian Terrier	25.4 cm (10 in)	6.34 kg (14 lb)
Bedlington Terrier	41 cm (16 in)	8.2-10.4 kg (18-23 lb)
Border Terrier	Dogs Bitches	5.9-7.1 kg (13-15.5 lb) 5.1-6.4 kg (11.5-14 lb)
Bull Terrier	(no height/weight limits)	
Bull Terrier (Miniature)	35.5 cm (14 in)	
Cairn Terrier	28-31 cm (11-12 in)	6-7.5 kg (14-16 lb)
Dandie Dinmont Terrier		8-11 kg (18-24 lb)
Fox Terrier (Smooth)	Dogs Bitches	7.3-8.2 kg (16-18 lb) 6.8-7.7 kg (15-17 lb)
Fox Terrier (Wire)	Dogs 39 cm (15.5 in) Bitches slightly less than above	8.25 kg (18 lb)
Glen of Imaal Terrier	35-36 cm (14 in)	
Irish Terrier	Dogs 48 cm (19 in) Bitches 46 cm (18 in)	
Kerry Blue Terrier	Dogs 46-48 cm (18-19 in) Bitches slightly less than above	15-16.8 kg (33-37 lb) 15.9 kg (35 lb)
Lakeland Terrier	Dogs 37 cm (14.5 in) Bitches	7.7 kg (17 lb) 6.8 kg (15 lb)
Manchester Terrier	Dogs 40-41 cm (16 in) Bitches 38 cms (15 in)	
Norfolk Terrier	25-26 cm (10 in)	
Norwich Terrier	25-26 cm (10 in)	
Scottish Terrier	25.4-28 cm (10-11 in)	8.6-10.4 kg (19-23 lb)
Sealyham Terrier	Dogs 31 cm (12 in) Bitches	9 kg (20 lb) 8.2 kg (18 lb)
Skye Terrier	Dogs 25-26 cm (10 in) Bitches slightly less than above	
Soft Coated Wheaten Terrier	Dogs 46-49 cm (18-19.5 in) Bitches slightly less	16-20.5 kg (35-45 lb) Bitches slightly less
Staffordshire Bull Terrier	Dogs 14-16 in Bitches	12.7-17 kg (28-38 lb) 11-15.4 kg (24-34 lb)
Welsh Terrier	39 cm (15.5 in)	9-9.5 kg (20-21 lb)
West Highland White Terrier	28 cm (11 in)	

Fig. 5.29—continued

NON-SPORTING BREEDS		
Breed name	Height at Withers (Top of shoulder) Ranges	Weight
Utility Group Boston Terrier		Lightweight: under 6.8 kg (15 lb) Middleweight: 6.8-9.1 kg (15-20 lb) Heavyweight: 9.1-11.4 kg (20-25 lb)
Bulldog		25kg (55 lb) 22.7 kg (50 lb)
Canaan Dog	Dogs 51-61 cm (20-24 in) Bitches - 48-56 cm (19-22 in)	18-25 kg (40-45 lb)
Chow Chow	Dogs 48-56 cm (19-22 in) Bitches - 46-51 cm (18-20 in)	
Dalmatian	Dogs - 58.4-61 cm (23-24 in) Bitches - 55.9-58.4 cm (22-23 in)	
French Bulldog	Dogs - 45.7 cm (18 in)	12.7 kg (28 lb) 10.9 kg (24 lb)
German Spitz	Klein 23-28 cm (9-11 in) Mittel 29-35.5 cm (11.5-14 in)	
Japanese Akita	Dogs 66-71 cm (26-28 in) Bitches 61-66 cm (24-26 in)	
Japanese Shiba Inu	Dogs 39.5 cm (15.5 in) Bitches 36.5 cm (14.5 in)	
Japanese Spitz	Dogs 30-36 cm (12-14 in) Bitches slightly smaller	
Keeshond	Dogs 45.7 cm (18 in) Bitches 43.2 cm (17 in)	
Leonberger	Dogs 72-80 cm (28.75-32 in) Bitches 65-75 cm (26-30 in)	
Lhasa Apso	Dogs 25.4 cm (10 in) Bitches slightly smaller	
Miniature Schnauzer	Dogs 35.6 cm (14 in) Bitches 33 cm (13 in)	
Poodles	Standard over 38 cm (15 in) Miniature 28-38 cm (11-15 in) Toy under 28 cm (11 in)	
Schipperke		5.4-7.3 kg (12-16 lb)
Schnauzer	Dogs 48.3 cm (19 in) Bitches 45.7 cm (18 in)	
Shar Pei	46-51 cm (18-20 in)	
Shih Tzu	26.7 cm (10.5 in)	4.5-8.1 kg (10-18 lb)
Tibetan Spaniel	25.4 cm (10 in)	4.1 kg-6.8 kg (9-15 lb)
Tibetan Terrier	Dogs 35.6-40.6 cm (14-16 in)	
Working Group		
Alaskan Malamute	Dogs 64-71 cm (25-28 in) Bitches 58-66cm (23-26 in)	38-56 kg (85-125 lb) 38-56 kg (85-125 lb)
Anatolian Shepherd Dog	Dogs 74-81 cm (29-32 in) Bitches 71-79 cm (28-31 in)	50-64 kg (110-141 lb) 41-59 kg (90.5-130 lb)

Fig. 5.29—continued

NON-SPORTING BREEDS		
Breed name	**Height at Withers (Top of shoulder) Ranges**	**Weight**
Australian Cattle Dog	Dogs 46-51 cm (18-20 in) Bitches 43-48 cm (17-19 in)	
Australian Kelpie	Dogs 46-51 cm (18-20 in) Bitches 43-48 cm (17-19 in)	
Bearded Collie	Dogs 53-56 cm (21-22 in) Bitches 51-53 cm (20-21 in)	
Belgian Shephed Dogs		
– Groenendael	Dogs - 61-66 cm (24-26 in) Bitches - 56-61 cm (22-24 in)	
– Laekenois	Dogs - 61-66 cm (24-26 in) Bitches - 56-61 (22-24 in)	
– Malinois	Dogs - 61-66 cm (24-26 in) Bitches - 56-61 cm (22-24 in)	
– Tervueren	Dogs - 61-66 cm (24-26 in) Bitches 56-61 cm (22-24 in)	
Burnese Mountain Dog	Dogs - 64-70 cm (25-27.5 in) Bitches - 58-66 cm (23-26 in)	
Border Collie	Dogs - 53 cm (21 in) Bitches slightly less	
Bouvier Des Flandres	Dogs - 62-68 cm (25-27 in) Bitches - 59-65 cm (23-25.5 in)	35-40 kg (77-88 lb) 27-35 kg (59-77 lb)
Boxer	Dogs - 57-63 cm (22.5-25 in) Bitches - 53-59 cm (21-23 in)	30-32 kg (66-70 lb) 25-27 kg (55-60 lb)
Briard	Dogs - 62-68 cm (24-27 in) Bitches - 56-64 cm (23-25.5 in)	
Bullmastiff	Dogs - 63.5-68.5 cm (25-27 in) Bitches - 61-66 cm (24-26 in)	50-59 kg (110-130 lb) 41-50 kg (90-110 lb)
Collie		
– Rough	Dogs - 56-61 cm (22-24 in) Bitches - 51-56 cm (20-22 in)	
– Smooth	Dogs - 56-61 cm (22-24 in) Bitches - 51-56 cm (20-22 in)	20.5-29.5 kg (45-65 lb) 18-25 kg (40-55 lb)
Dobermann	Dogs - 69 cm (27 in) Bitches - 65 cm (25.5 in)	
Eskimo Dog	Dogs - 58-68 cm (23-27 in) Bitches - 51-61 cm (20-24 in)	34-47.6 kg (75-105 lb) 27-41 kg (60-90 lb)
Estrela Mountain Dog	Dogs - 65-72 cm (25.5-28.5 in) Bitches - 62-68 cm (24.5-27 in) (with tolerance of 4 cm (1.5 in) above allowed)	
German Shepherd Dog (Alsatian)	Dogs - 62.5 cm (25 in) Bitches - 57.5 cm (23 in) (2.5 cm (1 in) above/below permissible)	
Giant Schnauzer	Dogs - 65-70 cm (25.5.-27.5 in) Bitches - 60-65 cm (23.5-25.5 in)	
Great Dane	Dogs - 76 cm (30 in) Bitches - 71 cm (28 in)	54 kg (120 lb) min 46 kg (100 lb) min
Hovawart	Dogs - 63-70 cm (24-27.5 in) Bitches - 58-65 cm (23-25.5 in)	30-40 kg (66-68 lb) 25-35 kg (55-77 lb)
Hungarian Puli	Dogs - 40-44 cm (16-17.5 in) Bitches - 37-41 cm (14.5-16 in)	13-15 Kg (28.5-33 lb) 10-13 kg (22-28.5 lb)
Komondor	Dogs - 80 cm (31.5 in) Bitches - 70 cm (27.5 in)	50-51 kg (110-135 lb) 36-50 kg (80-110 lb)

Fig. 5.29—continued

NON-SPORTING BREEDS		
Breed name	Height at Withers (Top of shoulder) Ranges	Weight
Lancashire Heeler	Dogs - 30 cm (12 in) Bitches - 25 cm (10 in)	
Maremma Sheepdog	Dogs - 65-73 cm (25.5-28.5 in) Bitches - 60-68 cm (23.5-26.5 in)	35-45 kg (77-99 lb) 30-40 kg (66-68 lb)
Mastiff		
Neopolitan Mastiff	Dogs - 65-75 cm (26-29 in) Bitches somewhat less	50-70 kg (110-154 lb)
Newfoundland	Dogs - 71 cm (28 in) Bitches - 66 cm (26 in)	64-69 kg (140-150 lb) 50-54.5 kg (110-120 lb)
Norwegian Buhund	Dogs - 45 cm (17.75 in) Bitches somewhat less	
Old English Sheepdog	Dogs - 61 cm (24 in) min Bitches - 56 cm (22 in) min	
Pinscher	43-48 cm (17-19 in)	
Polish Lowland Sheepdog	Dogs - 43-52 cm (17-20 in) Bitches - 40-46 cm (16-18.5 in)	
Portuguese Water Dog	Dogs - 50-57 cm (19.5-22.5 in) Bitches - 43-52 cm (17-20.5 in)	19-25 kg (42-55 lb) 16-22 kg (35-48.5 lb)
Pyrenean Mountain Dog	Dogs - 70 cm (28 in) Bitches - 65 cm (26 in)	50 kg (110 lb) min 40 kg (90 lbs) min
Rottweiler	Dogs - 63-69 cm (25-27 in) Bitches - 58-63.5 (23-25 in)	
St Bernard	Taller the better	
Samoyed	Dogs - 51-56 cm (20-22 in) Bitches - 46-51 cm (18-20 in)	
Shetland Sheepdog	Dogs - 37 cm (14.5 in) Bitches - 35.5 cm (14 in)	
Siberian Husky	Dogs - 53-60 cm (21-23.5 in) Bitches - 51-56 cm (20-22 in)	20-27 kg (45-60 lb) 16-23 kg (35-50 lb)
Swedish Vallhund	Dogs - 33-35 cm (13-13.75 in) Bitches - 31-33 cm (12-13 in)	11.4-15.9 kg (25-35 lb) 11.4-15.9 kg (25-35 lb)
Tibetan Mastiff	Dogs - 66 cm (26 in) Bitches - 61 cm (24 in)	
Welsh Corgi		
– Cardigan	30 cm (12 in)	
– Pembroke	Dogs - 25.4-30.5 cm (10-12 in) Bitches	10-12 kg (22-26 lb) 10-11 kg (20-24 lb)
Toy Group		
Affenpinscher	24-28 cm (9.5-11 in)	3-4 kg (6.5-9 lb)
Australian Silky Terrier	23 cm (9 in)	4 kg (8-10 lb)
Bichon Frise	23-28 cm (9-11 in)	
Bolognese	Dogs - 27-30.5 cm (10.5-12 in) Bitches - 25.5-28 cm (10-11 in)	
Cavalier King Charles Spaniel		5.4-8 kg (12-18 lb)

Fig. 5.29—continued

NON-SPORTING BREEDS		
Breed name	Height at Withers (Top of shoulder) Ranges	Weight
Chihuahua		
– Long Coat		1-2.7 kg (2.6 lb)
– Smooth Coat		1-2.7 kg (2.6 lb)
Chinese Crested Dog	Dogs - 28-33 cm (11-13 in) Bitches - 23-30 cm (9-12 in)	5.5 kg (12 lb) max
English Toy Terrier (Black and Tan)	25-33 cm ((10-12 in)	2.7-3.6 kg (6-8 lb)
Griffon Bruxellois		2.2-4.9 kg (5-8 lb)
Italian Greyhound		2.7-4.5 kg (6-10 lb)
Japanese Chin		1.8-3.2 kg (4.7 lb)
King Charles Spaniel		3.6-6.3 kg (8-14 lb)
Lowchen (Little Lion Dog)	25-33 cm (10-13 in)	
Maltese	25.5 cm (10 in) max	
Miniature Pinscher	25.5-30 cm (10-12 in)	
Papillon	20-28 cm (8-11 in)	
Pekingese	Dogs Bitches	5 kg (11 lb) max 5.5 kg (12 lb) max
Pomeranian	Dogs Bitches	1.8-2 kg (4-4.5 lb) 2-2.5 kg (4.5-5.5 lb)
Pug		6.3-8.1 (14-18 lb)
Yorkshire Terrier		3.1 kg (7 lb) max

Fig. 5.29. Sporting breeds.

For some breeds no data is available for height and weight.

Cats

There are more than 5 million non-pedigree cats in Britain. All types are seen due to the free range nature of the breeding of cats in this country and resulting mix of genes. Both long- and short-hair types occur naturally in the present population. All colours are found but the most common is tabby, of which there are two types: those with 'mackerel' stripes (narrow bands of colour similar to the coat of the Scottish wildcat) and those with the more common blotched tabby markings. The tabby colouring is followed in frequency by black and white colouring. More unusual colours like chocolate, colour point and chinchilla suggest that a pedigree cat has been involved in an individual ancestry.

Pedigree cat breeds are recognised and classified in the UK by the Governing Council of the Cat Fancy (G.C.C.F.), which is similar to the Kennel Club in that it:

- classifies breeds and issues breed standards by which cats may be judged;
- licenses cat shows and appoints judges;
- prepares and publishes the rules to control these functions;

- protects the welfare of cats and improves cat breeding;
- protects the interests of cat owners;
- exercises disciplinary powers.

In 1992 there was a major change in the GCCF's classification and grouping of cats, with the introduction of a new section, the 'semi long hairs'. The major groups are now:

- Long-hairs
- Semi long-hairs
- British short-hairs
- Foreign breeds
- Burmese
- Orientals
- Siamese and Balinese

The following lists are of breeds and colour variations recognised in each group. Note that some breeds are comparatively new to Britain and have only provisional or preliminary status.

PEDIGREE CAT BREEDS/COLOURS AS CLASSIFIED BY THE GCCF	
Long Hairs	Bicolour L.H. Black L.H. Blue L.H. Blue cream L.H. Cameo-Cream/Blue-cream/Red/Tortie Chinchilla Colourpoint-Cream/Blue/Lilac/Red/Red/Seal/Tabby/Tortie Golden Persian Pewter L.H. Self-Chocolate/Cream/Red Smoke L.H. Black/Blue/Cream/Blue-cream/Red/Tortie Tabby L.H.-Brown/Silver/Red Tortoiseshell L.H. Tortie. And White L.H. Blue Tortoiseshell and White White L.H.-Blue eyed/Orange eyed/Odd eyed Provisional breed status Long Hairs Chocolate tortie L.H. Lilac cream L.H.
Semi-Long Hairs	Birman-Blue point/Seal point Birman-Chocolate/Lilac/Red/Tabby/Tortie/Tortie tabby Turkish van Somali-Usual/Sorrel Main Coon Provisional breed status Semi-Long Hairs Somali – Silver Somali – A.O.C. Preliminary breed status (Assessment) Semi-Long Hairs Ragdoll Norwegian Forest Cat
British Short Hairs	Bicolour B.S.H. Black B.S.H. Blue B.S.H. Blue Cream B.S.H. Blue Tortie and White B.S.H. Colour Pointed B.S.H. Cream B.S.H. Manx Smoke B.S.H. Spotted B.S.H.-Blue/Brown/Red/Silver Tabby B.S.H.-Brown/Red/Silver Tipped B.S.H. Tortoiseshell B.S.H. Tortie and White B.S.H. White B.S.H.-Blue eyed/Orange eyed/Odd eyed
Foreign Breeds	Abyssinian-Blue/Sorrel/Usual Korats Rex-Cornish/Devon Russian Blue Provisional breed status Foreign breeds Abyssinians-Silver Asian-Smoke Asian tabby-Spotted/Classic/Mackerel/Ticked Burmilla Preliminary Breed Status (Assessment) Foreign breeds Asian-Tiffanie/Bombay Tonkinese Russian
Burmese	Blue Burmese Brown Burmese Chocolate Burmese Cream Burmese Lilac Burmese Red Burmese Tortoiseshell Burmese
Orientals	Foreign White Havana Oriental-Black/Blue/Lilac/Red/Tortoiseshell Oriental-Tabby/Classic/Spotted/Ticked

Fig. 5.30—continued

PEDIGREE CAT BREEDS/COLOURS AS CLASSIFIED BY THE GCCF	
	Provisional breed status – Orientals Oriental-Cinnamon/Cream/Red Oriental-Classic Tabby Oriental-Spotted Tabby/A.O.C. Preliminary breed status (assessment) – Orientals Angora Oriental-Non Self/Self
Siamese and Balinese	Siamese-Seal point/Blue point/Chocolate point/Lilac point/Tabby point/Red point/Tortie point/Cream point A. C. Balinese Preliminary breed status (Assessment) Siamese and Balinese Siamese-Cinnamon, Caramel and Fawn points/Tortie points/Tabby points/Tortie tabby points

Fig. 5.30. Pedigree cat breeds/colours as classified by the GCCF.

6

The Law and Ethics of Veterinary Nursing*

A. R. W. PORTER

Origins

Although veterinary surgeons have relied on the help of lay assistants of various kinds since time immemorial (and we are told that a Canine Nurses Institute was established in Great Britain at the beginning of this century) it was not until 1961 that the present veterinary nurse training scheme was set up by the Royal College of Veterinary Surgeons.

At that time, legislation designed to limit the title 'nurse' to those who were already trained and qualified to nurse human patients prevented its use in the veterinary field—even with the use of the word 'animal' as a prefix. Accordingly persons who qualified under the new RCVS scheme had to be content with the rather clumsy title of Registered Animal Nursing Auxiliary. They very soon became known as RANAs.

In the course of time the statutory position changed and it became possible for the title of nurse to be applied to those engaged in nursing animals, provided that the particular nature of their work was made plain. On 1 November 1984, the title of RANA passed into history and the new title of **Veterinary Nurse** came into being.

Students who pass both the Part I and the Part II examinations (formerly Preliminary and Final) for the veterinary nursing qualification, set by the RCVS, and fulfil the other requirements of two years' practical training at an Approved Training Centre, are entitled to have their names entered on the list of veterinary nurses maintained by the Royal College and, of course, to describe themselves as veterinary nurses (VNs).

Career Prospects

The scope of the work open to veterinary nurses can be quite wide but the main employment area is still in small animal practice. At present, the syllabus for training relates to small animals and does not yet relate either to the horse or to farm animals (though this situation may change). Nevertheless, some nurses now work in mixed or equine practices where they have been extensively involved with these larger animals.

Companion animals are treated and nursed not only in private veterinary practices but also in other centres such as university veterinary schools and animal welfare society clinics and kennels and so veterinary nurses will be found working there.

Other career opportunities are available with pharmaceutical companies, in teaching and in other establishments where animals must be well cared for, such as zoos. Many holders of the veterinary nurse qualification have found that it is highly regarded overseas, and have therefore gone to work permanently or for a time in other countries.

The Law Relating to Veterinary Nursing†

The Veterinary Surgeons Act 1966

The Veterinary Surgeons Act 1966 is the written law or 'statute' which governs the practice of veterinary surgery in the United Kingdom. It provides that (with certain specified exceptions) no one may practise veterinary surgery unless he or she is registered with the Royal College of Veterinary Surgeons. The title of **veterinary surgeon** is reserved by law to those whose names appear in the Register of Veterinary Surgeons maintained by the RCVS. Persons so registered are members of the Royal College and use the letters MRCVS, or FRCVS if they are qualified as Fellows. Veterinary surgeons may also be coloquially referred to as **veterinarians**, a title that was one of the earliest names used and is one widely recognised in North America and continental Europe. **Veterinary practitioner** is a title which the members of the Supplementary Veterinary Register may use. Those in this small group do not have formal qualifications in veterinary medicine and no further names may be added to this Register.

Veterinary surgery is defined in the Act as meaning:

the art and science of veterinary surgery and medicine and without prejudice to the generality of the foregoing, shall be taken to include:
(a) the diagnosis of diseases in, and injuries to animals, including tests performed on animals for diagnostic purposes;
(b) the giving of advice based on such diagnosis;
(c) the medical and surgical treatment of animals; and
(d) the performance of surgical operations upon animals.

The exceptions referred to give certain limited powers of treatment—under specified conditions—to doctors, dentists and animal owners and, under Statutory Orders, make provision for lay persons to

*The law contained in this chapter is the English law in operation at October 1993.

†See appendix for *Guide to Professional Conduct for Veterinary Nurses.*

carry out certain minor procedures which are applicable to farm animals.

Schedule 3 to the Veterinary Surgeons Act 1966

Veterinary nurses, like other non-veterinarians, may take advantage of those provisions in Schedule 3 to the Act which permit lay persons over the age of 18 to amputate the dew-claws of a puppy before its eyes open, and *allow anyone to render* **first aid** in an emergency for the purpose of saving life or relieving pain or suffering.

The question is sometimes asked as to the extent of the treatment which may be considered permissible under the term 'first aid'. Precise definition is impossible as to where first aid ceases to be life-saving etc. The RCVS has advised that:

> provided what is done, is done in order to save an animal's life or to stop its pain or suffering, and is done as an interim measure until a veterinary surgeon's services can be obtained, it is unlikely that, in most cases, there will be subsequent argument that what has been done has gone beyond first aid.

Since 1991, Schedule 3 has also included very special provisions which extended the rights and powers of veterinary nurses to do things which other non-veterinarians cannot do, and these provisions are dealt with below.

Schedule 3 provisions relating to veterinary nurses

The heading to Schedule 3 to the Veterinary Surgeons Act is 'Exemptions from restrictions on practice of veterinary surgery'. Part 1 of the Schedule is entitled 'Treatment and Operations which may be given or carried out by unqualified persons'. In this context, **unqualified persons** are those who are not qualified as veterinarians. If it were not for the special provisions written into the Schedule in 1991, veterinary nurses would be in the same position as any non-veterinarians.

Those special provisions for veterinary nurses consist of additions to Part 1 which make lawful:

> Any medical treatment or minor surgery (not involving entry into a body cavity) to a companion animal by a veterinary nurse if the following conditions are complied with, that is to say:
> (a) the companion animal is, for the time being, under the care of a registered veterinary surgeon or veterinary practitioner and the medical treatment or minor surgery is carried out by the veterinary nurse at his direction; and
> (b) the registered veterinary surgeon or veterinary practitioner is the employer or is acting on behalf of the employer of the veterinary nurse.
> In this paragraph, 'companion animal' means an animal kept as a pet or for companionship, not being a horse, pony, ass, mule, nor an animal used in agriculture, as

defined by the Agriculture Act 1947. 'Veterinary nurse' means a nurse whose name is entered in the list of veterinary nurses maintained by the RCVS.

Interpretation of the provisions

It should be noted that these provisions do *not* permit:

- the making of a diagnosis;
- the carrying out of any procedure which is neither medical treatment nor surgery;
- entry into a body cavity (e.g. a laparotomy);
- any medical or surgical treatment carried out on any animal that does not meet the definition of a companion animal.

Further, from 1 July 1993, by virtue of an amendment to Schedule 3, dogs' tails may no longer be docked by unqualified persons. The only persons now permitted by law to dock dogs' tails are veterinary surgeons.

But how should one interpret the positive aspects of these provisions? One can do no better than to set out in full the advice that the Royal College issued in 1992 in its Annual Report for that year:

> The amendment to Schedule 3 does not attempt to define what constitutes 'medical treatment or minor surgery' (which is a term used elsewhere in Schedule 3) but leaves it to the directing veterinary surgeon to interpret the phrase with common sense, allied to professional judgement. There should be less difficulty in construing the term 'medical treatment' than the term 'minor surgery', since it may be a matter of opinion as to what is minor or not. It may, however be helpful to note that Stedman's Medical Dictionary defines a minor operation as a 'surgical procedure of relatively slight extent and not in itself hazardous to life'.
>
> The Royal College Council gave very careful consideration (when the proposed amendment to Schedule 3 was being discussed with the Ministry of Agriculture) to the possibility of producing a list of procedures which veterinary nurses might carry out, and rejected this idea in favour of a more flexible system whereby each veterinary surgeon would decide not only what he or she considered could reasonably be described as 'minor surgery', but whether or not the experience and expertise of the veterinary nurse to whom he proposed to entrust the minor surgery, justified such a decision.
>
> The advice of the Royal College is therefore that veterinary surgeons, rather than seeking guidance as to what procedure should or should not be entrusted to veterinary nurses should ask themselves the following questions before directing the veterinary nurse to carry out any medical treatment or minor surgery:
> (a) how difficult is it to carry out the procedure in question competently and successfully and bearing in mind the risks of the procedure?
> (b) has the nurse who is to be asked to carry out the procedure in question been given training and gained experience in the performance of the procedure, and is she aware of the risks associated with the procedure and is she now competent to carry it out?

(c) does she have not only the expertise and general competence to carry out the procedure, but also the experience and good sense which will enable her to react appropriately in the event of any problem arising?

(d) if necessary, will a veterinary surgeon be available to respond to a request for assistance?

(e) does the veterinary nurse feel comfortable that she can competently and successfully carry out the procedure—or is she anxious that she may be asked to perform surgery beyond her capabilities?

When considering all these matters, in order to reach a judgement as to whether or not to give the proposed direction, the veterinary surgeon should also bear in mind that, should anything untoward occur, and the veterinary nurse carry out his direction incompetently and/or negligently, legal liability will rest with the employer, rather than with the veterinary nurse as the employee.

It will be appreciated that this advice was offered by the RCVS to veterinary surgeons and veterinary practitioners but it also serves as a clear guide to veterinary nurses as to their position. Incidentally, for legal purposes 'she' in these and other regulations also covers the actions of male veterinary nurses. Only a handful of men have sought the qualification of either RANA or VN and, without prejudice, texts (including this chapter) often assume that the VN is female.

The meaning of the word 'direction'

The amendment to Schedule 3 provides that a veterinary nurse may carry out medical treatment or minor surgery 'at the direction' of the employing veterinary surgeon. That means that it is sufficient for the veterinary surgeon to instruct the veterinary nurse to carry out the procedure in question. There is no requirement in law for the veterinary surgeon to be present and/or supervise the veterinary nurse.

The veterinary nurse in training

It must be clearly understood that Schedule 3 provisions as set out and explained above do not apply to student veterinary nurses. They apply only to veterinary nurses whose names appear on the RCVS's list of veterinary nurses. While in training, and not yet qualified, student nurses cannot take advantage of the special status conferred on qualified and listed veterinary nurses, and cannot lawfully be directed by an employing veterinary surgeon to carry out any of the procedures covered by the amendment to Schedule 3.

They can, however, still administer first aid in an emergency and also amputate dew-claws of a puppy before its eyes open provided they have reached the age of 18. These are rights granted to all lay persons.

They can also carry out nursing duties and assist veterinary surgeons in any way which does not involve an act of veterinary surgery.

Procedures that are not 'acts of veterinary surgery'

Some years ago the solicitors to the RCVS advised that there were certain common procedures which did not constitute even minor acts of veterinary surgery and therefore could be carried out by veterinary nurses, nurses in training or other non-veterinarians.

These procedures included the removal of sutures, the replacement of dressings, the cutting of nails and beaks (unless performed for the treatment of a pathological condition) and the scaling of teeth carried out for prophylactic or cosmetic reasons. The College was further advised that there were a number of 'borderline' procedures which might or might not be considered to be acts of veterinary surgery. These included the giving of enemata, oral and anal hygiene measures, and the administration of medical products (other than controlled drugs and biological products) by the subcutaneous, intramuscular, intravenous and intraperitoneal routes, following specific instructions from the veterinarian as to dosage.

The College solicitors advised even at that time (prior to the amendment of Schedule 3) that it would be unlikely that a veterinary nurse would be prosecuted for carrying out any such procedures if she did so at the direction of a veterinary surgeon. The advice would also apply to a student veterinary nurse although the veterinarian would wish to be particularly sure of her competence before directing her to carry out such a procedure.

A qualified veterinary nurse should now be on firm legal ground, since the carrying out of the procedure mentioned, on companion animals at the direction of an employing veterinary surgeon (or veterinarian acting on behalf of the nurse's employer), would be covered by the amendment to Schedule 3.

Insurance Cover for Nursing Duties

The employing veterinary surgeon carries responsibility for the incompetent or negligent actions of the veterinary nurse. Although a client who wished to bring an action in the courts could also sue the veterinary nurse, it is likely that the employer would be the plaintiff's target as being better able to meet any damages awarded.

All veterinary practices insured with the Veterinary Defence Society Ltd are covered for acts and omissions of not only themselves but also their nursing and other lay staff. The RCVS has advised its members insured with other companies to make certain that their policies provide equivalent cover.

Professional Ethics for Nurses

All veterinarians on the Register of Veterinary Surgeons or the Supplementary Veterinary Register of veterinary practitioners (both maintained in terms of the Veterinary Surgeons Act by the Royal College of Veterinary Surgeons) are subject to the investigative jurisdiction of the College's Preliminary Investigation Committee and the judgements of its Disciplinary Committee—both statutory committees. As an aid to the better understanding of the veterinary profession's ethical obligations, the College publishes (and revises triennially) its Guide to Professional Conduct, and any veterinarian whose ethical conduct is found by the Disciplinary Committee to be so seriously flawed as to amount to conduct disgraceful in a professional respect is in danger of having his or her name removed (or suspended for a stated time) from the Register.

The RCVS has no such powers in relation to veterinary nurses, and neither the British Veterinary Nursing Association nor any other body has powers of this kind either. Nevertheless, veterinary nurses must be aware that ethical misbehaviour on their part could be held to be the responsibility of the veterinarian for whom they work—particularly if it were to be considered that the misbehaviour was permitted, condoned or due to lack of adequate instruction or supervision. All veterinary nurses should therefore be aware of the main provisions of the Royal College's Guide to Professional Conduct in order that they may avoid acting in a way which might call their employing veterinarian's conduct into question.

Some of the most important obligations which veterinary nurses should bear in mind are as follows:

(1) Never to carry out any act of veterinary surgery other than those they are permitted to perform in terms of Schedule 3 to the Veterinary Surgeons Act or any other exemption order under the Act in terms of which they hold individual qualifications (e.g. the Veterinary Surgery (Blood Sampling) Orders).

(2) To respect client confidentiality in exactly the same way as a veterinarian must do in the terms of the RCVS Guide to Professional Conduct.

(3) At all times (again like veterinarians) to do all in their power to ensure the welfare of animals entrusted to their care.

(4) Not to make any adverse comment to a client or other member of the public regarding the treatment administered to an animal by a veterinary surgeon, whether a member of their own practice or organisation or any other.

(5) Not to participate in, or allow themselves or their qualifications to be used in relation to, the promotion of veterinary medicinal products, animal foods, or any other products directly associated with veterinary practice or animals.

All these obligations apply equally to veterinary nurses and to student nurses.

In regard to confidentiality (item 2 in the above list) there are a few specific exceptions which are clearly set out in the appropriate section of the Guide to Professional Conduct, and all veterinary nurses must familiarise themselves with this part (paragraph 20) of the Guide. These exemptions apart, the ability of a client to consult professional advisers, secure in the knowledge that their discussions and any information passing between them will remain totally confidential, is the hallmark of the profession. If there is no certainty of complete confidentiality, information relevant to the well-being and treatment of the animal in question might be withheld—to the disadvantage of the animal.

Second Opinions, Referrals and Specialists

The Guide to Professional Conduct lays down for all veterinarians the procedures that need to be followed when a case is being referred to another veterinarian for a second opinion or on a referral basis. As veterinary nurses are often the first people to be contacted by animal owners, they must familiarise themselves with the correct procedures and see that, in so far as any referral needs to be arranged by them, the correct procedures are followed.

Veterinary nurses must be aware that the description 'specialist' may only be applied to those veterinarians specifically authorised by the Royal College to use this designation and listed in the appropriate sections of the college's Register of Veterinary Surgeons. They should not, therefore, whether orally or in writing, refer to any member of the veterinary profession as a 'specialist' if that person is not recognised as such by the RCVS. Veterinarians who provide services of a particular nature, or for a particular species, simply have a special interest or particular skills: they are not 'specialists' until and unless those skills, allied to their qualifications and experience, have enabled the RCVS to endow them with specialist status.

Care must also be taken in referring to a veterinary surgeon as a consultant. He or she may be providing consultancy services in a practice, as a person with experience or expertise in a particular field, but should not be referred to in such a way (e.g. 'consultant in veterinary dermatology') as would suggest that he or she is authorised to use the title of specialist if that is not the case.

The Health and Safety at Work Act 1974

This Act applies to all persons at work (other than domestic servants) and covers every business (such as veterinary practice) and the self-employed. It has relevance to both employers and employees, and also to the health and safety of members of the general public who may come into contact with the business or work in question.

The objective of the Act is to ensure that all employers and self-employed persons carry on their businesses in such a way as to ensure that no one is exposed to risks to their health or safety. Employees, who will include veterinary nurses, must:

- take reasonable care for the health and safety of themselves and of other persons who may be affected by their omissions at work;
- co-operate with the employer (or other persons) as far as is necessary to enable any duty or requirement under the Act to be performed or complied with; and
- not interfere, recklessly or intentionally, with anything provided in the interests of health, safety and welfare.

The Health and Safety Executive, which has responsibility for enforcing and advising on the Act, has shown interest in health and safety in veterinary practice. Of particular relevance in this area are the regulations that have been in force since October 1989 on the control of substances hazardous to health (COSHH). These regulations, to quote the BVA COSHH Guide:

> require employers and the self employed to assess and then prevent or control the exposure to hazardous substances of all their employees and others who might be affected by exposure to hazardous substances at work. This includes microbiological agents, dusts of any kind in substantial quantities and all chemicals hazardous to health. Lead, asbestos and ionising radiation are covered by separate sets of regulations.

Chapters 11 (Occupational Hazards) and 13 (Pharmacology, Therapeutics and Dispensing) look at the Health and Safety at Work Act and the COSHH regulations in greater detail.

Environmental Protection Law

The Environmental Protection Act 1990 has a relevance to the work of veterinary nurses, especially in the handling of clinical waste. The Act imposed a duty of care upon all producers of clinical waste to ensure that waste is handled and stored safely on their premises, and also disposed of safely and legally by the producers and others to whom the waste is passed for this purpose. This very complex matter is considered in more depth in Chapters 11 (Occupational Hazards) and 26 (Theatre Practice). For a clear explanation of the provisions of the legislation, the article which appeared in the *Veterinary Record* (9 January 1993, pp. 43–45) under the title 'The veterinary surgeon's duty of care in handling and disposing of clinical waste' is essential reading.

In that article, the view was expressed that since the legislation allows waste producers to hand over waste for subsequent disposal only to an authorised person, pets which were put down or died at a veterinary surgery (and thereby became clinical waste) could not be returned to owners for burial or other disposal at home. Although that would appear technically correct, the British Veterinary Association was subsequently advised by the Environment Minister that the Act need not be interpreted so strictly. The pet owner retained ownership of the body in law, and therefore had a right to have it returned (*Veterinary Record*, 30 January 1993, pp. 99–l00).

The Environmental Protection Act 1990 is also the legislation which made it obligatory for all councils to provide a Dog Warden service from April 1992 and an offence for dogs to 'stray' on the public highway.

Other Relevant Legislation

Although the Veterinary Surgeons Act 1960 is the statute of principal relevance to veterinary practice and therefore to the work of veterinary surgeons and veterinary nurses alike, there are a number of other Acts of Parliament of which both must be aware. Within the compass of this chapter it is not possible to provide more than a very brief account of each Act: for a fuller understanding of the provisions of each, consult the Royal College's booklet *Legislation Affecting the Veterinary Profession in the United Kingdom*. The following are the principal statutes with relevance to companion animal practice, with which veterinary nurses should be familiar.

The Medicines Act 1968

This Act controls the manufacture, importation, sale and supply of medicinal products in the United Kingdom, for both human and veterinary use. Its purpose is to secure the safety, quality and efficacy of all such products.

Medicinal products are substances or articles manufactured, sold, supplied, imported or exported for use, wholly or mainly for administration to humans or animals for a medicinal purpose. A **medicinal purpose** is defined in the Act so as to include diagnosis, treatment or prevention of disease, contraception, inducing anaesthesia, and preventing or interfering with the normal operation of a physiological function.

Medicinal products are divided into three main categories:

- **GSL** products (on a general sales list).
- **POM** products (on prescription only).
- **P** products (pharmacy only medicines).

There is also a fourth category of veterinary medicinal products, which is commonly referred to as the Merchant's List and indicated as **PML**. These are mainly for sale to farmers and horse-keepers. Chapter 13 looks at this Act in more detail.

Misuse of Drugs Act 1971

Chapter 13 also considers this Act which, with its subsidiary legislation, controls the possession, supply and use of what used to be known as 'dangerous drugs'. In terms of the Act, these are now known as 'Controlled Drugs'.

The Act allows veterinarians to possess, use, supply and prescribe most controlled drugs, but for veterinary use only. It is important to note that all controlled drugs are also prescription-only medicines in terms of the Medicines Act (see above).

The Protection of Animals Acts

There is a group of statutes, beginning with the Protection of Animals Act 1911 and known collectively as the Protection of Animals Acts 1911–1988, which seeks to prevent cruelty to animals and alleviate suffering.

The Act of 1911 provides that the following actions constitute cruelty, punishable by a fine or imprisonment:

(a) Cruelly to beat, kick, ill-treat, over-drive, over-load, torture, infuriate or terrify an animal.
(b) To cause suffering by doing or omitting to do any act.
(c) To convey or carry any animal in such a manner as to cause it unnecessary suffering.
(d) To perform any operation without due care and humanity (in relation to which the provisions of the Anaesthetics Acts are relevant).
(e) The fighting or baiting of any animal or the use of premises for such a purpose.
(f) The administering of any poison or injurious drug or substance to any animal.

It should be noted that the legislation is not concerned with whether or not the cruelty was intended. It is the result of the relevant act or omission which is important. When an owner of an animal is convicted of cruelty, the courts may order:

- the destruction of the animal(s) either with agreement or on the evidence of a veterinary surgeon;
- the disqualification from having custody of a particular kind of animal or any animal at all.

The Protection of Animals (Amendment) Act 1988 has made it an offence either to be present, without reasonable excuse, when animals are placed together for the purpose of fighting or to publish, or to cause to be published, an advertisement for a fight between animals.

The Anaesthetics Acts

The Protection of Animals (Anaesthetics) Acts 1954 and 1964 are intended to prevent the infliction of unnecessary suffering on an animal during an operation. It provides that the carrying out of any operation with or without the use of instruments, involving interference with the sensitive tissues or the bone structure of an animal, shall constitute an offence unless an anaesthetic is used in such a way as to prevent any pain to the animal during the operation. An operation of this kind, performed without or with inadequate anaesthetic, is said to be performed 'without due care and humanity'—see subparagraph (d) of the previous section. Exceptions to this general rule (which may be relevant to companion animal practice) are as follows:

(1) The making of injections or extractions by means of a hollow needle.
(2) Experiments authorised under the Animals (Scientific Procedures) Act 1986.
(3) The rendering of emergency first aid for the purpose of saving life or relieving pain.
(4) The docking of the tail of a dog or the amputation of the dew-claws of a dog before its eyes open.
(5) Any minor operation performed by a veterinarian being an operation which, by reason of its quickness or painlessness, is customarily so performed without an anaesthetic.
(6) Any minor operation whether performed by a veterinarian or by some other person, being an operation which is not customarily performed only by a veterinarian.

The Animals (Scientific Procedures) Act 1986

This Act prohibits the carrying out of experiments on animals except under licence from the Home Office. This is a very specialised piece of legislation, and reference to Chapter II of the RCVS's legislation handbook is recommended. Nevertheless, the veterinary nurse in companion animal practice should be aware of the following three points:

- All establishments breeding and supplying the most commonly used laboratory animals are required to obtain a certificate of approval from the appropriate Secretary of State.
- The Act prohibits the use of cats and dogs unless they are obtained direct from the designated establishment where they were bred. The use of stray or stolen pets will not be allowed in any circumstances.
- Demonstrations using live animals will be permitted where absolutely necessary for professional training but the Act prohibits their use in the education of school children or others at the same level.

Legislation covering animals kept commercially

There are four statutes which are designed to control the premises on which companion animals are kept for commercial purposes and to ensure the welfare of such animals. These are:

- The Pet Animals Act 1951
- The Animal Boarding Establishments Act 1963

- The Breeding of Dogs Act 1973
- The Riding Establishments Acts 1964 and 1970.

The responsibility of enforcement of these Acts rests with the local authority, from whom licences to operate such premises must be obtained, but inspections are normally carried out on behalf of the authorities by veterinary surgeons. Environmental Health Officers and Dog Wardens may also be involved in the inspection of premises.

The Pet Animals Act relates to the keeping of pet shops and prohibits the selling of animals as pets in any street or public place. It also prohibits the sale of pets to children under 12 years of age.

The Animal Boarding Establishments Act relates only to establishments which board dogs and cats, and not to the boarding of other animals. It should be noted that the fact that a boarding establishment is kept and is run by a veterinary surgeon (as distinct from having cages for his patients) does not exempt him from the need to obtain a licence.

The Breeding of Dogs Act requires the licensing of any premises (including a private dwelling) where more than two bitches are kept for the purpose of breeding for sale.

The Riding Establishments Acts deal with ponies and horses used in riding schools for hire and riding tuition. Each of these Acts is concerned with making sure that the animals are properly accommodated, watered, bedded, exercised and protected against disease and fire. The Acts relate to the inspection by approved veterinary surgeons of horses let out for hire or where money is exchanged for riding lessons on a horse or pony not belonging to the rider. Pony trekking centres are also involved in inspections but both riding clubs and livery yards are exempt if no tuition is involved using hired horses.

The British Veterinary Association has published guide lines for the inspection of each type of establishment.

The Dangerous Dogs Act 1991

This Act, together with subsidiary legislation, is designed to stop people from keeping dogs which are bred for fighting. The dogs currently specified as falling within this category are the **Pit Bull Terrier**, the **Japanese Tosa**, the **Dogo Argentino** and the **Fila Braziliero**, but other types may be added by statutory order.

The Act prohibits the breeding, sale, exchange or gift of dogs of the specified types. The only such dogs which anyone may now lawfully possess are those which, by the appropriate date (now past), had been reported to the police by the owners and which the owners had ensured were neutered, permanently identified and made the subject of third party insurance. Even such a dog may be allowed in a public place only if it is muzzled and on a lead, securely held by someone of not less than 16 years of age. To abandon such a dog or allow it to stray is an offence. In the case of convictions for offences under the Act, the court has the power to order the destruction of the dog in question.

The Act also creates the separate offence of owning or being in charge of a dog of any type which is dangerously out of control in a public place.

Some other Acts of importance

Under the **Abandonment of Animals Act 1960** it is an offence for the owner or possessor of an animal to abandon it without good reason (whether permanently or not) in circumstances likely to cause unnecessary suffering. The **Animals (Cruel Poisons) Act 1962** prohibits the killing of any mammal by any cruel poison, which is specified as including red squill, strychnine and yellow phosphorus. The **Dangerous Wild Animals Act 1976** provides that no one shall keep a dangerous wild animal without a licence from the local authority. The question often arises as to whether an animal is dangerous and wild in terms of legislation. All animals covered by the Act are set out in a Schedule, which is repeated in Chapter II of the RCVS's legislation handbook.

The legislation regarding **wildlife** also affects veterinary practices, with regard to the care and rehabilitation of injured wildlife. This subject is relevant to Chapter 4 (Exotics and Wildlife).

Regulations on the Import and Export of Cats, Dogs and Birds

Generally, dogs and cats may not be **imported** into the United Kingdom without spending 6 months in quarantine in terms of the **Rabies (Importation of Dogs, Cats and Other Mammals) Order 1974**. Any queries in regard to importation and this order should be addressed to the Rabies Branch of the Ministry of Agriculture, Fisheries and Food (at Hook Rise South, Tolworth, Surbiton, Surrey KT6 7NF). From time to time a veterinary practice may be presented with a dog or cat which has been imported but has not met the quarantine requirements. Although the practice may consider there is a dilemma between reporting this serious breach of the law and the ethical requirements of preserving client confidentiality, the RCVS has resolved the problem by stating in its Guide to Professional Conduct that the exceptions to the confidentiality rule include this very situation. Accordingly the veterinary surgeon should at once report such a breach of the quarantine regulations to the Rabies Branch of MAFF or to the Divisional Veterinary Officer.

Special provisions have been made for the importing of cats and dogs from other member states of the European Community *provided that they are being imported for commercial purposes only.* Such animals may be imported without quarantine provided that they are accompanied by the necessary certificates testifying that they are at least 8 months old, were born and have remained in a single rabies-free establishment since birth, and are identified by microchip, have been vaccinated against rabies and blood tested to confirm immunity.

The import of any live poultry or other birds or hatching eggs is prohibited, except under licence, in terms of the **Importation of Birds, Poultry and Hatching Eggs Order 1979**.

With regard to the **export** of birds, cats and dogs to other countries, the veterinary certificates, vaccinations and other requirements will vary from one country to another. (It should be borne in mind that the formalities are not so much designed for the export from the United Kingdom as for the import into another country.) If information is required regarding the importation of a dog, cat or bird into another country, enquiries should be made of the Export Branch of the MAFF as far in advance of the proposed date as possible.

7
Practice Organisation

B. J. WHITE

Communication

Communication is the conveyance of information from one person to another and the establishment of whether the message has been received and understood. The message may be written, oral or visual. Methods of communication can be used formally (e.g. a letter) or informally (e.g. a telephone conversation).

A veterinary practice provides a service, therefore communications with clients, other business organisations and staff are of paramount importance. External communication is the conveyance of information to any organisation or person not employed by the practice itself; internal communication is the conveyance of information within the practice.

Clients and staff are the most important people in any practice. Unless old clients are kept and new clients are continually registering with the practice, it will not expand and prosper. Hard work and dedication by all members of staff is needed to win the loyalty of pleased and informed clients.

Rules for Good Communication

There are many reasons why communications fail to achieve their objectives. A few basic rules should ensure an accurate and effective system of internal and external communication:

- All forms of communication must be polite, clear and unambiguous.
- Information must be easily understood by both parties.
- Do not forget that the style and tone of a message or conversation can affect the response given.
- One of the most important aspects of communication is to be able to listen to others, to understand their viewpoint or requirements and to try to fulfil their expectations.

Communication Failure

Communication breaks down when either the sender fails to communicate properly or the receiver fails to grasp the true meaning. Any form of communication will fail to be effective if there is any form of barrier between the sender and receiver. Factors that act as barriers can be found at each stage, faults (as Fig. 7.1 suggests) being on the part of:

- Writer/speaker
- Reader/listener
- Senior staff
- Media used
- Difficult circumstances.

Receptionist's Role

The receptionist is usually the first person with whom a client or the general public have contact when they telephone or come into the practice. The image that the receptionist portrays at that point of contact will be what the person remembers and perceives as the image of the practice as a whole. It is essential that this first impression, be it by telephone, direct contact or letter, is the one the practice wishes to portray. Reception is often the hub of internal and external communication within the practice.

Those working in reception must understand the policies and procedures of the practice for greeting visitors and clients and for security, safety and emergencies, as well as policy relating to routine work such as neutering, vaccination, worming and dealing with second opinion or referral cases.

The reception area must be kept clean and tidy. With the use of plants, attractive and well-maintained posters or pictures, up-to-date reading material and comfortable seats, the area can project a warm, pleasant feeling which will encourage client confidence.

The personal appearance and hygiene of all members of staff are often perceived as representing the cleanliness and quality of the entire practice. Therefore it is important that a professional image is given. Clients like to know to whom they are talking and many practices now provide name badges.

Clients are like paying guests and they should be greeted as soon as they arrive. Ascertain the purpose of the visit and obtain all relevant details. Listen carefully and interpret the information that is given. Also look at the person who is communicating with you: non-verbal communication (body language) may tell you more than you are hearing.

Face-to-face communication has many advantages. It is fast, direct and two-way; it allows participation of all present and it also allows instant feedback. There are also disadvantages:

- No record.
- Lack of control of content (particularly if there are more than two participants).
- Difficulty in responding if put 'on the spot'.

195

BARRIERS TO COMMUNICATION		
Writer/speaker		
Content	Innaccurate; Irrelevant; Ill prepared;	Inadequate; Too technical; Outdated.
Presentation	Unclear; Ambiguous; Ill timed;	Illogical sequence; Age/educational background of receiver not taken into consideration.
Reader/listener		
Content	Non-comprehension; Inability to pass on an accurate message;	Inability to recognise the importance of the message; Failure to check details.
Receiver	Misinterpretation of information; Emotion;	Not taking notes; Messages taken down on scraps of paper.
Senior staff		
Content	Too technical; Insufficient information.	
Presentation	As for writer/speaker.	
Media used		
Unsuitable medium for information being given and/or person receiving it; Poor telephone techniques used; Inability to use the medium properly; Faulty equipment; Breakdown of equipment; Inadequate maintenenace of equipment; Inadequate facilities for workload or type of work.		
Circumstances		
Loss of documents; Inaccurate processing of information; Failure to follow procedures; Failure to set procedures.	Inadequate staffing levels; Lack of team work/co-operation between staff; Lack of communication between management.	

Fig. 7.1 Barriers to communication.

- Lack of security (compared with written communication).

Appointments and the Admission and Discharge of Patients

Appointments for consultation

Ensure that all those booking appointments know who is consulting and what length of consultation they require for certain procedures. Primary kitten vaccination consultations are sure to take longer than a post-operative check on a dog castration.

Nothing annoys clients more than surgeries that always run late. Try to ensure that surgeries start on time and that time is allotted for possible unexpected cases or emergencies.

Appointments for surgery

Ensure that all those booking animals in for operative or medical procedures are aware of the practice protocol for such cases. All animals should have been examined recently by the veterinary surgeon or be booked in for an appointment on the day of admission. Full details about the animal in question should be obtained from the owner plus a detailed list of procedures required to be undertaken whilst admitted into the practice.

Clients should be given accurate and detailed instructions on the preparation of the animal prior to admission.

Appointments for second opinions

When clients indicate to a veterinary surgeon that they are seeking referral for a second opinion from another veterinary surgeon, the original veterinary surgeon should make all the arrangements for such a consultation, including providing a full case history to the second veterinary surgeon.

Clients often telephone the practice themselves to arrange for a second opinion and it is essential that all staff dealing with such calls know what procedures should be followed to avoid the unethical situation of supersession. The original veterinary surgeon should be contacted by the practice and notified of the client's wish, so that both veterinary surgeons can discuss the case.

If the owner subsequently decides not to use the services of the original veterinary surgeon, the latter should be notified as soon as possible.

The following relevant definitions are given in the RCVS's *Guide to Professional Conduct* (1993 edn):

- **Second opinion**—when the original veterinarian or the client requests a second opinion from another veterinarian on diagnosis or on treatment, the intention being that the continued responsibility for treatment of the case should remain with the original veterinarian.
- **Referral**—when at the request of a veterinarian or client a case is referred to a second veterinarian or to another therapist for further diagnosis and treatment with the objective of return to the responsibility of the referring veterinarian at a mutually agreed time.
- **Supersession**—when a second veterinary surgeon assumes responsibility for diagnosis and treatment of the case without reference to the first veterinary surgeon or against the latter's wishes.

House calls

Ensure that the client's full name, address and telephone number are obtained when arranging a house call. It is helpful if the client gives suitable directions on how to reach the house. It is essential to obtain as full a description of the animal's condition as soon as possible to ensure that the veterinary surgeon takes not only the correct equipment and drugs but also support staff if necessary. Staff should be aware that the personal security of a veterinary surgeon going out on a visit may require that a nurse is taken along for safety in numbers. The time of the visit should therefore be arranged according to the urgency of the visit and the availability of staff.

Admission of animals

The admission of animals is best carried out by appointment in a separate room, allowing the owner time to discuss the case with the veterinary surgeon or nurse. This is usually done the evening prior to surgery, or at least 2 hours prior to surgery, thus giving time for the animal to settle and any preoperative procedures to take place.

Owners are frequently concerned about leaving a pet and often need the reassurance of a talk with a neatly dressed, friendly and knowledgeable person. There should be clear practice policies on who admits animals (if not the veterinary surgeon) and when an animal's preoperative check should take place. Owners often wish to see the premises where their animal will be hospitalised and there should be a clear practice policy on this matter also.

On admitting an animal, the nurse should write down routine details and ask relevant questions about the condition of the animal. These should include checking the owner's details and contact telephone number, the animal's details and an up-to-date weight. Ask the following questions:

- Have there been any changes since the veterinary surgeon last saw the animal?
- When did the animal last eat any food?
- When did the animal last take fluids?
- When did the animal last have any medication, particularly if on a current course prescribed by the veterinary surgeon?
- To the owner's knowledge, does the animal have any allergies or adverse reactions to particular foods or drugs?
- When was the last bowel movement/urine passed?
- If the animal is female and entire, when was she last 'in season'?
- Vaccination status?
- Temperament?
- Have any abnormalities been noticed?

Also take the following action:

- Make a note of all objects brought in with the animal, to ensure that they are returned with the animal when it is discharged.
- All cats should be brought into the surgery in some form of carrier—if not they should be placed in one immediately. For security, cats should always be carried in a carrier, even from one room to another.

- To ensure that dogs do not escape by slipping collars and leads provided by the owner, place practice slip leads on all dogs when transferring them to and from the kennels.
- It will depend on practice policy whether owners accompany their pets to the kennels. If not, it is best to ask the owner to leave the room before the dog is taken through.
- Any animal booked in for a procedure requiring the administration of a general or local anaesthetic should normally be admitted only after the owner or agent has read, understood and signed a fully completed anaesthetic consent form. Only some-one over the age of 18 year may sign this form.
- It is often practice policy that all operative and investigative procedures are paid for on collection of the animal. The veterinary surgeon admitting the animal should be able to give the owner some idea of the cost, but this can always be confirmed when the owner arranges an appointment on the date of collection.

Kennels. Kennels and cages must be labelled clearly and a system used to ensure that animals are not mixed up. It is possible to obtain identification collars for dogs and cats similar to the wrist bands placed on people when in hospital.

There must also be some method of correctly linking an animal in a kennel or cage with its full records, wherever these are kept. They might be on the front of the cage, or on clip-boards kept in a place corresponding to the appropriate kennel. If a compu-terised system is used, there must be a proper refer-ence on the kennel which can be used to access with certainty the right patient's data on the computer.

Think about the allocation of cages according to the species and the disease:

- Cats are best separated from dogs.
- Small animals need to be put in an appropriate place and type of cage.
- Birds and nocturnal animals prefer a secluded, dimmed area.
- Infectious animals must be isolated and their cages labelled with relevant information so that staff may handle and care for them accordingly.

The stress for a hospitalised animal can be reduced to a minimum with gentle, caring nursing and a little thought. Animals often settle very well if regularly visited by their owner, who may bring in a well-loved blanket or toy (as long as the animal is unlikely to eat it). Feeding an animal from its own bowls may also reduce stress. If this does not work, early discharge may need to be considered in the interest of the animal's wellbeing.

Discharging of animals

This process must be undertaken by someone who will be able to answer the owner's routine questions about the case.

No animal should be allowed to go home if the owner feels unable to care for it properly, be it wound management, stabilisation of an animal's fluid balance, digitalisation or diabetic stabilisation. Some animals are bright and well enough to go home but it is more convenient if the practice keeps the animal hospitalised—for example, when a dog has a discharging Penrose drain in a wound that needs flushing four times daily. A sleepy Pomeranian is easy enough to care for post-operatively, but this may not be the case with a Great Dane. Each case should be considered individually and discharged at an appropriate time that is convenient for the owner, but in the best interest of the animal.

Before discharging the animal:

- The owner should be given full details on the procedures undertaken and any results of investigative procedures carried out on the animal.
- Detailed information on immediate post-operative/investigative care with regards to wound care, diet, exercise and medication should be given.
- If the animal is present whilst this information is being given, the owner is likely to take in very little – it is better to give the information before the animal is brought through. Many owners benefit from being given these instructions in writing as well. They should always be reassured that they can contact the surgery staff if they have any queries.
- If any medication is being dispensed, owners are often very glad to be given a practical demonstration on how best to administer it, particularly if they have no previous experience.
- All drugs should be suitably packaged and labelled.
- Remember to return the animal's belongings and always ensure that they are clean before going out.
- Despite the animal's state on arrival for admission, every effort should be made to ensure that it goes out clean and well groomed. With certain animals the coat is in such a bad state on admission that it would require more than a good brush to remove the dirt and mats. Permission must be sought to go ahead with such a procedure.
- Finally, make an appointment for a return visit if required and deal with payment of the account according to the practice policy.

Forms of Communication

Communication can be divided into two kinds:

- Formal (approved or arranged by the practice management).
- Informal (unofficial or unplanned methods of communication).

Formal Communication

If a method of communication involves the **written** word, it can be regarded as **permanent**. Written communications include:

- Letters
- Written instructions
- Memoranda
- Messages
- Reports
- Wage slips
- Practice magazine
- Notices.

If the method does not involve the written word, it is not permanent and is open to misinterpretation unless confirmed in writing:

- Public address systems (broadcasting of messages).
- Staff meetings (unless minuted).
- Interviews/performance appraisals.
- Suggestion schemes.

Informal Communication

Informal communications are often swift and, if used effectively, they help in ensuring that work is done more quickly than by using some of the formal methods. However, they are not 'permanent' methods. They include:

- Casual conversation
- Telecommunications
- Body language
- Rumours (often inaccurate).

Methods of Communication

The main methods of communication are:

- Written
- Oral
- Telecommunications
- Computers/applications; word-processing.

Written Communication

For written communication to be most effective, it should be:

- clear and understandable;
- logical, using sentences and paragraphs that are concise and simple;
- in the correct style and tone to suit the circumstances;
- in the appropriate format and layout (e.g. letter, memo, message or report);
- punctuated accurately, with correct grammar and spelling;
- free from 'jargon'.

Before sending out any form of written communication, ensure that you or a senior member of staff proof-reads it to detect any errors. Poorly constructed written communications create a poor impression on the recipient.

Business letters

Business letters should be polite, brief, accurate and set out clearly. Figure 7.3 shows how the different components of such a letter might be set out. They are:

(a) **Date**—day/month/year
(b) **Reference**—the writer's and/or typist's initials and/or a reference number
(c) **Addressee**—name and address of the addressee
(d) **Salutation**—writer's greeting
(e) **Heading**—referring to the subject matter
(f) **Body of the letter** – sentences and paragraphs in a clear and understandable order.
(g) **Complimentary close**—the closing remark which is governed by the salutation used (e.g. Dear Sir/ Yours faithfully; or Dear Mrs Smith/Yours sincerely)
(h) **Description of signatory**—name and position of the writer.

Many organisations have a 'style' or display of letter to be followed by all staff members. In the modified full-block style illustrated in Fig. 7.3, all lines start at the left-hand margin, except the date which is on the right for ease of reference in files. The example also gives 'open' punctuation which is easy to read, giving an uncluttered appearance with no commas above or below the body of the letter, no full stops after abbreviations, no brackets around item numbers and no underscoring.

Envelopes. The postal town should be typed or written in capital letters and the postcode should be the last line of the address with one space between the two sections of the code.

Memoranda

'Memos' are used for internal communication. They include:

- To and from whom the memo is going.
- The date.
- A reference.
- A heading.
- The body of the memo.

Messages

Messages are best taken down using a preprinted sheet to ensure that all details are recorded in a logical and permanent manner and passed to the appropriate person. The following should be noted:

- Date and time of visit/call.
- Name of the person for whom the message is intended.
- Caller's name, address and telephone number.
- Full details of the message received.
- Whether the caller needs to be contacted or whether they will call back.

Reports

Reports vary in style, format, length and content depending on the audience and purpose of the report. For shorter more informal reports there are usually three parts:

- Introduction (background, description of the situation and reason for the report).
- Findings.
- Conclusion (and recommendations to be made).

Case recording. Within the practice, various reports may be produced in various forms—handwritten, typewritten or computer generated.

Medical records are usually handwritten or typed into a computer. These essentially hold all the owners' relevant details and information about the animals important to the veterinary surgeon, providing a history of previous medical and surgical treatment, laboratory and radiographic findings and vaccination status.

It is extremely important that all details are accurate and up to date. If a card system is employed the filing of these and any radiographs and laboratory forms should be conscientious and accurate. Despite tradition, this is not a job for the most junior member of staff and is best done by a limited number of people to avoid the misplacement of records. On removal from the system, records should be replaced by a marker card indicating when and by whom the report was taken (as described in the Filing section of this chapter).

FORMAL COMMUNICATION	
Written	Letters Written instructions Memoranda Messages Reports Wage slips Practice magazine Notices These are "permanent" methods of communication.
Public address systems	Broadcasting of messages. This is open to misinterpretation as the information is NOT a permanent method of communication.
Staff meetings	Unless information is confirmed in writing (minutes of the meeting) it is not a "permanent" method of communication.
Interviews/ performance appraisals	Unless information is confirmed in writing this again, is not "permanent" and open to misinterpretation.
Suggestion schemes	If done in writing these are a "permanent" method of communication.

Fig. 7.2. Formal methods of communication.

Taking a case history. For each case handled a summary of the following facts need to be collected:

- Client: title, name, initials, full address, business and home telephone numbers, date.
- Animal: species, breed, description, sex (neutered or entire), age, temperament.
- Details of vaccinations, medical or surgical procedures undertaken by a previous veterinary surgeon, if applicable.
- Reason for the visit.
- Brief description of the owner's observations of the animal's condition.

When administering first aid prior to the arrival of the veterinary surgeon, obtain as much of the above information about the animal as possible before proceeding. The information must be taken down in a clear and legible form—something that is made easy with the use of computers.

Oral Communication

Person to person

This may be between a member of staff and a client, or staff communicating with each other. This 'non-permanent' method of communication is open to inaccuracy and misinterpretation if not used carefully but it can be a most effective, efficient and rapid method of transmitting information.

Tone of voice, facial expression, body language and the selection of words have a massive impact on the message being transmitted.

Veterinary nurses spend a considerable amount of time talking to clients when taking case histories, when admitting and discharging patients and when making appointments whilst working on reception:

- Dress neatly and cleanly.
- Be pleasant, kind, patient, understanding, prepared to listen and when necessary sympathetic.
- Maintain a dignified, knowledgeable, efficient but friendly manner at all times.
- Show no sign of annoyance or fear, despite the occasional angry client or vicious patient.
- If clients are kept waiting for any reason (on the telephone or in the waiting room) keep them informed regularly.
- Learn to read people's body language. They will certainly pick up information from your body language, particularly if what you are saying is not what you feel or mean.

Messages

Oral messages should always be transcribed into an accepted written format as a permanent form of communication. Listen carefully and extract the relevant and appropriate information from the conversation, preferably filling in a message sheet to ensure that all information is recorded. To ensure

accuracy, read the message back to the deliverer, then pass it on as appropriate. Notify the deliverer of the approximate time/date this will be given to the receiver, remembering to find out what they wish the receiver to do on obtaining the message.

Always ensure that client, colleague and practice confidentiality is maintained at all times.

Meetings

Meetings are direct but not permanent methods of communication and can be ineffective if held too frequently or for too long.

An agreed agenda and an elected chairperson will help to produce an active and informative meeting. Minutes will confirm in writing what was said and recommendations agreed at the meeting.

Telecommunications

Developments in the field of telecommunications are so rapid that any description of equipment rapidly becomes out of date. It includes a wide range of telephone, facsimile ('fax') and telex systems; intercom, paging and public address systems; and

---

LAYOUT FOR A LETTER

a)   14th April 19...

b)   Our Ref: TTH/PM/123

c)   Mrs A Brooke
      42 Springvale Road
      Tollgate
      UPPINGTON
      South Yorkshire
      S42 2SS

d)   Dear Mrs Brooke

e)   **Abbeyvale Veterinary Hospital Open Day**

f)   As a valued client of long standing you are invited to attend a tour of our Veterinary Hospital complex.
      A complete tour has been planned to allow you to see what facilities we have and to give you an opportunity to understand about our Veterinary Hospital care.
      If you would like to take part in the tour, please indicate your preference of dates and times listed below. For safety reasons, numbers are limited, so please apply early. The tour will be rounded off with coffee and biscuits, providing time for members of staff to answer any questions you may have. The tour will take approximately half an hour.
      Friday 3 May 19...   7.30 pm
      Monday 6 May 19...   7.30 pm
      Saturday 11 May 19...   2 pm
      Saturday 11 May 19...   4 pm

g)   We look forward to hearing from you.

      Yours sincerely

h)   Theresa T Hanson BVSc MRCVS
      Practice Manager

Fig. 7.3. Layout for a letter.

LAYOUT FOR A MEMORANDUM

Memo

To: _____ Date: _____

From: _____ Ref: _____

Subject: _____

Fig. 7.4. Layout for a memorandum.

computer systems. Figure 7.5 briefly describes some of the telecommunications equipment that veterinary nurses might be required to use.

Answering the telephone

The telephone should be answered promptly, confidently and efficiently, saying good morning (or afternoon or evening) and giving the name of the practice. Speak clearly and remember that your greeting will create a favourable or unfavourable impression of the practice as a whole.

Some practices may require that you then state your name and ask, 'How may I help you?' however this will vary. Always ask who is calling. If you are unable to deal with the enquiry yourself, obtain as much information as possible and notify the caller that you are placing them 'on hold' while you see if someone else is able to assist.

Pre-empt any queries or lapses of memory by surgery staff about the waiting caller by giving them the relevant information before putting the call through. This will also create a favourable impression with the client. In the meantime, keep going back to a caller 'on hold' to apologise for any delay. They may be required to call back at a more appropriate time or you may need to obtain details from them so that the call can be returned. All telephone messages should be recorded in writing.

The practice should have a clear policy about the information that may be given over the telephone to clients and non-clients. All staff must be aware of these policies and then the relevant information can be given out in a clear and informed manner. If there is any doubt, the veterinary surgeon should be consulted and the client asked to bring the animal into the practice for examination.

A client may require telephone advice on animal first aid procedures. This should be given in a clear, calm manner by someone who has received training or instruction in the aims and procedures of animal first aid. Chapter 3 (First Aid) gives a checklist of questions to ask. You may need to advise the owner on how best to transport the animal to the practice or alternatively arrange a visit depending on the situation.

Computers

The use of computers is growing rapidly and they are playing an increasingly important role in the day-to-day running of veterinary practices in a number of areas, including:

- Client records
- Sales and purchase control
- Stock control
- Costing and budgetary control
- Personnel records
- Wages/salary systems
- Market research
- Cash flow analysis
- Word processing
- Desktop publishing.

All users of computers must be aware of the Data Protection Act 1984, which is supervised by the Data Protection Registrar. All employers holding computerised data including personnel records need to register as 'data users' and must state the following before registering:

- The types of data held.
- Why the data is held.
- From whom and how the information is obtained.
- To whom the information will be disclosed.

Employees and clients have a statutory right to access all computerised information held about themselves. Reference to any manual records from the computer system are not covered by this Act provided that any such manual records contain purely factual information.

Eight principles within the Act govern the processing of computerised personal data:

- Data must be obtained fairly and lawfully.
- Users are required to register the personal data held with the Data Protection Registrar and it must be held only for specified and lawful purposes.
- Data must only be disclosed and used for the purpose registered.
- Data must be relevant, adequate but not excessive for its requirement.
- Data must be accurate and up to date.
- Data must not be held any longer than necessary.
- Individuals have a right to be granted access to their own personal data at reasonable intervals without undue expense and must be provided with a copy of it, in a understandable form. Data must be amended or removed where appropriate.
- Necessary precautions must be taken by data users to ensure security in order to prevent unauthorised access, disclosure, alteration, or removal of personal data and accidental loss of data.

Computer hardware

The physical parts of a computer are described as hardware:

TELECOMMUNICATIONS EQUIPMENT	
Cellular 'phone	**Portable** Hand-held battery-operated – can be used anywhere. **Mobile** Permanently fitted in cars. Some allow "hands free speech" and will accept voice activated dialling. **Transportable** Battery operated and can be used in or out of a car. Costs include a monthly airtime rental charge.
Cordless 'phone	Enables telephone to be used within 100 metres from base unit.
Intercom	Enables communication between 2 or more locations, often within the same building, without interfacing with the main telephone system.
Public address system	Useful if not overused when it can become irritating, distracting and subsequently ignored.
Paging system	Used to attract attention of an individual and direct them to particular location to collect message or receive further instructions.
Bleeper system	**(personal radio receiver)** Pocket-sized, battery-operated, giving out a high pitched signal usually activated from switchboard. Holder of "bleep" then telephones the switchboard to collect message. Care must be taken to ensure used within range of central control point.
Radio paging	Similar to "bleep" but operates over wider area.
Telephone answering machine	Includes those that: – answer call and play recorded message; – answer recorded message left by caller; – (dual purpose telephones and answer machines) enable personal answering of calls or leaving the machine to record; – have a bleeper or voice-activated remote control facility enabling off-site user to contact own machine and listen to messages.
Telemessage	Telegram-type printed message delivered by first class post if message sent before 2200 hours from telephone or telex machine.
Telex	Quick means of transmitting messages, using teleprinter, to another subscriber of telex system. Standard rental charge for hiring line to telex exchange. Charges based on distance and duration of calls therefore messages should be as short, clear and unambiguous as possible. Messages should contain: – Sender's answerback code – repeated at end of message – Correspondent's telex number – repeated at end of message – Date and time – Reference Do not use: – Salutation/complementary close – Non-essential words Do use: – Common abbreviations – Repetition of numerical information in words. Messages are typed and corrected before transmission (using visual display screen). Messages can be copied by printer ensuring both sender and receiver have hard copy. If printer is in use, incoming messages are stored in memory and printed out as soon as it is free. Can be used to store information for later recall and for transmitting same message to multiple addresses.
Facsimile (fax)	Transmits exact copies of documents (including graphics, photographs) over telephone lines to other fax terminals quickly and accurately. Charges based on time to transmit message at same rate as telephone calls. All faxes compatible, grouped by speed of transmission. Groups 1 and 2 slowest; Group 3 transmit A4 document in approximately 20 seconds; Group 4 (used with digital telephone networks) capable of transmitting same message in approximately 3 seconds. Fax machines can be fitted into cars.

Fig. 7.5. Telecommunications systems.

- Terminal—a visual display unit and a keyboard linked to a computer, in effect the point of use for the operator.
- Peripheral device—any input or output device that is used to communicate with the computer; a typical set includes keyboard, mouse, VDU and printer.
- **Central processing unit (CPU)**—controls the operation of the computer.
- **Keyboard**, through which the operator enters data into the computer.
- **Visual display unit (VDU)**—displays data on a screen.
- **Mouse**—portable input device on a rolling ball; it is used to move a pointer on the screen, the position of which is activated when the mouse button is 'clicked'.
- **Printer**—data printed out on paper by the printer is described as **hard copy**. The wide choice of printers currently fall into two main categories:—character printers, which print one character—i.e. letter or number—at a time (e.g. dot matrix or

inkjet);—page printers, which print a complete page at a time (e.g. laser).

Computer disks

Hard disks, normally of metal, might be:

- Fixed (Winchester) type—fixed inside a micro-computer and able to store from 20 to more than 1000 megabytes of data.
- Exchangeable type—in stacks of up to 6 disks enclosed in a plastic case (generally used only by large organisations).

Floppy disks are of thin, flexible plastic protected by a hard or soft plastic cover and are in two sizes: 3.5 in or 5.25 in. The size and the density of the disk determines the volume of data that can be stored on it. A 3.5 in disk holds more information than a 5.25 in disk; high density (HD) disks hold more than single density (SD) or double density (DD) disks. The choice of size and density is dictated to some degree by the CPU.

Floppy disks are placed into the appropriate **disk drive** mounted on the computer when required. They can be used as a method of filing computer data but for large volumes (as in a veterinary practice system) it is more usual to store the information on hard disk and perhaps use a tape back-up system. Different types or sources of data can be stored on separate disks but these must be clearly labelled and stored safely in a disk box.

Computer tapes are similar to those used in music systems. The density of a tape is a measure of the amount of data that can be stored on its surface (measured in bits per inch). To locate information in the middle of the tape it is necessary to play the tape through to that point. Thus access is relatively slow, but tapes are cheap and tend to be used for back-up storage where quick access is not required.

Optical disks include computer disk (CD) Read Only Memory (ROM) disks that look like compact disks and are designed as bulk storage systems for information that does not require changing. They are usually produced commercially and hold data such as textbook information—they have a role in teaching. 'Floptickal' disks are similar to CD-ROMs but can accept information; they are similar in size to floppy disks but with a huge capacity.

Computer systems

Single-user systems include personal computers (PCs)—one VDU, one keyboard and one CPU—usually with one person accessing the information. Some of these are 'dedicated' as word processors.

Network systems are groups of single-user PCs linked (by cable) to a terminal so that data and expensive resources such as printers can be shared.

Multi-user PCs, using special software, allow a number of terminals to operate a single computer (one CPU and a number of 'dumb' terminals). This is the system most commonly used in large, fully computerised veterinary practices.

Software

The program that dictates what the hardware does is described as the 'software'. The process of switching on the computer and loading the software into its memory is described as 'booting up'.

Software application packages are written for particular functions. For example:

- Games
- Drawing or painting
- Design drawings
- Management information systems (appointment system/meetings)
- Database (sales/purchases/wages systems)
- Word processing
- Spreadsheets (calculations and accounts).

Database programs are designed to manage and store large quantities of data. They are often custom-written and a veterinary practice's database program might include information on vaccinations, species, coat colours etc. The program allows the creation, amendment and deletion of records so that client and animal information is kept up to date.

Spreadsheets are powerful calculating tools used in managing numerical information quickly and efficiently. For example:

- Plotting graphically the values of monthly vaccination sales.
- Calculating the costs of an operation by inputting figures—for example, if you enter the number of hours an animal is under an anaesthetic, the flow rate of the gases and the unit cost of the gases, the computer will calculate how much it costs to provide the gases for that particular operation.
- Calculating averages and standard deviations—for example, calculating the average transaction fee. If the practice price list is stored on a spreadsheet it is very simple and quick to increase prices by the rate of inflation without having to calculate and change each price individually.
- Accounts and VAT records can also be kept.

Desktop publishing is a facility for preparing documents containing both text and graphics of a quality adequate for use in publications—incorporating pictures with the text, laying out pages with multiple columns etc., as required for a practice newsletter.

Word processing

A variety of documents can be produced using a word processing applications program on a PC or stand-alone (dedicated) word processor (WP). The screen displays typed input or text, either with codes that control its design and layout, or as straight text on the basis of WYSIWYG ('what you see is what you get').

There are many word-processing applications:

- Processing articles, letters, reports, minutes etc.
- Amending and updating documents without retyping all of the information (e.g. drug lists, mailing lists, price lists, telephone numbers).
- 'Merge-printing' standard letters with a mailing list so that each letter is individually addressed and detailed (e.g. booster reminders).

More sophisticated WP programs have extended capabilities such as database, spreadsheet and desktop publishing facilities.

Data safety

Floppy disks are prone to damage which can corrupt the information stored on them unless they are handled and stored correctly:

- Do not handle the exposed parts of a floppy disk.
- File disks in a dust-free box when not in use.
- Do not drop them.
- Keep coffee and other liquids well away from disks (and keyboards).

Information held on the computer in a veterinary practice is irreplaceable. It is essential to have a **back-up routine** that will minimise the loss of information in most eventualities. Each practice should devise a regular back-up routine and should ensure that the routine is followed rigorously. The essence of backing up is to copy data on to a separate disk or tape, stored separately from the originals.

- Back up daily (or more frequently in a very busy practice). Daily back-ups are often performed automatically overnight.
- In addition, back up weekly to ensure that data is saved in case corruption of information goes unnoticed for a number of days.
- For added insurance, back up on a monthly basis as well. (This is a 'belt-and-braces' system—many practices follow only a daily back-up routine.)

Intelligent tills

Intelligent tills incorporate some of the elements of a computer. They may be able to read item prices, using a bar-code reader, or have dedicated buttons for items and services sold. Some also have the capacity to check stock levels and create automatic orders. Certain intelligent tills can be used to update vaccination reminder information. If a practice uses a manual medical record-card system, an intelligent till provides a cheap and effective way of automating certain routines such as stock control and vaccination reminders.

The future of electronic technology

Increasingly, computers are replacing manual filing systems. Digital data may be stored (filed) 'on-line' in a computer, or 'off-line' on disks or other magnetic media. Advances in technology are likely to result in significant changes in the way that data is generated, stored and utilised, particularly in the fast-moving world of veterinary medicine. In the near future it is possible that one or more of the following will be used in the day-to-day running of many practices:

- Storage of ECGs on computer.
- Interpretation of ECGs by computer.
- Storage of radiographs on computer.
- Scanning of radiographs by computer.
- Digital cameras linked to the computer to take and store information such as skin conditions.
- Electronic drug-ordering, the order to the wholesaler is transmitted direct from the computer.
- Laboratory reports transmitted electronically from the laboratory directly to the practice computer.

The management of information may be in the form of one or a combination of the following increasingly sophisticated systems:

- Card systems and an ordinary till.
- Card system and an intelligent till capable of stock control.
- Card system and an intelligent till capable of stock control and producing vaccination reminders.
- Word processor and intelligent till holding clinical data as well as controlling stock and producing vaccination reminders.
- Multi-user system.
- Computer system at the main surgery linked to the branch surgeries by dedicated land lines, ensuring access of information gathered at all sites.

Clinical information held on a card system at a practice that runs more than one site can be difficult to access when, say, an animal normally seen at a branch is brought into the main surgery out of normal working hours. Practices that encounter this problem will probably favour the computer-link system described above.

Filing Systems

Filing is often an unpopular job but it is a vital one. A poorly managed system will produce hours of extra work spent looking for misfiled or lost material. If the filing of records is carried out regularly and accurately, a fast efficient system for the retrieval of information can be developed.

The storage system must be suitable for the information being stored and accessibility required. The storage of radiographs in labelled envelopes or cardboard sleeves placed in suspension filing cabinets is more appropriate than stacking them all on top of one another in a box.

The ideal filing system should incorporate the following features:

- Guaranteed fast retrieval of information.
- Easy identification of misfiled material.
- Easy identification of active material and archive material.
- Allowance for expansion of the system.
- Determination of the period of retention of documents.
- Consideration of security and safety.
- Identification of file users by a system of tracer cards or 'out' guides showing users' names and date borrowed, placed in position of file removed.
- Suitable system of indexing.
- Index and cross-references if necessary.
- Colour coding for awareness of misfiling and for ease of identification.

Commonly used indexing systems include:

- Alphabetical
- Numerical
- Alpha-numerical
- By subject
- Geographical.

The alphabetical system is most commonly used in practice for client files. However, misfiling can occur when staff are not aware of the rules of such a system.

- Identifying by surname. If the surnames are identical, determine the position by the spelling of the christian names:
  —SMITH James
  —SMITH John
- For hyphenated names, start with the first part of the name and ignore the hyphen; treat the surname as one word:
  —PYGOTT-SMITH Jennifer
- Place short names before long (the 'nothing before something' rule):
  —MOOR
  —MOOR A
  —MOOR Alan
  —MOORE Alan
- Treat compound names as one name:
  —DE LA MOTTE Phillip
  —DE LA RUE Phillis
  —LE MESURIER John
- File all names written St. or Saint under Saint.
- File all names beginning with Mc or Mac as Mac and place in the appropriate sequence:
  —MCADAM
  —MACE
  —MACKINTOSH
  —MACNAIR
- Titles are placed after the surname and ignored as indexing units:
  —HIBBLE (Dr) Alice
  —HOLTE (Lady) Phillipa
  —SALTER (Maj) John
  —THOMAS (Prof) Jayne
- Use the first name of an organisation with several names:
  —JAMES, Alan and Smyth Veterinary Surgery

- Commonly abbreviated names should be treated as if written out in full:
  —BRITISH OXYGEN COMPANY—BOC
  —NATIONAL RADIOLOGICAL PROTECTION BOARD—NRPB
  —PEOPLE'S DISPENSARY FOR SICK ANIMALS—PDSA
- Treat any number as if it were written out in full:
  —1st Street Cat Shelter—FIRST Street Cat Shelter
  —33 Restaurant—THIRTY THREE Restaurant
- Government ministries and departments should be filed under the key word:
  —AGRICULTURE FISHERIES & FOODS, Ministry of
  —EDUCATION & SCIENCE, Department of
- Ignore 'the', conjunctions and prepositions when filing company names:
  —PET FOOD COMPANY (The)
  —PET FOOD COMPANY LTD
  —PET FOOD COMPANY (of) DERBY (The)
  —SMITH (and) JONES.

Storage of Documents

Due to the nature of the work carried out in a veterinary practice, a variety and large volume of documents and correspondence need to be stored. Each practice should draw up an appropriate retention and disposal policy to ensure that essential, irreplaceable information is protected and non-essential documents and records are disposed of at appropriate intervals. Depending on the subject matter and legal obligations, certain correspondence and documents must be kept for certain periods:

- Accident records: 3 years
- VAT records: 3 years
- PAYE records: at least 3 years after the income tax year to which the earnings relate.

There is no statutory obligation to keep the following records but the Veterinary Defence Society recommends that they are kept for a minimum of 2 years; if there is any possibility of dispute about a case, keep them for longer:

- Anaesthetic consent forms
- Medical/hospital records
- Laboratory reports
- Radiographs
- ECG/EEG traces.

The Royal College of Veterinary Surgeons recommends that records are kept for a minimum of 6 years. In disputed cases that are taken to the Veterinary Defence Society, the Society is advised to keep papers and documents with reference to the case, for court purposes, for 6 years and 364 days.

Many practices keep documents and records for longer than is legally required. These are termed 'dead files' and it is important to ensure that the storage system is both cost-effective and easily accessible.

Security

Security in a veterinary practice covers many areas and all members of staff should be aware of the implications of a lax system with reference to theft, damage and personal safety.

Premises

Burglaries are not uncommon and it is wise to ask the local Crime Prevention Officer for advice on how best to secure the premises. All doors, windows, skylights and shutters should be locked and checked before the building is left unattended.

Personal Safety

It is unwise for anyone on their own at the practice to open the surgery door to a caller who may appear to be the owner of an animal in distress. A telephone intercom may be fitted so that you may speak directly to the person without opening the door. Then contact the veterinary surgeon on call before proceeding any further. A good source of light should make it easier to see and identify the caller and their vehicle (write down its make and number).

To minimise the risk of personal danger to a nurse, arrangements can be made with known clients to call at the surgery at a specified time. They should have given a description of themselves, their vehicle and the animal. Ensure that all staff are aware of practice policy on this matter and that they all **think** before putting themselves in potentially dangerous situations. The fitting of 'panic buttons' in strategic places within the practice can make staff feel more secure.

Tills

Never leave an open, unlocked till unattended, even if you are staying in the same room. Never place the money tendered by the client into the till until you have counted out and given them their change and receipt.

It is very easy to accept into the till a £10 note for a small transaction only to be told, on giving the person their change, that they had given you a £20 note. Unless there is a detailed list of what was in the till, it is very difficult to prove that they did not in fact pass over £20.

Dangerous Drugs Cupboard

Only veterinary surgeons and nominated staff should hold keys to the dangerous drugs cupboard and these should never be left lying around or lent to unauthorised staff. Nor should the cupboard be left unlocked.

Staff-only areas should be well signposted and clients should never be left unattended in areas that contain anything other than GSL drugs.

Prescription pads and headed paper should not be left lying around. Stolen pads have sometimes been used by drug users trying to obtain prescription-only medicines or controlled drugs.

Animals

Always ensure the security of the animals in your charge and lock cages if necessary to prevent escape.

Emergency situations with animals are considered in detail in Chapter 3 (First Aid).

Further Reading

Blaney, D. *Information Technology*, Institute of Administration Management.

Denyer, J. C. *Office Management*, Pitman Publishing.

Graham, H. T. *Human Resources Management*, M & E Handbooks.

Harding, H. *Secretarial Procedures Theory and Applications*, Pitman Publishing.

Harrison, J. *Office Procedures*, Pitman Publishing.

Lysons, K. *Manpower Administration*, Institute of Administration Management.

Osuch, D. *Administration in the Office*, Institute of Administration Management.

Guide to Professional Conduct, Royal College of Veterinary Surgeons (1993 edn).

8
Bereavement Counselling

D. S. MILLS

Coping with the Grieving or Anxious Client

The loss of a loved pet will always be a painful experience for an owner and may result in considerable disturbance within a veterinary practice. There is, however, much that a veterinary nurse can do to help both the client and the practice during this time. It is essential that the veterinary nurse should be mentally prepared to cope with this emotionally charged situation.

All staff must appear sincere and interested in anything that causes a client distress. This is achieved by making eye contact, listening carefully to what owners have to say and letting them know that you are concerned and will take the appropriate action. When talking to owners, make sure that the pet's name is correct, identify the pet's sex with the accurate use of he or she (never 'it') and try to avoid technical jargon. There should be as few interruptions as possible. Any laughter from an adjacent room will cause suspicion in an owner about the sincerity of the practice.

> A client is often more impressed by a sympathetic approach by the nurse in a stressful situation than by the best treatment a veterinary practice can offer.

Handling the Situation for Animal Euthanasia

This situation is critical to the owner and it should never be seen to be rushed. The decision to end a pet's life is inevitably the decision of the owner, who accepts the responsibility though perhaps not understanding the medical situation. Any uncertainty about what is happening is likely to increase the intensity of the grief process and so it is important to take time to listen and answer any questions the client may ask. In some instances only the veterinary surgeon may be able to answer these but communication is essential and the contact should be personal. The clients should appreciate that the recommendation is made in the best interests of their pet. They should not be blinded by scientific terminology.

It is essential that the pet owner is given consistent information from every person they respect in the practice. Where there are several veterinary surgeons who have dealt recently with the animal, the nurse may be the one person who has been present throughout a course of treatment and the owner will turn to the nurse for assistance when a decision on euthanasia becomes necessary. A casual or ill-chosen word or comment may have long-lasting or devastating effects and this will affect their ability to cope with the situation. Comments such as 'I understand how you feel' or 'I can appreciate that this is a very painful decision/sad moment' will help to support the owner emotionally. In some instances reference to the loss of the nurse's own animal can establish a bond of sympathy. The stress in a euthanasia consultation may be reduced if the nurse prepares for it beforehand:

- Prepare and complete as far as possible all documentation before the event. Where necessary, give assistance in the completion of consent forms. Details for cremation will need to be known. The payment for treatment should be discussed in advance if possible. If a bill has to be sent on later as a special arrangement, it should be made clear that all services have to be paid for. The phrase 'veterinary services' is preferable to words such as 'euthanase and dispose' when charging the client.
- Avoid using the words 'put to sleep,' as an owner might understand only that an anaesthetic is about to be given to treat a particularly painful condition. If children are present, these words could cause distress, anxiety or even psychological problems in some children, as the same word may be used at a later stage in a different context (e.g. to go to bed or to have a general anaesthetic in hospital).
- Try to book the appointment at a quiet time of day, when staff will have time to spend with the client and there will be a minimal number of onlookers.
- Do not keep clients waiting unnecessarily when they arrive. If any delay is likely, explain this to the owner. Try to talk in a light manner about their family etc. The response may alert you to the emotional state of the owner and indicate the especially vulnerable client to whom the pet is their only friend.
- Do not jump to conclusions: agitation or the smell of alcohol on the owner's breath may show that the person has until then lacked the courage to bring in a terminally ill animal. There may be other reasons for euthanasia of a pet that the nurse may not be aware of.
- Be sensitive to a client's needs. Some owners may wish to spend a last few minutes sitting quietly

alone with their pet. Respect their privacy. Other owners may feel the need to talk and explain their actions to the nurse.

- When it comes to the euthanasia injection time, find out if the owners want to be present. Find out their wishes: some may like to hand over the animal to the veterinary surgeon and nurse, whilst others may wish to leave and then return after the euthanasia injection to see their dead animal for the last time. If an owner wishes to remain with the body or take it home, explain that even if the animal is no longer alive (i.e. its heart has stopped and there is no brain activity) it is still possible for muscles to twitch which may appear like gasping actions. Be prepared for the bladder to empty after death by arranging suitable absorbent material.

- If the patient is already hospitalised and it seems likely that the parting with the owner present is likely to be difficult, arrange for a preplaced canula in the vein or have a drip running. Sedation before the euthanasia may help but sometimes the owners wish their animals to recognise them and respond to their voice.

- A plentiful supply of tissues, seating close at hand and a glass of water may all be needed. Tears should be anticipated and often crying is the best immediate response to death. Owners should have time and privacy to recover before appearing in public or having to drive themselves home.

- When discussing the arrangements for the after-care of the body (cremation, burial etc.), it may help if the body is retained for a short time on the surgery premises until the owner has come to a decision, as other members of the family may have to be consulted. If a client asks the nurse about what happens to the bodies at the surgery, you must be honest but diplomatic. Saying that 'the bodies are all cremated together' is preferable to saying that 'they're all incinerated'. Individual cremation of a body with the return of the ashes is an option that owners should be offered as a service.

- When moving a body after death, in the owner's presence, do not appear immediately with a black plastic bag. If the owner wishes to remove a pet for burial, they may use their own basket or a cloth wrapping. The risk of soiling from faeces or urine should be assessed and sometimes the rear end of the body can be placed in the bag if you explain the reason for this first.

- Where possible, escort the owner out of the surgery by a route that gives as much privacy to their grief as possible. Some may need help, especially if they have come to a surgery on their own.

- It is often better to say nothing, remaining quiet if you are not sure of a situation. Saying the wrong thing may create a long-lasting adverse impression. A friendly touch on the arm and the offer of help, or suggesting a friend the owner can talk to about their pet, is often very consoling if made in a sincere manner.

- Finally, make sure that all records are amended so that an owner is not sent booster reminders or other communications about a deceased animal. Being active after an unpleasant experience is the best antidote to the veterinary nurse becoming over-involved in the death of an animal.

Bereavement and the Grief Sequence

Whilst there is obviously considerable variation in how people react and cope with grief, there are five well-recognised stages in a grieving process:

- Shock.
- Anger.
- Bargaining.
- Depression.
- Acceptance.

It should be noted that not all these events occur as distinct episodes. They often overlap, so that the bereaved person feels more than one emotion at the same time. The stages may be interchanged or displayed in a different sequence, or some stages may not be seen at all. Some people progress through the stages quickly; others become permanently halted at any time.

Shock

The signs of a grieving owner in a state of shock include a refusal to accept the death or a disbelief at a grave prognosis. Watch for responses such as: 'Surely not!', 'It can't be true,' or 'You seem very serious about it!' Owners may demand a second opinion before accepting that a pet is in terminal stages, or ask about alternative treatments long after help of this nature will be of benefit. When describing an animal's illness, they may focus on minor ailments in order to blot out the reality of the situation—asking about overgrown claws or the presence of a small wart, for example.

The shocked person may look pale, dazed or confused when they realise that euthanasia may be the only outcome of the consultation. An owner might even arrive at the surgery with an obviously dead animal, refusing to believe that death has occurred and then asking the veterinary surgeon or nurse to 'look for a spark of life'.

This stage of shock is often brief and should not last more than a day.

Nurse's action

When clients express disbelief at the situation, do not contradict them directly. Sympathise with their shock but be direct about the situation. Statements such as 'I know it is hard to believe but. . . .' are helpful.

If a client wishes to seek a second opinion, this should not be refused but travelling a long distance with a dying animal may not be in the best interests of the shocked client or the pet. Another veterinary surgeon in the same practice who knows the client and the pet may be the best person to consult.

Anger

This is commonly directed at the practice, as the owner feels an injustice. The anger may be directed at individual members of staff or the procedures used to determine the diagnosis. Questions such as 'Why don't you . . .' and 'Why didn't you. . . .' may be asked when the veterinary surgeon was only being kind and trying to avoid needless expense. If owners direct the anger at themselves, it will result in feelings of guilt.

Nurse's action

Do not take a verbal attack by a client personally but stay calm. Always be courteous and do not aggravate a situation or be too defensive. It does not help angry clients to have their own faults and previous wrong-doings pointed out. The nurse should be under-standing but firm.

An expression such as 'I can understand that you are very upset by what has happened but I can assure you this is a normal procedure' may defuse a situation before explaining (or offering to find someone in a better position to explain) the reasons for any procedure.

Explain those reasons if you can but the veterinary surgeon is better equipped to answer any accusations. (If a client complains about someone, that person should not go out of their way to avoid the client.) When asking a veterinary surgeon to explain, make sure that he or she is properly briefed before they speak to the client and that case records are available.

Avoid making any statement that could be inter-preted as an admission of carelessness, neglect or error.

Bargaining

At this stage of the grieving process, some clients may offer something in exchange for a more favour-able situation. The nurse may even receive a small gift, which should be accepted gracefully. Clients may even express a revival in religious beliefs or an intensity of prayer not previously experienced.

Nurse's action

It is important to be the guardian of the pet's welfare and support whatever recommendations have already been made by the veterinary surgeon. Do not take advantage of the owner in this situation. Do not advise or suggest treatments for a pet that may be expensive and have little chance of success.

Depression

Most clients will feel sad about the situation but the intensity varies with individuals, according to the nature of the relationship (the pet may have been a substitute for a child or a close friend) and the length of the relationship—but an owner can very quickly become attached to a dependent animal such as a puppy or kitten. The owner's current interests, work and any domestic disturbance, or a sudden death of a close associate may be mirrored in the subsequent death of a pet and similar feelings will be aroused all over again.

In depression, a person may become physically ill, be unable to eat or sleep properly and lose interest in a normal daily routine. Bereaved animal owners sometimes appear confused about events and easily distracted, or imagine that they can still sense their pet's presence in the home. They may experience periods of unaccountable crying or 'grief pangs'. These are all normal signs of depression and may be seen a few hours or a few days after the event, often reaching a peak of intensity about two weeks later.

Nurse's action

Sometimes a client telephones the surgery but often the depression is only heard about when a third party contacts the surgery for help. If the client does not appear to know anyone who can appreciate their loss, the practice staff are in the best position to provide initial support as they will often have known the pet as well as the client. If asked, the nurse should try to make discreet enquiries and be prepared to provide support—often by discussion over the telephone. Talking things over with a depressed person may alleviate some of the suffering but often being a good listener whilst making sympathetic interjections can be very valuable. It is important to establish effective communication with a grieving client, who should be reassured that there is nothing unusual about the feeling of depression or the disruption in interests and normal routine. Encourage the client to make a memorial gesture, e.g. give a donation to a charity, plant a tree, or a similar act to remember the lost pet, as this helps the grieving process.

Sometimes a client needs to be directed to a suitable support group, who will be far more skilled in handling the situation.*

If there is a local group, it is important that the practice be aware of it and be the one to recommend it rather than the client hearing of such a group through others—they may think that the lack of

*The Society of Companion Animal Studies (SCAS) offer a Befriender Service in the U.K. for telephone counselling (0891 615285).

information from the practice represents a lack of care.

If the depression is very intense or it continues for more than three weeks or there are any suicidal overtones, professional medical advice should be advised immediately.

Acceptance

This is a recovery stage, when the client can again talk about the pet without the distress shown before. They will be more objective about the assessment of the circumstances of the pet's death. Any new pet or other interest is accepted on its own merits.

Nurse's action

The nurse can be relieved that this stage has been reached. Until then, any new pet is likely to form an association with lost love and may prolong the grief chain or inhibit acceptance. The premature suggestion of a replacement animal may be misinterpreted as disrespectful to the lost pet or as a failure of others to appreciate the special relationship that existed between the original pet and its owner. It is best not to encourage a client to obtain a replacement before this acceptance stage has been reached.

An offer to help in choosing a new addition to the household at this time is often appreciated, even if it is not accepted. A dog or cat from a 'rescue' kennels may make the bereaved person feel that they are now able to help an unfortunate abandoned animal to find a new home in the better circumstances that their former pet enjoyed.

Guilt

Many clients feel some guilt after the death of a pet for a variety of reasons but especially if they have chosen euthanasia or the pet died in an accident that might be due to human carelessness. They may feel guilty about something they did or failed to do that contributed to the pet's death—perhaps they left a gate open and that led to a road accident. Sometimes these feelings are unfounded; for example, no one would know that the first yelp of pain was a sign of a terminal illness, and contacting the practice immediately may not have altered the outcome. They may blame themselves for previous episodes of punishment or minor neglect. It is important not to intensify these feelings with ill-chosen comments such as: 'If only we had seen him two weeks earlier.' Equally, a well-meaning remark ('You always did your best for . . .') may trigger these guilt episodes as the owner then remembers the times when they did put their pet in second place. If an owner expresses guilt feelings in conversation, give reassurance that this is a normal reaction for someone who has lost a friend in such tragic circumstances and that it is an expression of an inner desire to undo what has happened.

> The greatest need for clients at this time is a reassurance that what they feel is normal.

Assessing the Client's Needs

Every situation will be different and the student or newly qualified veterinary nurse may not have had many personal experiences of handling these situations. It is often helpful to identify clients who are least able to cope and then bring them to the notice of a more senior member of staff. Preparation can then be made for any extra support that may be needed.

Some of the factors that suggest an owner will cope less well with pet loss, and that indicate the need for professional assistance, can be identified quite easily:

- Lack of time for an owner to prepare for the event or come to terms with it.
- The owner lives alone and has few close friends.
- It is the owner's only pet or has been nursed through a period of intense care and dependency.
- The pet is seen not only as a member of the family but it has acquired special status, e.g. it may have stayed with the owner through a domestic crisis or been present when a close friend or relation has died.
- The pet is a symbol of some other intense feeling or relationship, e.g. it was the deceased spouse's favourite.
- The owner is forced to elect for euthanasia for reasons of change of status, financial hardship or other circumstances despite the fact that the pet could be treated.
- The owner is aware of someone who is suffering a similar disorder to their sick pet and studying the symptoms of each illness may be too close a parallel when one has already died.

All clients who appear to be at risk should be contacted or visited a few days after the pet's death. A reason may be found for the nurse to phone or call at the home. Any contact should be sincere, provide reassurance to the client and at the same time try to establish the stage or depth of any grief shown. Solicitous enquiries about health or sleeping patterns may indicate if there is any deep depression and support can then be suggested. If the client appears to be in danger of developing a pathological depression, medical help is necessary but a further call after a few weeks may be helpful to find out how the situation has developed. Some people will feel embarrassed at the suggestion they need additional help, such as a trained counsellor or joining a support group, but often they can be persuaded to see their own doctor if they are not sleeping or eating properly. They will need extra reassurance that their condition is not unusual and that help is available. If they refuse help, do not be forceful but say that you are always available to talk—they might change their minds later about asking for assistance.

The euthanasia of a pet can also be a stressful occasion for the veterinary surgeon and for other staff. This may be more apparent if a patient has been nursed for a long time in a hospital, for intensive care facilitates a strong emotional bond between carer and patient.

Nursing care in veterinary practice should include the staff taking care not only of themselves but also of less experienced colleagues, as it is normal to be upset in such circumstances. Older colleagues may show less emotion: their experience has given them a coping mechanism which may include the ability to adjust rapidly to death in their patients, but they still care.

9
Problem Behaviour and Animal Training

D. S. MILLS

Problem Behaviour

Any action by an animal which causes an owner concern may be considered to be a behavioural problem. This may be a normal or abnormal behaviour pattern (Fig. 9.1).

Behaviour problems are the problems of what the animal does. **Temperament problems** are problems arising from what an animal thinks or feels. Both may be affected by a number of factors, including:

- The genetic make up of the individual.—Genotype.
- The current state of the animal's internal environment—hormone and metabolite levels.
- The current external environment.
- Previous experience and learned behaviour.

Genetic Factors

These may determine and affect the behaviour of the species, the breed or the individual:

- It is essential to be well versed in the normal behaviour of the **species** in order to appreciate if something is genuinely abnormal (e.g. an owner thinking that a cat in oestrus, rolling on the floor, is abnormal or in pain).
- A good knowledge of **breed** characteristics will help in the appreciation of what is normal (e.g. vocalisation of the Siamese). Breed behaviour tendencies may indicate what problems may be likely in a given breed (e.g. noise phobias in bearded collies). An understanding of the breed is an aid to giving advice on the suitability of a possible pet for a specific home.
- **Individual** behaviour is seen in the animal's character.

The Animal's Internal Environment

Some abnormal behaviours are more frequent or only occur in one sex. For example, in the case of urine spraying in male cats, neutering may help in both the prevention and the treatment of the problem. It is important to realise that not all aggressive behaviours are driven by male hormones;

castration should not be recommended in all these individuals as it may in fact be contraindicated.

Other disorders may be due to disease (e.g. aggression in the hyperthyroid cat). Poisons such as chronic lead poisoning in the dog can be the cause of anxiety and reduce a working dog's obedience.

Drug therapy may be considered as a way of altering the internal environment as the presence of certain chemicals in the body affects receptors which may alter an animal's behaviour.

> **WARNING**
> As behaviour problems may be caused by disease and/or require medical therapy, it is essential that any case requiring more than obedience training is given a thorough clinical examination by a veterinary surgeon, who will take responsibility for the case. The need to consult a veterinary surgeon should be explained by the veterinary nurse to any clients seeking advice and to those considering referral to behaviour experts.

The External Environment

A problem may arise with an animal's behaviour because of the situation in which it finds itself, so that altering the environment may avoid the problem. Such measures include rehoming a dog with separation anxiety to a family where it will not be left on its own. Whilst this may resolve the situation, and save the animal's life, it is important to realise that the problem still exists even if it is no longer expressed. Alternatively, the environment can be changed temporarily so that the problem does not arise whilst the animal is trained not to exhibit the undesirable behaviour.

Previous Experience

In early life, dogs and cats have 'sensitive periods' when they learn more readily or form impressions which will affect their behaviour and temperament.

CLASSIFICATION OF BEHAVIOUR PROBLEMS		
	Example of normal behaviour	Example of abnormal behaviour
Behaviour problems	Spraying (male cat) Lack of obedience	Obsessive-compulsive disorders
Temperament problem	Fear biting	Aggressive behaviour due to the effect of a brain lesion

Fig. 9.1. Classification of behaviour problems.

The **socialisation period** largely determines how an animal will react to other individuals (of the same and different species), groups and the surrounding environment for the rest of its life. This period is roughly between the 4th and 10th week of age in the puppy and between the 2nd and 5th week in the kitten (but it is less clearly defined in the feline species). It is vital that pets receive pleasant experiences at this time, associated with things that are to be accepted later, and that they are not overstressed by early weaning. This is the stage at which most temperament problems are developed: damage done at this time is much harder to undo later.

The next stage is the **juvenile period**, when the animal matures sexually. Cats and dogs are still capable of forming strong attachments to new owners at this time if they have already been socialised with people.

Many behaviour and temperament problems arise because the animal has not been properly socialised when young. The veterinary practice has an important role in this aspect of preventive medicine:

- Advice should be given to breeders and potential new owners on suitable weaning, handling and exposure procedures.
- Practices should run 'puppy classes' or be able to recommend local ones. These classes combine basic obedience training with socialisation, plenty of handling and lots of novel stimuli provided in a controlled and pleasant environment. Puppies are taught what is acceptable and what is not (e.g. biting). All vaccinated puppies can be exposed to other puppies.
- All visits to the practice at this time should be made as pleasant as possible. When injections need to be given, as for vaccination, distract the animal during the procedure and then reward it afterwards. Overindulging a crying animal will make it more fearful.

Principles of Animal Training

DEFINITIONS
Psychology—the study of mind and behaviour.
Psychiatry—the study of disease of the mind and behaviour; this is more of a medical subject than psychology.
Ethology—the study of the function and development of animal behaviour.
Stimulus—any influence or action that produces a response.
Conditioning—the learning of association between stimuli and between a stimulus and a response.
Cognition—the ability to think or reason and the processes necessary to do so.

Conditioning and cognition represent ways in which animals can learn.

Training Requirements

Training or retraining an animal often requires a vivid imagination and a flexible approach by the trainer. What may be suitable for one client and their pet may not be appropriate for another with the same problem. Before offering any advice, it is important to consider not only the pet but also the nature of the relationship between the pet and owner.

Communication and a good client manner are essential. Owners are often uncomfortable about seeking professional advice in dealing with a problem and to many it is as painful as admitting failure as a parent. They often feel guilty about a pet's predicament, whether or not they are to blame, and they need to be reassured and given time to explain the problem. The veterinary nurse may be the most suitable person to do this in the practice.

It is important to define the problem fully—not only what is happening but where, when, with whom and why. Some owners hold back information either because they think it is not important or because they feel guilty about some action. It is essential to build up trust and to listen patiently, without making judgements about a situation. Both the adviser or trainer and the client must be relaxed. When talking about any treatment, talk about what 'we' will do rather than telling the owner what *they* should do.

Training Approaches

The situation should be viewed and explained from the animal's point of view. Learning is greatest when motivation is highest, therefore the nature of the bond between owner and pet should be considered and modified accordingly. The owner should be respected and obeyed by the pet but force is not necessary to establish this.

Rather than criticise an owner for using an ineffectual technique, suggest that it may be better to try an alternative method, explaining what the chosen method is expected to achieve and why. Do not let the client expect too much too soon, as unrealistic expectations often lead to abandonment of the plan. The goals set must be both manageable and effective.

It is often helpful to suggest an initial period of a week or two to try to crack a problem with quite intense treatment. The thought that it is only a temporary measure gives the owner a greater motivation to break previous habits or to follow what may be an inconvenient plan of action. Once this has been done it is much easier to continue.

Training Techniques

When training an animal the following points should be noted:

- The subject must be attentive to the trainer. This may require the use of a whistle or other aids to interrupt the animal's current activity. It is also important not to exceed the animal's attention span.

- In order to motivate an animal to comply, any reward must be truly rewarding compared with available alternatives. There is no point in offering a food reward just after the animal's main meal.
- Initially, do not give commands that cannot be enforced. This may mean leaving the lead attached if it is safe to do so.
- Training sessions should always finish on a positive note, even if it means returning to a basic command.

There are many training methods but the most common in use are extinction, punishment, negative reinforcement and positive reinforcement.

Extinction

This method involves neither reward nor punishment of the behaviour, in the hope that it will pass away. Doing nothing is not necessarily easy, especially if an owner enjoys stroking the pet. The technique is most commonly used to address attention-seeking behaviour. In such cases, any attention (good or bad) rewards and reinforces the behaviour. Physical punishment is contraindicated as the trainer is unwittingly giving the animal a version of what it is seeking: attention. Ignoring or isolating the individual may be effective but it is essential not to give in as this will reward the undesirable behaviour.

Punishment

This method can be misused and overused so that it becomes a euphemism for abuse. There are three forms: interactive, remote and social punishment.

Interactive punishment is seen to come directly from the owner. If it is to be used properly it is important that the animal is informed in such a way that it can understand that it has done wrong and preferably be told what it should be doing. If a whistle is used prior to a punishment, then the whistle will eventually become a way of informing a dog it has done wrong (classical conditioning) and may be used in other training situations. An instructive reprimand (such as 'Off') may be used, which not only tells the animal that it has done wrong but also tells it what it should be doing instead. *It is essential that the animal knows from previous training what the command means*—for example, it has already been taught the 'Off' command.

It is also essential that any punishment is effective, being of a suitable but not excessive intensity, and is associated with the misbehaviour. This usually means that it must occur instantly—within half a second of the action that is to be punished. A common mistake with a dog that does not come when it is called is to punish the animal when it finally returns. The punishment thus becomes associated with the return, instead of with the failure to recall, and so the dog is even less keen to return the next time.

Remote punishment is not seen to come from the owner but from the behaviour. It includes such devices as specially constructed 'boobytraps' and remote-control collars to stop barking in dogs.

Social punishment is when things the pet enjoys are withdrawn. These may be physical (e.g. toys) or psychological (e.g. attention). If the owner becomes the provider of good things which have previously been taken for granted, this will often serve to strengthen the bond between the owner and the pet.

WARNING
Both interactive and remote punishments are contraindicated in the treatment of phobias or the nervous animal. This also includes most cats.

If any punishment is to be used properly it must be delivered consistently. If the punishment is not delivered every time, the animal will start to look for occasions when it is not punished. This may exacerbate the problem or limit the expression of the behaviour to when the owner is absent, so that it becomes even harder to correct.

There are normally more ways to get something wrong than to get it right. If only on welfare grounds, punishment has no place in 'explaining' new behaviour (i.e. the early training stages). For the average pet it may be used with caution to correct activities. If it needs to be used a lot of the time to correct a behaviour that the trainer thinks that the animal should understand, the trainer should always ask: 'Where have I gone wrong?'

Negative reinforcement

This means making a behaviour unpleasant for as long as it continues (in contrast with punishment, which is a single unpleasant experience used to terminate the behaviour). Many of the problems inherent in the use of punishment also apply to negative reinforcement. It is most succesfully used in the prevention of certain behaviours (e.g. scent marked boobytraps where the scent acts as a negative reinforcement warning). Before using negative reinforcement, ask: 'Why does the animal want to behave like this? How strong are the necessary drives?' The use of negative reinforcement to force an animal to learn obedience commands cannot be justified.

Positive reinforcement and rewards

This technique involves motivating the animal by means of pleasant lures and rewards. The technique is relatively easy and humane and it helps to strengthen the trainer–animal bond. This makes it very effective, as it also increases motivation and social stability. Social stability is particularly important to dogs and many problems in this species would not occur if the dog respected its owner; therefore the teaching of basic obedience, if not already present in the problem dog, is to be recommended. Applications of positive reinforcement are:

- To teach obedience commands.
- To teach a whole new action (e.g. a dog is taught to sit to greet rather than jumping up). The new behaviour is incompatible with the problem behaviour.
- To put an existing behaviour on a cue (classical conditioning). The expression of behaviour can then be limited, as with certain types of barking.
- To shape an existing behaviour pattern towards another (more desirable) behaviour pattern, e.g the training of complex activities, socialisation and desensitisation.

Desensitisation is used to reduce an animal's response to a stimulus. The animal is distracted or exposed to the stimulus at an intensity that does not produce a response and is then rewarded accordingly. The process is repeated and the intensity increased until the animal learns to accept the stimulus. It is essential not to rush this process but to proceed at a pace that the animal can accept. It is most frequently used in the treatment of phobias and other overexciting stimuli.

Positive reinforcement may be:

- **continuous**, when every response is rewarded (this is often used to lure or explain to the animal a new action but it is easy for the animal to get bored with the activity and so its motivation is reduced);
- **variable**, when the reward is sometimes given and at other times not (this is most useful in shaping a behaviour—only those behaviours nearest to that which is desired are rewarded);
- **differential**, when both the size and the frequency of the rewards are varied (once an animal knows what is required, this is very effective in improving

the speed and nature of the response to any command—the unpredictable nature makes the training actively addictive).

Some Common Behaviour Problems

The most widespread condition is lack of obedience, and another major problem is aggression. House-soiling and house destruction are also of concern for some owners, and reasons for these two problems are shown in Fig. 9.2.

Aggression

Aggression in the dog is a sign, not a diagnosis. The owners of aggressive animals must be informed of their special responsibility to prevent injury to others.

Aggression can be categorised into eleven different types, some of which have very different treatments:

- Dominance (asserting position).
- Possesiveness.
- Territorial or protective aggression.
- Play.
- Predatory.
- Fear-induced.
- Pain-induced.
- Maternal (occasionally paternal).
- Intermale or interfemale (a form of competitive aggression).
- Redirected (inhibition of aggression in one direction results in expression in another).
- Pathophysiological (due to medical disorders).

> All problems of behaviour in the dog and cat reported to the veterinary nurse should be considered seriously and, if necessary, referred to a more experienced colleague.

REASONS FOR HOUSE-SOILING AND HOUSE DESTRUCTION		
	Causes in the dog	**Causes in the cat**
House-soiling	Lack/loss of house training Separation anxiety Fear-induced Submissive Scent-marking Excitement Disease	(First distinguish between marking and inappropriate elimination) Disease Territorial Sexual Genetic tendency to spray Litter box unsuitability (position, Type of container or contents)
House destruction	Boredom Separation anxiety Phobias Escape attempt Play Extension of puppy teething Disease Enjoyment Hunger	

Fig. 9.2. Reasons for house-soiling and house destruction.

10
Basic Training

E. M. WILLIAMS

Clients consult veterinary practices for advice on all aspects of pet care, preventive as well as curative—including behavioural development. Concern may be expressed and advice sought regarding two important aspects: house training for puppies and kittens, and obedience training for dogs. The veterinary nurse is in an ideal position to give advice on both but should be aware that there are many different theories about training methods.

Basic House Training for Puppies

Puppies up to 12 weeks old have little control over the urge to urinate or defecate. They may go anywhere at any time and in these situations it is pointless to blame the puppy — owners should not have unrealistic expectations. Time and patience are essential.

To minimise the incidence of 'accidents', the owner should provide a convenient confined area near the pup's sleeping quarters where newspapers are readily available for elimination purposes. To encourage evacuation, use a consistent command and lavishly praise the result so that the puppy associates the command with the action. Gradually move the newspaper nearer the door, and then outside to the designated toilet area, finally dispensing with the newspaper. By then urine will have seeped through to the soil: the pup will sniff and be able to identify the toilet area, and will continue to use it on command.

This training to command is increasingly important today. Local authorities are justifiably taking steps to ensure that dogs do not foul public open spaces and streets, and owners should encourage their pets to relieve themselves in appropriate areas before exercising them in public places. It should be noted that dogs prefer to relieve themselves on surfaces similar to those they used as puppies, which is often grass. Many dogs are trained not to use concrete surfaces, as part of their 'pavement training'.

The owner of a puppy should aim to identify times when the pup is most likely to urinate and defecate—for example after meals, on walking, or during exercise or play. Signs of a puppy's wish to relieve itself include whimpering, restlessness, sniffing the floor and going to the door.

Most animals will not soil their sleeping quarters unless they are genuinely incapable of self-control. Many owners, instead of constant supervision, use a crate or indoor kennel in which the puppy can be confined after it has been given every opportunity to defecate or urinate. Such a kennel also satisfies the puppy's natural desire for its own 'den' and can be its place of refuge in a household of children.

Prevention of 'Accidents'

- The puppy should be confined in the owner's absence.
- It should be observed at all times.
- It should not be punished, or it will associate punishment with soiling. It is far better to reward good results.
- To discourage the puppy's further use of an unsuitable area, clean the area thoroughly after an accident.

Problems

If house training is not straightforward, the nurse might seek relevant information from the client:

- **Type of diet fed:** The diet needs to be scientifically formulated without excessive amounts of nutrients or salt—raised salt levels encourage excessive drinking, and hence urine production, making it difficult for the pup to gain bladder control.
- **Amount of food:** Feeding fixed amounts of food at particular times limits the amount of food the puppy consumes (in contrast with free-choice feeding) and regulates the amount of waste produced. Free-choice feeding not only hinders development of a regular defecation pattern but also may encourage the pup to become overweight.
- **Timing of feeding and exercise:** Feeding late in the evening is inadvisable, as the puppy will need to defecate during the night. Exercising late is also inadvisable, as the puppy will drink excessively after exercise and will therefore need to urinate during the night.
- **Availability of the owner:** The owner must not have unrealistic expectations. Until control is well established, someone should be available at all times to supervise the puppy.
- **Confinement when unsupervised:** If the puppy must be left alone, it must be confined to a small area with plenty of newspaper available.
- **Health problems:** Any suspicion of a health problem in the puppy, such as urinary incontinence or diarrhoea, should be investigated by the veterinary surgeon at the earliest opportunity.

Feline House Training

The basic principles of house training for puppies can be applied to kittens. The cat is normally fastidious in its personal hygiene, digging a hole for its eliminations and then covering its faeces. This behaviour is so characteristic in cats that it is usually relatively easy to house train a kitten.

The owner should provide a readily accessible litter tray of appropriate size, in a convenient quiet place. The litter should be cleaned out on a regular basis. Initially the animal should be confined to one room until it is reliable in using the litter tray. It may be necessary to use slightly soiled litter, the odour of which will attract a kitten. Gradually the tray can be moved outside if required, and the animal encouraged to use loose soil in the garden. The tray may be needed indoors again if the weather is bad or the animal is ill.

Problems

- In multi-cat households there is often a problem of dominance: more submissive cats are deterred by others from using the litter tray.
- Infrequent cleaning of the litter tray deters use.
- Individuals may have an aversion to a different litter, e.g. if it contains a deodorant.
- A fright whilst in action on the litter tray can deter use.
- Failure to clean soiled 'accident' areas thoroughly encourages further use of those areas.

Obedience Training for Puppies

When a puppy is presented for vaccinations, there is an ideal opportunity to advise the owner on various aspects of puppy training. The veterinary practice, by modelling some of the behaviour characteristics of its future patients at this stage, helps to make them happy, confident, well-behaved pets and easy to handle under practice conditions. This early training also helps to avoid the development of undesirable habits which may need referral to a behavioural specialist later on.

Basic training should start as soon as the puppy arrives in its new home and all members of the family should be encouraged to take part—though care should be taken not to confuse the puppy with a variety of commands. Each puppy is different in character but the ground rules must be laid down early so that the animal learns its place in the family home. All owners want a dog that will be a pleasure to own and it is essential that they receive sound guidance not only to be firm with a dominant pup but also to encourage a more submissive one that may lack confidence.

At this young age most puppies are extremely biddable and eager to please, and this should be exploited. Praise and play reinforce the association of a particular sound with a particular act. Simple command words such as 'come', 'sit' or 'down' should be used when the puppy naturally assumes these positions, and then the praise should be lavish so that the puppy associates the act with the word. Soon it will respond automatically to the word, in anticipation of praise.

Socialisation at a very early age is crucial to the later behaviour of dogs, and the puppy should be allowed to mix with humans and animals frequently. Although it should not mingle with other dogs until its course of vaccinations is complete and immunity achieved, it can become used to travelling in vehicles, playing with children, meeting new people and being introduced to cats, horses, livestock and similar aged puppies in a safe environment. In the earliest months of its life the puppy is particularly receptive to socialisation and indeed is likely to develop behavioural problems if it is deprived of such opportunities at this stage.

Owners should be encouraged to attend specialist puppy-training classes as soon as the vaccination course is effective. At these classes puppies are gently and sympathetically introduced to basic commands and also gain by early socialisation with other dogs and people. The classes are followed by more formal tuition when the pup is 5–6 months old.

It should be impressed on owners that all dogs are capable of learning basic exercises which will make them a pleasure to their owners but that this will involve time and effort. It is all part of the commitment of owning and caring for a dog.

Puppy training guidelines

- Puppies can only concentrate for a very short time. Their lessons at home should be brief and should be incorporated into the daily routine. If the puppy shows signs of boredom or tiredness, the training session should be stopped. Gradually, as the puppy grows older, it should be able to tolerate four short training periods daily, of perhaps 5–10 minutes each.
- Training should take place in a quiet area, without distractions.
- Lessons should be fun for both the puppy and the owner—they should incorporate play as well as learning.
- Patience is essential: it is important not to rush through the various learning steps of each exercise. The puppy needs to learn and understand every step of each command, otherwise it will easily be forgotten. The necessity for regular practice cannot be overstressed to an owner: a puppy learns quickly but also forgets quickly.
- Instructions must be clear and concise. Many of a puppy's mistakes are because the handler has not made the commands clear or has not attracted the puppy's attention before issuing a command. To avoid confusion, use only the puppy's name and a command word.

- Give the command in a firm but kind voice. The tone of voice is important: the dog's hearing is finely tuned to hear the sounds of the command and it needs to associate the sound with the act required. The tone should indicate firmness, in order to gain the puppy's respect, and pleasure when the puppy understands and complies with the command.
- Puppies should not be scolded for their mistakes. It is much more important to keep trying and to lavish praise for success. If a puppy does something totally unacceptable, use the 'No!' command to correct it but *never* lose your temper or show anger to the animal. The emphasis in training today is based on reward rather than punishment and training sessions should always finish with fun and play. The necessity for regular practice can not be overstressed to an owner, it is essential to practice commands, otherwise the puppy will quickly forget the correct response to them.

Dog Training Aids

Collar and lead

A collar with a name-and-address tag is required for all dogs by law, regardless of other training aids used.

It is important to choose the correct size of collar and length of lead for the individual dog. A puppy should be introduced gently to a light collar and lead, being allowed to trail it around the house or wear it at feed times until it is tolerated. Chain leads, as opposed to collars, are not recommended as they are uncomfortable on the hand.

Slip leads and check collars

Figure 10.1 shows a continuous lead and collar that allows slight checking to take place. The dog can be walked on a loose lead and it is a useful control once a dog is accustomed to walking at heel.

Check chain

This chain-link collar (Fig. 10.2), when placed correctly over the dog's head and attached to a lead, will effect a check-and-release mechanism so that the handler can correct a dog's undesirable behaviour. When applied incorrectly, however, it will not release after checking and will cause the dog an unnecessary choking effect and discomfort. Some trainers strongly dislike the use of check chains, and some dogs are highly nervous of the sound of the chain so close to their ears.

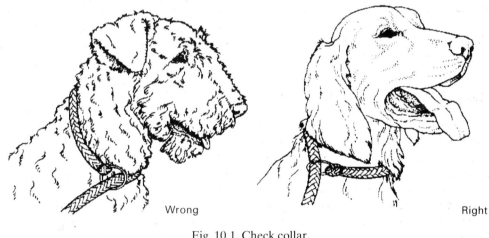

Fig. 10.1. Check collar.

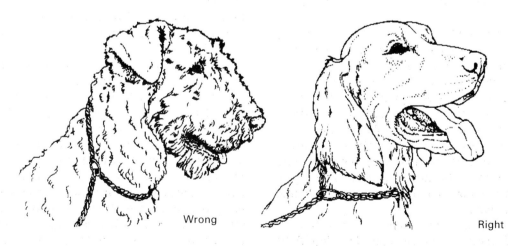

Fig. 10.2. Check chain.

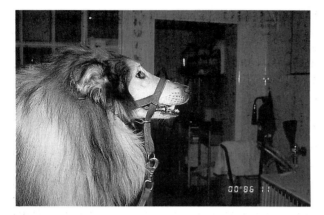

Fig. 10.3. Head halter.

Head halter

There is a special type of head halter (Fig. 10.3) which exerts a self-correcting influence on the head (without applying uncomfortable pressure around the neck) when a dog attempts to pull forward, to lunge and bite. It can also be used as a muzzle during examination procedures.

Teaching Commands

There are different attitudes towards training and owners should be made aware that there are a variety of training methods to suit all types of dog and their possible problems. Whichever method is used, commands should be clear and concise and should always be preceded by the dog's name in order to gain its attention.

Come

This command is most easily taught when a young puppy is first introduced into the home. Most

puppies naturally follow their owners at this age. In a confined area, run a short distance away from the pup and then call it by name with the command 'Come!', using a happy and encouraging voice. When the puppy bounds after the owner it should be praised, and perhaps rewarded with a titbit. If necessary a lead can be left on the puppy and given a gentle tug as a reminder.

(b)

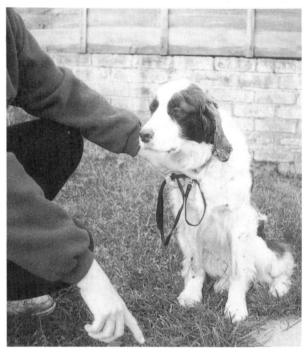

(c)

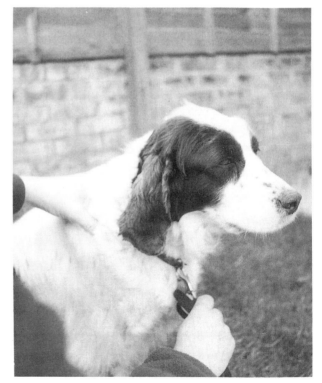

(a)

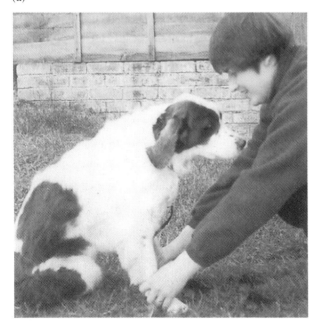

Fig. 10.4. Teaching the 'Down!' command.

Sit

Most puppies sit naturally and the command 'Sit!' should be given at the same time, so that they associate the action with the word. There are other methods of teaching this command. In training classes the dog might be placed at the owner's left side on a short lead held in the right hand. The left hand pushes the dog's hindquarters down gently; the 'Sit!' command is repeated several times and the dog is praised in the sitting position.

Down

Figure 10.4 shows one of several training methods used to teach this position.

Heel

The teaching of this command requires time and patience but is well worth the initial effort while a puppy is small enough to be manageable. A puppy which has accepted a light collar and lead is placed to one side of the handler (traditionally the left), level with the knee, and is expected to walk on a loose lead without pulling. The treat, either in the hand or in a pocket, is an invaluable aid to encourage its attention. If it pulls ahead, the handler stops walking and, giving the command 'No!', places the puppy in the correct position again with the command 'Heel!'. If it does not pull on walking forward, it should be praised.

Stay

With the dog sitting in the 'Heel' position, give a firm 'Stay!' command, reinforced by showing the dog the palm of the hand. Keeping the lead loose, take a step either to the side or to the front of the dog. If it moves, put it back in the sitting position and repeat the command. Leave the dog for only a few seconds initially, until it understands the command, after which the distance and the time can be increased slowly. When the dog completes its short-time stay, return to its side and praise it lavishly.

*The reader should be aware that a variety of dog training methods are in use and in the Assistance Dog movement, training is entirely by the 'reward' system with positive reinforcement methods practised by disabled persons using dogs—*Editor.*

11
Occupational Hazards

R. BUTCHER

The Laws Relating to Occupational Health

The very nature of veterinary practice means that staff, clients and visitors can be exposed to potential hazards and the work situation is such, that accidents are possible. Recent Health and Safety legislation attempts to make the workplace as safe an environment as possible, by ensuring that practices examine their working procedures to reduce to a minimum the risk of exposure to hazardous materials, or circumstances in which accidents can occur. Even so, accidents will happen and practices should draw up contingency plans to deal with them. The legislation also makes provision for the recording and reporting of diseases and injuries that occur in the workplace.

It is important that veterinary nurses are familiar with this legislation, not only because they have specific obligations as employees but also because they may become involved in formulating the practice policy or ensuring that other staff adhere to it. The most important Health and Safety legislation relating to veterinary practice include:

- The Health and Safety at Work Act (1974).
- The Control of Substances Hazardous to Health (COSHH) Regulations (1988).
- The Ionising Radiation Regulations (1985).
- The Control of Pollution Act (1974).
- Collection and Disposal of Waste Regulations (1988).
- Environmental Protection Act (1990).
- Reporting of Diseases and Dangerous Occurrences Regulations (RIDDOR) (1980).

In addition to these major regulations, a number of others have relevance to practice Health and Safety and some of these are considered in Chapter 6 (Ethics and Legislation).

The Health and Safety at Work Act (1974)

This Act applies to all businesses, however small, and relates to all persons in the workplace, whether employers, employees or visitors. It sets out the specific duties of both employers and employees, and indicates that the ultimate responsibility rests with the senior partner of the practice.

The general provisions of the Act dictate that every *employer* should ensure that:

(1) Proper provision is made to establish safe systems of work. These should be written down as '**Local Rules**' and be displayed on Health and Safety notice boards at the appropriate work stations.
(2) All equipment is adequately maintained to the manufacturer's specification.
(3) The premises (including vehicles) should be kept in a good state of repair and adequate attention given to providing safe access or exit in times of emergency.
(4) All articles and substances used within the practice should be handled, stored and transported in a safe manner.
(5) Information, instruction and supervision of employees should be carried out regularly.
(6) All appropriate protective clothing is provided free of charge.
(7) A satisfactory working environment is maintained with adequate facilities and arrangements for employees' welfare at work. This should include adequate washing and toilet facilities as well as a separate hygienic area for rest and refreshment.
(8) Appropriate first aid facilities are available. In addition all accidents should be recorded, and the more serious ones reported to the Health and Safety Executive (see below).

In addition, an employer with five or more employees must prepare, and when necessary revise, a written **Health and Safety Policy Statement**. This must outline the general policy of the practice, as well as listing the general duties of all members of the practice. It may be necessary to appoint (in writing) individual members of staff to jobs with special responsibilities (e.g. practice safety officer, fire officer, first aid officer etc.), providing written job specifications for these posts. It is essential that this statement, and any revision, is brought to the attention of all employees.

The Act also highlights the responsibilities of all *employees*, who must:

- take reasonable care for the health and safety of themselves and of other persons who may be affected by their acts or omissions;
- co-operate with the employer so far as it is necessary to enable any duty or requirement under the Act to be performed or complied with;
- not interfere, recklessly or intentionally, with anything provided in the interests of health, safety and welfare.

These broad guidelines to the Act are highlighted on a poster and leaflet produced by the Health and

Safety Executive (HSE) entitled *Health and Safety Law – What you should know*. The poster should be displayed on the practice notice board, and the leaflets should be provided to all staff.

The Control of Substances Hazardous to Health (COSHH) (1988)

These Regulations were introduced to cover areas that were not dealt with adequately by the more general Health and Safety at Work Act. They require that all practices should make an assessment of all the potential hazards that are in the work place (**COSHH Assessment**—see below). This will involve the development of written **Standard Operating Procedures (SOPs)**. In reality, there is often much overlap between these and the 'Local Rules' as required by the Health and Safety at Work Act so that it may be preferable to write a single document, combining:

- Local Rules
- SOPs
- COSHH Assessment
- Healthy and Safety Policy Statement (if applicable).

Hazards and risks

A **hazard** is defined as something with the potential to cause harm. A **risk**, however, is something that is likely to cause harm. The essence of the COSHH Regulations is to identify all the hazards to which the staff are exposed and then to develop work protocols that reduce the risks from these hazards to a minimum.

The range of potential hazards within a veterinary practice is vast, but can usefully be classified into:

- Pharmaceutical products.
- Laboratory reagents.
- Cleaning materials.
- Miscellaneous (non-laboratory) solvents.
- Explosive/flammable agents.
- Laboratory micro-organisms.
- Zoonotic infectious agents.
- Hypersensitivity to animal tissues.
- Unidentified allergens.
- Sharps.
- Inhalation of fumes.
- Radiation.
- Direct injury inflicted by animals.

Warning labels. All hazardous chemicals have clear warnings on the bottle and are classified as:

- Toxic.
- Highly flammable.
- Corrosive.
- Harmful.
- Irritant.

Examples of warning labels are shown in Fig. 11.1.

Maximum Exposure Limit (MEL). The Maximum Exposure Limit of a hazardous substance is assessed in relation to a specific reference period when calculated by a method approved by the Health and Safety Commission. Exposure should not exceed this level.

Occupational Exposure Standard (OES). Where an OES has been approved for an inhalation agent, control can still be regarded as adequate if the level is exceeded and yet the employer identifies the reasons and takes the appropriate action to remedy the situation as soon as is reasonably practical.

The COSHH Assessment

A detailed discussion of how to perform a COSHH Assessment is beyond the scope of this chapter (see Further Reading). Very broadly, the assessment can be approached in three stages:

(1) Consideration of the individual hazards.
(2) The production of Standard Operating Procedures (SOPs).
(3) An overall assessment of the safety within each work station, in the light of (1) and (2).

Individual hazards. The veterinary nurse should consider each hazard in relation to:

- **The nature of the hazard**—What symptoms are seen if exposure occurs? Is there a published MEL or OES?
- **Route of exposure**—Remember that there may be more than one for each substance, and that accidents may result in unexpected routes of exposure (for example, injectable drugs could enter the body by accidental self-injection, but also via the skin or eyes if the bottle is broken).
- **First aid**—Are there any specific first aid measures if accidental exposure occurs?

Fig. 11.1. Hazard warning labels.

- **Preventative measures**—Does this particular substance need to be used, or is a safer alternative available? Will strict SOPs, possibly involving the use of protective clothing, greatly reduce the risk?
- **High-risk staff**—Are there any members of staff who may be at a greater risk (for example, those with known allergies or at risk during pregnancy)? In this regard it is important that staff feel able to notify the practice safety officer or senior partner in confidence if they consider there is any chance of being pregnant, or if they have any disease condition that might increase the risks when working in a particular environment.
- **Recording of exposure**—Are there any monitoring schemes available to record exposure? This would include dosimetry for X-ray radiation exposure and any monitoring for halothane and nitrous oxide in the operating theatre.

Many of the individual hazardous substances can be grouped together since the hazards are similar. Further subdivisions can then be made within the major groupings (e.g. pharmaceutical drugs can be split into smaller groups such as: injectable antibiotics, topical steroid creams, cytotoxic drugs, organophosphate insecticides, etc.). Much of the technical data can be gleaned from the *COSHH Hazard Data Sheets* that should be available for each product from the manufacturers. (Note that these are not the same as the standard Product Data Sheets.)

Standard Operating Procedures (SOPs). Written SOPs should be produced to cover the range of all work performed at the surgery. They must above all be clear and concise, and be tailored to the work protocols of each individual practice. Copies should be posted at the appropriate work stations, so that the group of SOPs in that area forms the basis of the Local Rules as required by the general Health and Safety legislation. A pictorial component would give more impact to SOPs posted on notice boards. Specimen SOPs are available as part of the BSAVA Members' Information Service.

The actual SOPs required by each practice may vary, but suggested topics (some of which are discussed in greater detail in relevant chapters of this book) include:

- Radiation protection
- Accidents and first aid
- Health surveillance
- Laboratory procedures
- Postage of laboratory specimens
- Safe prescribing and handling of medicines
- Injections
- Restraint of animals
- Spillages
- The dental scaler
- Waste disposal
- Disinfectants and floor cleaning
- Kennel management
- Anaesthetic gases—scavenging and monitoring
- Fire precautions
- Mortuary/post-mortems
- X-ray processing
- Sterilisers
- The practice vehicle
- On the farm/stable

Overall assessment of each practice work area. This builds on the information collated above, and is basically a critical look at the safety of each work station within the practice. The format discussed below is that suggested in *COSHH: BVA guide to the initial assessment in veterinary practices.*

At each work station (or room or department) the assessment involves methodical listing:

(1) Hazardous substances/pathogens that may be encountered in that area. For each one the practice must assess the degree of risk and allot a hazard code (H = high; M = moderate; L = low; N = negligible). If the substance has a known MEL or OES, this too should be recorded.
(2) All the members of staff present in this area. This should include their sex, official job title, and a brief summary of their involvement in this area.
(3) All the practice SOPs that may be of relevance in this area.
(4) The control measures in use in the area. This may simply require reference to specific SOPs.
(5) Safety clothing provided and used.

Having completed this stage of the assessment, it is important to record a comment that represents an overview of the exposure and actual risks in that area. It is possible that various deficiencies are highlighted. These should be listed and a note made when they have been corrected.

An important part of the assessment is to ascertain where further staff training or instruction is required. This too should be planned and a note made when completed.

Finally, the date of the next assessment should be set (at least annually). The COSHH assessment is therefore an on-going process promoting continual improvements to the practice's safety standards.

Ionising Radiation Regulations (1985)

These apply specifically to the hazards associated with radiography and are dealt with fully in Chapter 28 (Radiography).

Clinical Waste Regulations

The principle regulations relating to this subject are:

- Control of Pollution Act (1974).
- Collection and Disposal of Waste Regulations (1988).
- Environmental Protection Act (1990).

Together they regulate the correct segregation, storage, transfer and eventual destruction of waste products produced at the surgery. The waste produced at veterinary practices must be classified by the veterinary nurse (clinical waste, 'sharps', special waste, cadavers, industrial waste) and disposed of correctly.

Clinical waste includes all waste that consists wholly or partly of animal tissues, blood or other body fluids, excretions, drugs or pharmaceutical products likely to be hazardous to health. It should be collected and stored in approved colour-coded plastic sacks (yellow with the words 'Clinical waste' clearly printed on the outside).

'Sharps' is a special category of clinical waste that includes used needles, scalpel blades or other sharp instruments. These should be discarded *immediately* after use, into special yellow plastic tubs that can be sealed once full.

Special waste, a further category of clinical waste, includes bottles and vials contaminated with pharmaceutical products. These too are stored in specific plastic bins.

Cadavers are technically clinical waste. Strict interpretation of the law would cause problems for owners who wish to bury their pets in their garden. The Department of Environment Management Paper No. 25 states: 'Pets deceased at a veterinary practice remain the property of the owner and may be disposed of by the owner within the curtilage of their dwelling in their capacity as a private individual without breach of duty of care. Where the pet suffered from an infectious disease or for other reasons may be significantly hazardous, then it should be dealt with by the veterinary surgeon as clinical waste. Low hazard deceased pets should be classed as non-clinical commercial waste where the owner requests disposal by the veterinary surgeon, who will be subject to the duty of care'. This is of importance to the owner who wishes to bury their own pet in their garden.

The remainder of the practice waste is regarded as **industrial waste**. This is non-hazardous and can be removed by the local authority or other registered carrier (an appropriate charge may be levied for the service).

Segregation and storage within the practice

The practice must have a strict policy on the segregation of waste. To be practical this must allow for the immediate disposal of material after use, and hence there must be sufficient receptacles to allow for segregation at each work station. This should also apply to practice vehicles. Prior to collection, clinical waste should be stored in a secure place within the practice.

Transport and disposal

Clinical waste is collected by a registered carrier in a 'dedicated' vehicle, licensed specifically for the transport of clinical waste. It is transferred to a licensed plant where final disposal is achieved, preferably by high temperature incineration. Each collection (or batch of collections) should be accompanied by the appropriate certification, copies of which should be kept by the practice.

The regulations place a duty of care on the producers of clinical waste to ensure that, from production to ultimate disposal, the waste is dealt with according to the law. The practice itself is responsible for checking that both the carrier and incineration plant have the appropriate licenses (ideally keeping photocopies for its own records).

General Maintenance and Care

It is important that all buildings are kept in a good state of repair, especially with regard to electrical or gas installations and fittings.

All equipment (X-ray machines, anaesthetic machines, autoclaves etc.) should be regularly serviced according to the manufacturer's recommendations, and service records should be kept.

Fire Precautions

Adequate precautions should be taken to avoid or combat fires. This is covered by the Fire Precautions Act 1971 and may involve:

- The provision of adequate fire fighting equipment. Advice needs to be taken on the correct extinguishers for different work stations, and these should be checked regularly.
- An alarm system, regularly maintained.
- Well sign-posted emergency exits.
- Emergency lighting.
- Clear local rules stating what to do in case of fire. These should be posted in strategic places, and reinforced by regular fire practices.
- Care in the storage of inflammable and explosive material.
- The provision of fire doors where appropriate.

The practice should appoint a fire officer to oversee these precautions. Very valuable advice can be obtained from the local Fire Prevention Officer.

Protection of the Person Against Physical Attack

Unfortunately, veterinary practices are not immune from the attentions of criminals. Nurses or veterinary surgeons 'on call' at night and weekends are especially vulnerable, and it might be worth incorporating personal 'panic buttons' into the practice alarm system. The local Crime Prevention Officer may give useful advice on this matter. Staff should always state where they have been called out to and obtain phone numbers.

First Aid and Reporting Accidents

First aid

Despite every precaution, accidents will occur. The practice must keep an approved first aid box, the size and contents of which reflect the number of staff. The practice's first aid officer should ensure that this is regularly checked and re-stocked as necessary. It would be valuable to train one or more members of staff in basic first aid techniques, perhaps on a course run by the local Red Cross or St John's Ambulance groups.

It is worth considering (in relation to the COSHH Regulations) that the blood from another member of staff, or a client, is potentially hazardous and so adequate precautions (disposable gloves etc.) should be taken by those administering first aid.

Recording accidents

It is the duty of the practice to record all accidents and injuries that occur. An accident book approved by HSE (Form B1 510) is available from HMSO. The information that is to be recorded includes:

(1) The full name, address and occupation of the person who had the accident.
(2) The signature (with date) of the person filling in the book. This must also include the address and occupation if the person is different from (1).
(3) When and where the accident happened.
(4) Details about the cause of the accident. Record details of any personal injury.
(5) Indicate whether the injury needs to be reported under RIDDOR.

Reporting accidents

Under the provisions of the Reporting of Injuries, Diseases and Dangerous Occurrences Regulations (RIDDOR), the practice is obliged to report certain serious events direct to the HSE. These can be broadly divided into three categories:

- Major or fatal accidents.
- 'Three-day' accidents.
- Dangerous occurrences and near misses.

Major or fatal accidents must be reported as soon as possible by telephone, followed by written confirmation within seven days on Form 2508. Major accidents are defined as:

- A fracture of the skull, spine or pelvis.
- A fracture of a long bone of the limb.
- Amputation of a hand or foot.
- Loss of sight of an eye.
- Any other accident which results in an injured person being admitted into hospital as an in-patient for more than 24 hours, unless only detained for observation.

Fatal accidents include those instances where a fatality occurs within one year as a result of an original accident at work.

'Three-day accidents' relate to absences from work for a minimum of three days as a result of an accident at work. The DHSS will notify the HSE, who in turn will require a written report from the practice.

There is a list of **dangerous occurrences** that should be reported to the HSE (Form F2508) whether or not an injury occurs. These include:

- Explosion from a gas cylinder or steriliser.
- Uncontrolled release of substance (including gases, vapours and X-rays) liable to be hazardous to health.
- Any escape of substances that might result in problems due to inhalation or lack of oxygen.
- Any cases of acute ill health that could have resulted from exposure to pathogens in infected material.
- Any unintentional ignition or explosion.

Practical Health and Safety in the Practice Environment

The following section indicates the veterinary nurse's responsibility for looking at some of the areas that should be of concern when formulating the practice's Health and Safety policy statement and COSHH assessment. These can only act as hints, as each practice will have its own particular hazards and work practices.

General points

Many items covered by the SOPs will be common to all parts of the practice (e.g. first aid, fire precautions, floor cleaning and disinfectants, etc.) and will not be mentioned below.

In all work areas where hands are likely to become contaminated, it is worth considering the use of elbow taps on sinks and disposable towels.

Waiting room/reception

Probably the major potential hazard in this area is injury from unrestrained animals. Clients should be made aware (ideally by a sign outside the building) that all animals must be suitably restrained. Leads and cat baskets should be available in reception for clients who arrive without them.

Recently washed floors must be dried well or 'wet floor' warning notices displayed.

The consulting room

A special consideration here is the potential hazard of children becoming injured by contact with sharps or pharmaceutical products. Ideally drugs should be stored outside the consulting room. Where this is not practical, they must be kept well out of the reach of children.

Clinical waste, including sharps, should be disposed of in the appropriate manner immediately after use.

The dispensary

The correct storage and dispensing of drugs (as recommended by the RCVS), including special provisions for controlled drugs, is an important factor and is discussed fully in Chapter 13 (Pharmacology, Therapeutics and Dispensing).

Care must be taken when dispensing drugs that can be absorbed through the skin (e.g. cytotoxic drugs). Some individuals show skin hypersensitivity to antibiotics and so disposable gloves should be considered when handling tablets. The use of automatic tablet counters avoids direct handling altogether.

Care must also be taken when dispensing small quantities of powdered material that could be a hazard if inhaled. Face masks should be worn. Similarly, precautions may be needed if dispensing small volumes of liquid from a larger stock solution.

Stores

In most practices space is at a premium and so storage often involves high shelving. Avoid putting heavy material on the highest shelf and provide non-slip stools in each store room where they may be required. Where heavy items need to be transported within the practice (e.g. trays of petfood or anaethetised dogs), a trolley should be available to avoid back injury. It is important to keep corridors free from stored material as this could impede rapid exit in the case of fire.

The practice laboratory

There are many potential hazards in the practice laboratory and strict attention to SOPs is required. This is considered in more detail in Chapter 12.

In practices without a laboratory, it is important to adhere to the regulations for the postage of pathological specimens.

The X-ray room

The problems associated with radiation hazards are discussed fully in Chapter 28 (Radiography). It is worth considering here the problems of disposing of spent developer and fixer solutions. The appropriate protective clothing should be worn when dealing with these chemicals and good ventilation is essential to avoid inhalation of fumes. Consideration should also be given to the extraction of silver from spent developer before this is discharged into the normal waste water supply.

The preparation area

The problems related to anaesthetic gas scavenging and monitoring are of significance in this area. In addition, the amount of animal hair should be reduced to a minimum, not only to improve general hygiene but also to reduce the risk of hypersensitivity reactions in some individuals.

Dental scalers are often used in this area, and an SOP should be formulated to cover the use of masks and eye protection. It is also recommended that chlorhexidine is added to the coolant water.

In practices using oscillating saws to remove plaster casts, thought should be given to the control of the amount of dust, which could be hazardous if inhaled.

The operating area

There are no specific problems here not already dealt with elsewhere but it is worth considering the transport of animals to and from the theatre using trolleys to avoid heavy lifting.

The level of waste anaesthetic gases in the recovery area is likely to be high as the animals exhale it on recovery. Good ventilation is therefore essential in this area.

Hospital kennels and catteries

Thought should be given to hygienic kennel protocols that reduce the risk of infection from zoonotic agents. The practice might consider the provision of isolation facilities (Chapter 5) in cases where there is a known risk of zoonosis.

There should also be clear instructions to staff relating to the handling of animals and their transport within the building to avoid physical injury from bites and scratches.

Mortuary

Correct protective clothing and disinfection regimes are essential in this area. Special thought should also be given to precautions taken if post-mortems are performed on parrots, since there is the additional risk of the inhalation of the agent causing psittacosis from feather debris.

Staff rest room

Adequate rest room facilities should be provided to allow refreshments to be enjoyed away from the working areas. A sink should be provided specifically for the supply of drinking water and for washing up crockery.

Office

There are guidelines relating to the minimum temperatures and lighting conditions for the workplace. There are also regulations associated with the use of computer screens.

Car park/entrance

The Health and Safety legislation extends to the limit of the practice boundaries. Ensure adequate lighting at night, and consider providing bins for the disposal of dog faeces.

Practice vehicles

Within vehicles, ensure that all drugs are stored safely and securely. Also make provision for the immediate disposal of clinical waste and sharps. The habit of bringing trays of used syringes and needles back to the surgery for others to dispose of greatly increases the risk of accidental self-injection (especially important in relation to drugs like prostaglandins).

On the farm

The same principles of Health and Safety apply when working on the farm. Many potential hazards relate to zoonotic infections, and the BVA guidelines are very useful in this regard. Farmers also have responsibilities under the Health and Safety at Work Act and the COSHH Regulations, and the veterinary surgeon's advise is very important in helping farmers

to formulate their own SOPs with regard to zoonotic infections.

Further Reading

BSAVA Members' Information Service (1993) *Guides to Local Health and Safety Rules.*

BVA (revised 1989) *Health and Safety at Work Act—A Guide for Veterinary practices.*

BVA (1991) *COSHH: BVA Guide to the Initial Assessment in Veterinary Practices.*

HMSO (1986) *A Guide to the Reporting of Injuries, Diseases and Dangerous Occurrences Regulations 1985.*

HMSO (1988) *The Guidance Notes for the Protection of Persons against Ionising Radiation arising from Veterinary Use.*

HMSO (1989) *COSHH Assessments—A Step-by-Step Guide to Assessment and the Skills Needed for it.*

HMSO (1989) *Essentials of Health and Safety at Work.*

HMSO (1989) *Writing your Health and Safety Policy Statement.*

HMSO (1991) *Fire Safety at Work.*

NOAH (1990) *The Safe Storage and Handling of Animal Medicines.*

RCVS Guidelines (1988) *Dispatch of Pathological Specimens by Post* (reprinted by BSAVA Members' Information Service).

12
Running a Small Animal Practice Laboratory

P. A. BLOXHAM

Veterinary nurses are now expected to be able to provide the practice with the technical skill and ability to operate a small in-house laboratory. They therefore need to understand the equipment currently available and to know how to use it to produce good quality, reliable results and to perform basic diagnostic tests safely. Appendix 16.6 of the RCVS's Guide to Professional Conduct (1993 edition), relating to Practice Standards, advises that the practice must:

Either provide laboratory facilities; or have access to one or more other laboratories which are adequately equipped to perform routine clinical pathology rapidly and accurately.

If the practice provides laboratory facilities it must ensure that:
(a) Laboratory procedures are performed in a room or a designated area used specifically for that purpose.
(b) Laboratory procedures are undertaken only by designated persons or persons under their supervision.
(c) Persons designated to undertake laboratory procedures are adequately trained for the tasks performed by them.
(d) Local rules are drawn up to cover cleanliness, tidiness, disinfection, first aid boxes, outbreaks of fire, the safe handling of equipment and reagents, the use of protective equipment and clothing, the dispatch of specimens by post, the disposal of laboratory waste and that the rules are displayed on a notice board in the laboratory.

This chapter considers the management of a practice laboratory and the understanding, use and maintenance of its equipment. Chapter 22 (Diagnostic Tests) explains how to collect and examine specimens, or how to prepare them for submission to a pathology laboratory for professional examination.

Laboratory Apparatus

Cleaning and Disposal

Chemically clean glassware is essential and although more glass is being replaced by disposable plastic it is important to know how to clean and dry glassware. The use of commercial laboratory detergents is advisable and instructions should be followed carefully. As a matter of routine, put all reusable glassware into disinfectant containers as soon as it has been used. The cleaning procedure is as follows:

(1) Soak any dirty glassware in suitable disinfectants.
(2) Using disposable gloves, remove any surface material with the aid of test-tube brushes or other soft bristle brushes so as not to scratch the glass.
(3) Transfer to fresh solution of detergent and leave to soak, or use ultrasonic bath.
(4) Once the glassware is physically clean, rinse it thoroughly in distilled/deionised water, with two or three changes of fresh water, to ensure complete removal of any residue detergents.
(5) Allow to drain.
(6) Then dry in a drying oven or in air, ensuring that the atmosphere is free from dust and chemicals.

```
Checklist
• Soak in detergent.
• Soak in disinfectant.
• Rinse 2–3 times in distilled/deionised water.
• Drain and dry.
```

It should be routine practice to clean all equipment and work-surfaces daily following use. Equipment should be wiped down with suitable disposable cloths impregnated with disinfectant. Any tubes, cuvettes and pipes should be flushed through with disinfectant solutions. Some manufacturers recommend and supply special cleaning and flushing solutions for their machines and they should be used as appropriate.

Put disposable 'sharps' into sharps bins and all other disposable waste into yellow bin bags as soon as they have been used. They should then be disposed of as clinical waste.

Pipettes

Graduated pipettes have a series of lines or marks engraved on the side to indicate the volume of their contents. A 10 ml pipette of this type is graduated in 1 ml divisions; each ml is subdivided into ten 0.1 ml units. The meniscus of the fluid in the pipette should be at the level of the line required.

One-mark volumetric pipettes have only a single mark on them indicating the level for a specific volume.

Both of these pipettes are usually filled by attaching a rubber tube and plastic mouth piece to the top and applying gentle oral suction. Care is needed not to suck up the fluid into the mouth and cotton plugs may be inserted into the top of the pipettes to restrict fluid into the tube. For safety reasons, it is preferable not to 'mouth-pipette' but to use a large-volume, flexible rubber bulb to create the suction.

Micro-pipettes come in various styles, with single or adjustable volumes and disposable pipette tips. For some (particularly the very small volume types), positive displacement is achieved using a probe which comes into contact with the fluid; other micro-pipettes operate on the principle of air displacement. The disposable tips are usually colour coded for the various volumes. Accurate and reproducible pipetting requires care and practice. Tips should be discarded into sharps bins and most pipettes have an ejection system so that the tips do not need to be handled.

Automatic pipettes are becoming more common and two basic types are in use:

- **Single-shot reservoir**—dial the volume required and fill the reservoir; an electronic button then dispenses the required volume, one shot at a time.
- **Multihead** pipettes—often used for ELISA plate work and normally have eight tips so that eight wells can be filled at the same time (electrically) with the same amount of fluid from a single reservoir.

Pasteur pipettes were originally made from soda glass tubes pulled to a fine point over a Bunsen flame. They have a rubber bulb on the other end. The technique is to press the bulb and then immerse the tip in a liquid; as the bulb is released, fluid passes up the capillary section of the pipette into the lumen of the tube. The fluid in the tube can then be released into a separate container by squeezing the bulb again. This system was commonly used for the removal or separation of serum or plasma from a blood sample. Currently most Pasteur pipettes are of moulded flexible plastic with integral bulbs.

Bottles

Chemicals and reagents are often supplied in plastic containers or in glass bottles. The original amber glass **winchester**, a tall bottle, has been replaced by a more dumpy, wider based bottle with a lower centre of gravity, which is less likely to be knocked over. Many acids are supplied in this type of bottle and should be kept in a metal safety cupboard with lockable doors and at floor level. Never put concentrated acid bottles on high shelves.

Common **reagent** bottles for use in the laboratory have either a screw top or a glass stopper and are made from clear glass, clear or opaque plastic, or amber glass. If making up reagents it is important to label the bottles clearly (using a waterproof marker) showing details of contents and date made, together with any storage details. Any **hazardous substances** should be clearly identified with the correct symbols and stored in accordance with the Control of Substances Hazardous to Health (COSHH) regulations. Various adjustable **volume dispenser systems** are available to aid in the transfer of fluid from the bottles.

Smaller reagent bottles with integral pipettes in the lid are used for dispensing reagents and stains. Some **dropping bottles** have grooved glass stoppers so that drops can be dispensed. Many modern versions of the dropping bottle are of polythene, with an elongated, tapering nozzle that may be cut at the tip to allow a single drop at a time or, if cut lower down at a wider diameter, to dispense a stream.

Universal bottles are small, wide-mouthed, screw-top plastic or glass 30 ml bottles, often used for urine or faeces samples. They are usually supplied as sterile containers.

Microscopes

A good compound microscope (Fig. 12.1) is an essential piece of equipment for every veterinary practice. It is advisable to use a binocular microscope

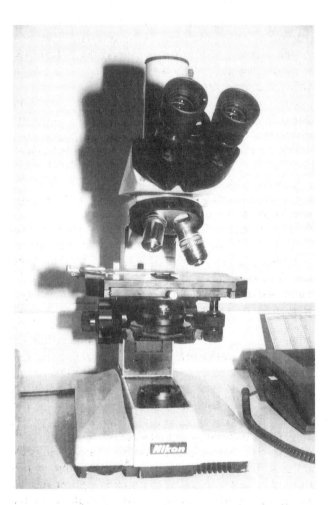

Fig. 12.1. The compound microscope.

with an integral **light source** (usually a 6 volt halogen filament bulb) in the base or foot. A **transformer** controlled by a **rheostat** modifies the intensity of the light source. The light passes through a **lens** and **field diaphragm** to a **mirror** that directs the light up from the foot to the **substage condenser**. The condenser consists of two lenses that focus the light source on the object being viewed: the condenser is moved up or down by turning the **condenser knob**. Before the light reaches the condenser it passes through the **iris diaphragm**, which is a lever-controlled aperture that modifies the amount of light passing through the condenser. Below the iris there are often glass **filters**, e.g. a blue daylight filter to reduce the amount of red or yellow components of the light spectrum.

Above the substage condenser is the **stage**, which holds the slide being examined. It is mounted on a mechanical assembly referred to as the **mechanical stage**. This enables the slide holder to be moved left or right, up or down.

> **TIP**
> When viewed through a compound microscope an object appears to be upside down and reversed. Movement of the mechanical stage is also reversed, so that as the stage is moved to the left the image moves to the right.

Each **axis** (there are two of them) has a **vernier scale** on it so that the position of any particular item on the object slide may be recorded. Tradition demands that the position is recorded in the same way as grid references on a map.

Above the stage is the **nose piece**, with a rotating turret holding normally three or four **objective lenses**, each with a different magnification. The most common objective lenses are: 4× (scanning), 10× (low power), 40× (high dry) and 100× (oil immersion). The stage is racked up and down by means of an outer **coarse focus** and an inner **fine focus** knob on the limb of the microscope.

As light passes through the selected objective lens it travels up the **optical tube** mounted in the body of the microscope to a series of **prisms** in the binocular head (body) which deflect the light path through the **ocular lenses** mounted in the **eye-pieces**. The eye-pieces may be adjusted to the interpupillary distance of the person using the microscope and one of the ocular tubes in the eye-pieces is adjustable to correct for individual differences between the two eyes. The inclined binocular head may increase the actual magnification 1.5× and the factor is engraved on the head. The lenses in the eye-pieces are usually low powered with a magnification of 4× or 6×, while 8× is the maximum for practical use.

Some binocular microscopes have interchangeable bodies so that a monocular **photographic tube** can be attached. Others have a permanent photographic tube as well as the binocular head. Specially designed teaching heads have two binocular sets.

The purpose of a microscope is to magnify, and the size of the object can be measured if a **measuring scale** is put into one of the eye-pieces. The amount of magnification is calculated by the magnification of the eye-piece × magnification of the binocular head × the objective magnification.

Care, cleaning and maintenance of microscopes

The microscope is a precision instrument.

- It should be located in a convenient position and not moved unnecessarily.
- If it does have to be moved it should be carried in both hands, one under the base or foot and the other holding the limb.
- Do not place it near centrifuges or other sources of vibration, and keep it away from sinks and direct sunlight.
- Keep it covered when not in use.
- To maximise the life of the bulb, turn the rheostat down before switching it off or if the light is left on for any period when not in use.
- Keep extra light bulbs in stock but do not handle the actual bulb when replacing it.
- Only lens paper should be used to clean the lenses and eye-pieces. It is designed for the job and will not scratch the lenses.
- Remove oil from the oil immersion objective after use and ensure that solvents do not remain in contact with the objective as they may loosen the cement holding the lens in place.
- When finished with the microscope, turn off the light (after turning down the rheostat), then lower the stage and turn the lowest power objective into position. Clean the oil immersion lens and cover the microscope.
- If dirt appears in the field of study it is likely to be on the eye-piece. Rotate it: if the dirt also rotates, clean the eye-piece with a lens paper.

Using the microscope

(1) Check that the lowest objective is in position and that all lenses and eye-pieces are clean.
(2) Check that the rheostat is down low.
(3) Place the slide or counting chamber firmly into the mechanical stage and centralise below the object lens.
(4) Switch on and then turn up the rheostat to increase the brightness.
(5) Adjust the distance between the two eye-pieces so that each field appears identical and that both fields are viewed as one.
(6) Using the course and fine focus knobs, bring the object into clear view.
(7) Adjust the position of the condenser and diaphragms for optimal illumination.
(8) Using the mechanical stage travelling knobs, examine the field on the slide under low power.

(9) If a specific area under view requires higher magnification, rotate the objective nose turret until the $40\times$ high dry objective lens clicks into place and then adjust the fine focus to obtain a clear image. The diaphragm and condenser may require readjustment as more light may be needed at the higher magnification.

To view under oil immersion:

(1) First view the field under low power.
(2) Then place a drop of immersion oil on the field and rotate the oil immersion objective into position.
(3) If the field does not come into view, stop looking down the eye-pieces and look directly at the position of the oil immersion lens in relation to the surface of the slide and the oil. The lens of the objective should be in the oil but not touching the slide.
(4) Slowly adjust the position with the fine focus knob so that the slide is moved away from the lens but the lens remains in the oil. Careful focusing while returning to view the object via the eye-pieces should bring the field into view.
(5) Adjust the iris diaphragm and condenser to ensure adequate illumination.

Never allow the high dry or other non-oil immersion lenses to come into contact with the oil. When finished with oil immersion viewing, lower the stage, rotate the lenses so that the lowest power is in position, turn the light down and then off, clean the oil immersion lens and remove the slide from the stage.

Colorimeter

Colorimetry is the measurement of light absorbed or transmitted by a substance. A **colorimeter** is the apparatus or analyser which measures the light absorbed (**inverse colorimetry**) or transmitted (**direct colorimetry**) by a solution at a wavelength. The selection of a wavelength in a colorimeter is achieved by use of filters; however, most modern analysers are in fact **spectrophotometers**, which use prisms or monochromatic gratings to separate the light path into a single wavelength. This is then passed through the solution (normally held in a **cuvette**) and the emergent light is then detected and converted into electrical energy and displayed by means of an **analogue meter** or, more commonly, by means of **digital read-out**.

Colorimeters and spectrophotometers are 'wet' **chemistry systems** that require the use of various liquid reagents which are commercially available in kit form. Detailed methodology for use of the kit in conjunction with a particular analyser is provided by the manufacturer or supplier. The analysers normally found in a veterinary practice are of the manual or semi-automated type allowing one test to be performed on one sample at a time. The systems used in commercial laboratories are larger automated ones allowing a variable number of tests to be performed on batches of samples.

More recently, **'dry' chemistry systems** have become available for practice use. With these a sample is put on to a prepared slide or reagent strip and the analyser determines the reflective light (usually as the reaction occurs) and displays the results. Whichever system is used, it is important to follow the manufacturer's operating rules fully and to ensure that the machine is kept clean and is serviced regularly.

Temperature control

Enzymes are totally dependent on temperature. In the veterinary world, the recommended temperature for performing determination of enzyme activity is $30°C$. It is essential that the temperature is controlled. Machines should not be placed in positions with direct exposure to sunlight and the ambient operating temperature must be maintained constantly.

Quality control

Storage of kits, reagents and samples must be carefully monitored and regular use of internal quality control samples and external quality assessment samples is essential if the practice is to comply with the RCVS standards. Operators should be adequately trained by the supplier and if necessary receive further professional training in order to become and remain competent.

Centrifuges

These machines spin at speed to produce a high gravitational force referred to as the **relative centrifugal force (RCF)**, which is measured in G forces. Acceleration due to gravity (G) is $981\,cm/second/second$. The objectives are:

- to separate the cells from fluid;
- to partition different density (size and mass) of material; and
- to concentrate the material.

The deposit is termed the **sediment**; the fluid is the **supernatant**.

Standard centrifuges are of two types according to the style of rotor head: a swing-out and an angle-head.

A **swing-out head** consists of a rotor with specimen buckets suspended vertically from the arms of the rotor. As the rotor turns, the buckets swing out into a horizontal position. When the rotor slows down and stops, they fall back into a vertical position. The swing-out head generates air friction and it heats up at speed, which may be a problem and restricts the speed at which the centrifuge may be operated. The swinging is likely to remix the samples slightly at the end of centrifugation.

An **angle-head** rotor has a series of holes drilled around the rotor at a fixed angle (normally 52° from the perpendicular). Samples are placed in these holes. The angled head can be operated at higher speeds without heat build-up but the deposit is laid down at the fixed angle of the head and may be disturbed as the tubes are removed and stood upright in test tube racks.

The **inner bowl** of the centrifuge is a very solid piece of metal designed as a **guard** to retain the rotor buckets and samples should they become detached, or should metal fatigue lead to fracture of the rotor. It is good laboratory practice to wipe out, clean and disinfect the entire bowl as a matter of routine.

Modern centrifuges have a number of inbuilt safety devices, including an **integral lid-lock** that prevents opening of the centrifuge while the rotor is still spinning, nor can the rotor begin to operate until the lid is securely closed. A **safety plate** is present on many machines either as a separate screw-on lid behind the main lid or as an integral part of the main lid; like the guard bowl, it prevents penetration from inside in case of accidents.

Samples, usually in glass or plastic tubes, are put into **buckets** or carrier tubes which have rubber cushions at the bottom to prevent the bases of the sample tubes from damage or breakage. For safety, the buckets should be able to be removed for washing (and if necessary autoclaving) in case of breakage or spillage. To prevent aerosol dissemination, especially from potentially pathogenic samples, always use bucket guards or lids (these are autoclavable). It is important to ensure that buckets are balanced and so tubes of equal volume and weight should be placed opposite each other. Water-filled tubes may be used to balance the buckets if necessary.

Most centrifuges now have variable **speed control** and a gauge to show the speed, a **timer** to dial up the required period of centrifugation and a **brake** to slow down the rotor once the timer switches off. To increase the gravitational force, the rotor's turning speed is controlled and so is the duration. If the radius of the centrifuge from the centre of the shaft to the tip of the bucket is R (cm) and the number of revolutions of the rotor per minute (RPM) is N, then the G force is calculated using the following equation:

$$G = 1.118 \times 10^{-5} \times R \times N^2.$$

Routine cleaning, lubrication and general service maintenance are essential for reliable and safe operation and the manufacturer's instructions should be followed. The motor is powered by electricity and it is important that the wiring (including the plug and correct fuse) is checked regularly under the Health and Safety rules for the inspection of electrical apparatus. The motor's brushes should be replaced when they wear down. It is advisable to keep a log of the usage of the centrifuge and to relate this to regular servicing by the manufacturer, in the same way that vehicles are serviced on the basis of mileage.

Microhaematocrit

A microhaematocrit is a special type of centrifuge (Fig. 12.2) for separating whole blood in capillary tubes to enable assessment of packed cell volume (PCV). It has a special type of rotor consisting of an almost flat, horizontal surface with slots for capillary tubes. There is a rubber cushion on the outside of the lip of the rotor. A safety plate is screwed down on top of the rotor to hold the tubes in place and then the lid is closed to operate. Sometimes capillary tubes do not seal properly and sometimes there may be breakages, so that the rubber cushion is likely to be covered with blood and may be damaged by fragments of capillary glass. It should be wiped clean after use and the rubber replaced regularly. The entire head, rubber cushion and the safety plate should be disinfected as a matter of routine.

Incubator

Electric incubators are used to culture bacteria. These enclosed units of various sizes have removable

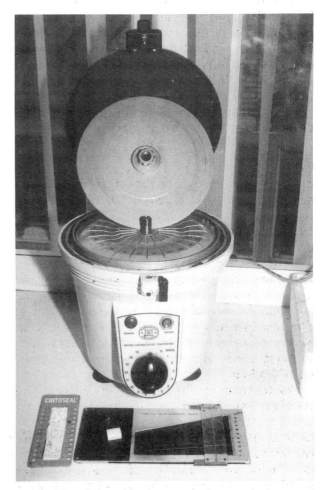

Fig. 12.2. Microhaematocrit centrifuge.

shelves and impervious smooth surfaces of metal or plastic. They are well insulated with a gasket sealed door so that the air inside is maintained at a set temperature (37°C is the optimal temperature for almost all pathogenic bacteria). It is important to check the wiring and thermostat and to maintain a daily record of the temperature to ensure that the operation is as desired. Because potentially dangerous bacteria may be grown, it is essential to have a set procedure for cleaning and disinfecting or perhaps fumigating the incubator.

Safety in the Laboratory

The laboratory is a dangerous place.

- It should be accessible only to authorised people.
- Smoking, eating or drinking must never be allowed in the laboratory.
- Protective laboratory coats should be donned on entry and removed on departure from the laboratory area.
- Disposable gloves should be worn.
- Surfaces should be kept clean and tidy.
- Books and papers should be kept away from the working bench area and should be kept separate from any samples or reagents being handled.

Training and complete understanding of the Health and Safety at Work Act 1984 as it relates to laboratories are essential, as is knowledge of the Control of Substances Hazardous to Health (COSHH) regulations (discussed in Chapters 6 and 11). Safety training courses are available and every person should have attended such courses and also be familiar with simple first aid procedures.

If glass is broken or liquid spilled, it is essential to know how to protect everybody from risk. Take appropriate action and record what happened. If in doubt, report to a senior person and follow instructions.

ACCIDENT BOOK
The minimum information to be recorded in relation to accidents at work, in order to satisfy the regulations in the Social Security Act 1975 and Reporting of Injuries, Diseases and Dangerous Occurrences Regulations 1985 (RIDDOR).
1) Give full name, home address and occupation of the person who had the accident.
2) The person filling in the book must sign and date it. If they did not have the accident then they must also give their name, home address and occupation.
3) Record time and date of accident and where it happened.
4) State how the accident happened. Give the cause if you can. If any personal injury, state what it is.
5) If the accident is reportable under RIDDOR then employer must initial and report.
6) Accident books must be retained for three years after the date of the last entry.

Fig. 12.3. Accident book headings and information required.

In case of accidents

- If something is splashed in the eye, wash it out immediately with a deionised water eye-bath (which should be readily to hand).
- Acid or alkaline spillage must be correctly neutralised.
- Any infectious agents must be killed by means of bacterial or viricide disinfectants.
- All accidents should be reported to a responsible person and entered into an accident book in a standard format such as that shown in Fig. 12.3.

Disposal of Clinical Waste

Because it is possible that significant pathogens may be isolated in the practice laboratory, attention to Health and Safety codes is important at all times when working with bacterial samples in particular. Attention to the control and disposal of clinical waste is very important and current legislation places the responsibility for it on the person who generates the waste.

- Glassware should be soaked in suitable disinfectants and detergents to kill micro-organisms.
- Disposable plastic items should be put into discard bins or sharps bins, as appropriate.
- Culture plates should be placed into autoclave bags and sterilised in autoclaves before being put into yellow clinical waste bags for incineration.
- Samples should also be autoclaved where possible before being placed in the yellow bags.

It is the responsibility of the staff in a practice laboratory to ensure that the material is made as safe as possible and that the yellow bags are collected regularly and transported by licensed clinical waste carriers to approved incineration facilities and disposed of correctly under the legislation. The local authority may be able to provide these facilities and some commercial operators also offer a service. Record-keeping and adherence to the regulations are important.

One final aspect of laboratory practice is to ensure at all times that the staff:

- keep the laboratory neat and tidy;
- follow the local Health and Safety rules;
- dispose correctly of clinical waste (used reagents and equipment);
- clean up and disinfect working surfaces;
- act immediately to control spillage;
- record any accident;
- ensure adequate training;
- if in doubt—ask.

These aspects are very important. Quality results depend on good working practices; safety and care in the laboratory also depend on adherence to standard operating procedures.

13

Medicines: Pharmacology, Therapeutics and Dispensing

J. ELLIOTT

Pharmacology, the science of drugs, can be divided into two parts. Firstly it is concerned with the study of the way in which the functions of the living body are affected by drugs **(pharmacodynamics)** and secondly, with the absorption, metabolism and excretion of drugs by the body **(pharmacokinetics)**. Much of the understanding of the pharmacology of drugs is derived from studies in normal healthy animals; the study of **clinical pharmacology** attempts to transpose this information to the diseased clinical patient.

Therapeutics can be defined as the rational and optimal use of drugs in the management of disease states or in the manipulation of physiological functions. In order to use drugs in a 'rational' and 'optimal' way, an understanding of the nature of the disease process and of the pharmacology of the drug to be used is required. Without such an understanding, the clinical use of drugs is 'empirical'.

The subject of **pharmacy** can be defined as the **preparation** of drugs and their formulation into medicines followed by their **dispensing** (giving out) to the owner of a sick animal. Nowadays, most medicines are formulated by the pharmaceutical companies and are ready for dispensing. In many veterinary practices, medicines are dispensed to owners of sick animals from the practice premises. They can also be dispensed by pharmacists when presented by the owner of the animal with a written instruction **(prescription)** from the veterinary surgeon who is responsible for the care of the animal in question.

Drug Classification

Definitions

Drugs are often classified according to:

(a) the way in which they bring about their effect on the body, and
(b) which body system (or infective agent) they affect.

This is the most useful form of classification for the practice pharmacy as, in many instances, it determines what the drugs are used for in clinical cases (i.e. their **major desired effect** on the body). In addition, a knowledge of the mode of action of drugs may enable the prediction of **side effects** (effects which occur in addition to the desired therapeutic effect). However, it is important to recognise that side effects of drugs cannot always be predicted from the way in which they cause their desired effect. When the side effects of a particular drug compromise the health of an animal they are termed **undesirable** or **adverse drug** reactions. Any suspected adverse drug reactions encountered in veterinary practice should be reported to the Veterinary Medicines Directorate on special reporting forms. Any drug which is administered at dosages above those recommended for therapeutic use (accidentally or deliberately) may cause **toxic effects** in the animal. The **therapeutic index** of a drug is the ratio between the dose which causes toxic effects and the dose required to produce the desired therapeutic effect. The lower this ratio the more dangerous a particular drug may be to use and the smaller the margin of error allowed when determining the dose for a particular animal.

Most drugs produce their desired effects by interacting with a defined target in the body or in the infective organism. This target may be a receptor for a naturally occurring hormone or neurotransmitter, which the drug may **mimic** by stimulating the receptor or **block** by occupying the receptor without stimulating it (receptor **antagonist**). Other targets for drugs include enzymes which serve physiological functions in the body or the infective organisms and which may be inhibited by drugs.

The categorisation of drugs set out in the rest of this section is used by both veterinary and medical formularies and would be a logical basis for organising a practice pharmacy into groups of drugs. In each case, examples of drugs used in small animal practice are given. The name used is always the **generic** (approved or official) name rather than a **proprietary** (brand or trade) name. Where possible, examples will be given where a product exists which has been approved **(licensed)** for use in small animals.

Drugs Used in the Treatment of Infections Caused by Micro-organisms

The micro-organisms include bacteria, fungi, viruses and Protozoa. Drugs used to treat infections caused by these organisms can be termed **antimicrobial agents**. If the drug is a natural product of another micro-organism (as many are) then it is called an **antibiotic**. These drugs show the property of **selective toxicity**, targeting and damaging processes which are essential to the micro-organism but which do not take place in animal cells.

Antibacterial drugs

These are some of the most commonly used drugs in small animal practice. If they are capable of killing bacteria they are described as **bactericidal**; whereas if they just prevent division of bacteria they are called **bacteriostatic**. An antibacterial drug is described as **narrow spectrum** if it is active against a narrow range of bacteria (usually either Gram-positive or Gram-negative organisms) and **broad spectrum** if it is active against a wide variety of bacteria (or other micro-organisms such as protozoans). Some antibacterial drugs when used in combination produce more than the additive effects of the two drugs when used alone. In these cases, the drugs are said to **potentiate** each other (e.g. *potentiated sulphonamides* are a combination of a *sulphonamide* plus *trimethoprim*). Anti-bacterial drugs are classified into families of drugs which are chemically related. The family of *penicillins*, for example, have the same mode of action and so are all bactericidal and share common side effects (all can induce allergic reactions in sensitive animals) for the animal being treated. Small changes in structure, however, may change their spectrum of activity. Figure 13.1 summarises the main families of antibacterial drugs used in small animal practice, giving examples of each.

Antifungal drugs

These will kill or stop the growth of fungi (and could be described as **fungicidal** or **fungistatic**). *Griseofulvin* is used to treat dermatophytosis ('ringworm') in the dog and cat; *nystatin* is contained in some topical ear preparations to treat yeast infections.

Antiviral drugs

These are infrequently used in veterinary medicine. *Idoxuridine* is used topically in the eye to treat feline herpes virus infection.

Antiprotozoal drugs

These are used to treat infections caused by protozoal organisms such as *Toxoplasma gondii*. Example: *pyrimethamine*.

Drugs Used in the Treatment of Parasitic Infections

Endoparasiticides

These are used to treat infections of internal parasites. The majority of such infections in veterinary medicine are caused by helminths (nematodes, cestodes and trematodes) and so the drugs are termed **anthelmintics**. The internal parasites of the dog and cat are **nematodes** (round worms) and **cestodes** (tape worms). As with antibacterial drugs, anthelmintics can be broad or narrow spectrum. Figure 13.2 gives examples of commonly used drugs and their spectrum of activity.

Ectoparasiticides

These are used to treat infestations of fleas, lice, ticks and mites and are often administered topically in the form of sprays, baths, dusting powders or impregnated collars. The organophosphate compounds (e.g. *dichlorvos*) and synthetic pyrethroids (e.g. *permethrin*) are commonly used in small animal medicine. An understanding of the life cycle of the parasite involved is important for the successful treatment of parasitic infestations.

Drugs Acting on the Gastrointestinal System

These are shown in Fig. 13.3.

ANTIBACTERIAL DRUGS			
Family	Example	Spectrum of activity	Bactericidal or bacteriostatic
Penicillins*	Benzyl penicillin	Narrow (G +ve)	Bactericidal
	Amoxicillin	Broad	Bactericidal
Tetracyclines	Oxytetracyline	Broad	Bacteriostatic
Aminoglycosides	Neomycin	Narrow (G -ve)	Bactericidal
Lincosamides	Clindamycin	Narrow (G +ves and anaerobes)	Bacteriostatic
Sulphonamides	Sulphadiazine	Broad	Bacteriostatic
Potentiated sulphonamides	Sulphadiazine plus trimethoprim	Broad	Bactericidal
Nitroimidazoles	Metronidazole	Narrow (anaerobes)	Bactericidal
Chloramphenicol	Chloramphenicol	Broad	Bacteriostatic
Fluoroquinolones	Enrofloxacin	Broad	Bactericidal

Fig. 13.1. Antibacterial drug families.

*Penicillins and cephalosporins (e.g. Cephalexin) are related chemically and collectively called beta lactams.

Drug	Tape worms			Round worms		
	Echinococcus	Taenia	Dipylidium	Toxocara/ Toxascaris	Hookworms (Uncinaria)	Whip worms (Trichuris)
Bunamidine	1	2	2	0	0	0
Fenbendazole	0	2	0	2	2	2
Mebendazole	1	2	0	2	2	2
Nitroscanate	1	2	2	2	2	0
Piperazine	0	0	0	1	1*	0

ANTHELMINTIC DRUGS FOR SMALL ANIMALS

*Effective at 1.5 x the normal dose.
2 – excellent activity; 1 – very good activity; 0 – poor or ineffective.

Fig. 13.2. Examples of anthelmintics.

DRUGS ACTING ON THE GASTROINTESTINAL SYSTEM

Main drug class	Class	Mode of action	Examples
Antidiarrhoeal agents		*Suppress diarrhoea non-specifically**	
	Adsorbents	Coat the gut wall, adsorb toxins	Charcoal, kaolin, bismuth
	Modulators of intestinal motility	Reduce gastrointestinal motility	Loperamide, diphenoxylate
	Chronic antidiarrhoeals	Anti-inflammatory agents	Sulphasalazine, prednisolone
Anti-emetic drugs		Prevent or suppress vomiting (emesis)	Metoclopramide (vomiting due to gastritis) Acepromazine (motion sickness)
Emetic drugs		Stimulate vomiting	Washing soda (orally) Xylazine (by injection)
Laxatives		*Increase defecation*	
	Lubricant laxatives	Lubricate faecal mass	Liquid paraffin
	Bulk forming laxatives	Increase volume of faeces	Isphagula husk
	Osmotic laxatives	Hypertonic solutions, poorly absorbed	Phosphate (enemas)
	Stimulant laxatives	Stimulate local reflex gut motility	Danthron
Antacids		Neutralise acid secreted in stomach	Aluminium hydroxide
Ulcer-healing drugs		Inhibit acid secretion in the stomach and allow ulcers to heal	Cimetidine
Pancreatin supplements		Contain protease, lipase and amylase activity to aid digestion in EPI**	Pancreatin

*Specific treatment relies on identifying the underlying cause. In some cases, for example, antibacterial drugs or anthelmintics may be indicated
**Exocrine pancreatic insufficiency

Fig. 13.3. Drugs acting on the gastrointestinal system.

Drugs Used in the Treatment of Disorders of the Cardiovascular System

These work primarily on the heart, the blood vessels, the blood coagulation system or the kidney.

Drugs acting on the heart

The heart can be stimulated to beat more strongly by drugs which are called **myocardial stimulants** (or positive inotropes)—examples include *digoxin* and *etamiphylline camsylate*. Other drugs also increase the rate at which the heart beats and may be used in an emergency to treat complete heart block. The **sympathomimetic** *isoprenaline* (mimics the action of the sympathetic nervous system on the heart) is an

example of such a drug. When the heart beats very fast with an abnormal rhythm it is said to be *arrhythmic*. Cardiac arrhythmias can be suppressed by **antidysrhythmic drugs** such as *lignocaine* (for ventricular arrhythmias) and *diltiazem* (for atrial arrhythmias). (The preparation of lignocaine used to treat ventricular arrhythmias must *not* contain adrenaline.)

Drugs acting on the blood vessels

Vasodilators relax the smooth muscle of blood vessels and lower resistance to blood flow, so reducing the work the heart has to do. Some act primarily on arterial smooth muscle (**arterial dilators**;

hydralazine); some act primarily on venous smooth muscle (**venodilators**; *glyceryl trinitrate*); and others act on both sides of the circulation (**mixed dilators**; *enalapril*). A potential side effect of these drugs is excessive lowering of arterial blood pressure (*hypotension*). Indeed, some are used in man to treat *hypertension* and are called **antihypertensive** drugs.

Drugs acting on the kidney

Diuretics increase the volume of urine produced by an animal and the amount of salt excreted. Many are used in the treatment of congestive heart failure because in this condition the kidney tends to retain salt and water which contributes to the problem. The *loop diuretics* (e.g *frusemide*) and the *thiazide diuretics* (e.g. *hydrochlorothiazide*) are most commonly used. Both give rise to excess potassium loss. Use of potassium-sparing diuretics (e.g. *spironolactone*) with these drugs will counteract this effect.

Drugs acting on the blood clotting system

Anticoagulants prevent blood clotting (*heparin*, *warfarin*) whereas **fibrinolytic agents** break down clots once they have formed (e.g. *streptokinase*). **Haemostatics** arrest haemorrhage and are usually applied topically to local bleeding areas (e.g. *calcium alginate*).

Drugs Used in the Treatment of Disorders of the Respiratory System

Inhalation of infective agents or allergens (e.g. pollen) stimulate inflammation and tissue damage leading to reflex stimulation of coughing and bronchoconstriction. The sites at which drugs may counteract some of these disease processes are shown in Fig. 13.4. Examples of the drugs acting at these sites are given in Fig. 13.5.

Drugs Acting on the Nervous System

Sedatives

Sedatives produce calmness, drowsiness and indifference of the animal to its surroundings and are often used as **premedicants** for animals which are to be anaesthetised. Examples include *acepromazine* and *medetomidine*. The action of medetomidine can be reversed by the **sedative antagonist** *atipamezole*. The degree of drowsiness produced depends on the the particular agent or agents used, the dose and the

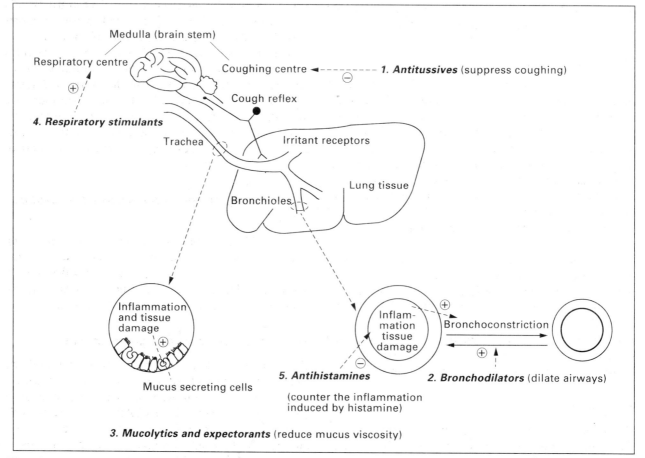

Fig. 13.4. A schematic representation of the respiratory system showing the sites at which drugs act in the treatment of respiratory disorders ($\oplus$ = stimulation, $\ominus$ = inhibition of the processes indicated). Inhalation of allergens or infective agents initiate inflammation, bronchoconstriction, increased mucus secretion and coughing (via the cough reflex which stimulates the coughing centre in the medulla).

DRUGS USED IN THE TREATMENT OF RESPIRATORY DISEASES	
Drug class	**Example**
Antitussive	Butorphanol
Antihistamine	Diphenhydramine
Bronchodilator	Theophylline, terbutaline
Mucolytic/expectorant	Bromhexine/ipecacuanha
Respiratory stimulant	Doxapram

Fig. 13.5. Drugs used in the treatment of disorders of the respiratory system.

route of administration. A mild sedative is sometimes referred to as a **tranquilliser**, whereas drugs used to produce deep sedation (*narcosis*) can be called **narcotics**.

Opioid analgesics

These relieve pain by acting on opioid receptor sites in the brain and spinal cord. Examples are *morphine* and *buprenorphine*.

Combinations of sedatives and opioid analgesics can be used to produce deeper and more reliable sedation than sedatives alone. Such combinations are termed **neuroleptanalgesics**, an example being *fentanyl* with *fluansinone*. Sedation can then be reversed using an **opioid antagonist** such as *naloxone*.

General anaesthetics

These produce unconsciousness so that surgical or other procedures can be carried out painlessly. Pre-anaesthetic medication with sedatives and analgesics will allow a reduction in the dose of general anaesthetic required and produce a smoother induction and recovery from anaesthesia. **Injectable general anaesthetics** may be used for induction of anaesthesia (e.g. *thiopentone*) and maintenance of anaesthesia is often achieved by the use of **inhalational** (or **gaseous**) general anaesthetics (e.g. *halothane*).

Antimuscarinic drugs may be given before anaesthesia to counteract the salivation and increased bronchial secretions which, in small dogs and cats, may obstruct the airway. In addition, some surgical procedures may increase vagal nerve stimulation of the heart, reducing heart rate (causing bradycardia). Anti-muscarinic drugs will prevent bradycardia. Examples are *atropine* and *hyoscine*.

Muscle relaxants

These prevent the message from the nerve reaching the skeletal muscle and so paralyse the muscle. *Pancuronium* is an example of such a drug which is used with general anaesthesia for intrathoracic surgery. Its effects can be reversed by the **muscle relaxant antagonist** *neostigmine*.

Local anaesthetics

These temporarily prevent conduction of an impulse along a nerve fibre. Tissues are infiltrated with drug around sensory nerve fibres to produce analgesia of an area. Motor nerve fibres can also be affected if the injection is made around them. Vasoconstrictors are often included in such preparations to reduce blood flow to the area and so prevent the local anaesthetic being removed from its local site of action. Example: *lignocaine* with *adrenaline*.

Anti-epileptics

These drugs are used to treat epilepsy, a condition of the central nervous system characterised by the spontaneous occurrence of convulsions or seizures. Examples: *phenobarbitone, diazepam*.

Drugs Used in the Treatment of Disorders of the Endocrine System

Disorders of the endocrine system result either from lack of production or overproduction of a hormone. Drugs are used either to replace the natural hormone or to prevent overproduction of the hormone in question (Fig. 13.6). Anterior pituitary hormones (or their analogues) are used in diagnostic tests for endocrine diseases. For example, *tetracosactrin* (an adrenocorticotrophin analogue) is used in the ACTH stimulation test which is performed in the diagnosis of both Cushing's disease and Addison's disease.

Steroid hormones share a common chemical structure and are produced by the adrenal cortex (**adrenal corticosteroids**) or by the ovary and testes (**sex steroids**—see below). **Anabolic steroids** are derivatives of the male sex hormone, testosterone, and are used to increase muscle mass and to promote tissue repair in convalescing animals. Examples: *Boldenone, nandrolone*.

Drugs Acting on the Reproductive and Urinary Tract

Figure 13.7 describes sex hormones (sex steroids), luteolytic agents (prostaglandins), myometrial stimulants (ecbolics) and drugs used to treat urinary tract disorders. Drugs used in the management of disorders of urination are presented in Fig. 13.8.

Drugs Used to Treat Malignant Disease

Cytotoxic drugs kill actively dividing cells and are used in the **chemotherapy** of some forms of cancer which can not be removed surgically (e.g. malignant lymphoma). As normal cells in the body are actively dividing, these drugs have a low therapeutic index and need to be used with great care. They are also a hazard to people handling them (as are some other drugs already discussed), a subject which will be dealt with below. Examples: *cyclophosphamide, vincristine*.

DRUGS USED IN THE TREATMENT OF ENDOCRINE DISORDERS			
Gland	**Disease state**	**Drug class**	**Example**
Adrenal gland	*Deficiency:* Hypoadrenocorticism (Addison's disease)	Adrenal corticosteroids Mineralocorticoids (sodium conserving) Glucocorticoids	Fludrocortisone Prednisolone, dexamethasone
	Excess: Hyperadrenocorticism (Cushing's disease)	Adrenolytic agent Glucocorticoid synthesis inhibitor	Mitotane Ketoconazole
Thyroid gland	*Deficiency:* Hypothyroidism *Excess:* Hyperthyroidism	Thyroid hormone replacement Antithyroid agent	Levothyroxine Carbimazole
Endocrine pancreas	*Deficiency:* Diabetes mellitus (hyperglycaemia) *Excess:* Hypoglycaemia (low blood glucose)	Insulin Oral hypoglycaemic agents Glucose (intravenous) Anti-insulin agents	Protamine zinc insulin Tolbutamide Dextrose solution Dexamethasone (glucocorticoids)
Posterior pituitary gland	Diabetes insipidus (deficiency of ADH)	Posterior pituitary hormone (ADH analogue)	Desmopressin

Fig. 13.6. Drugs used in the treatment of endocrine disorders.

DRUGS ACTING ON THE REPRODUCTIVE AND URINARY TRACT		
	Examples	**Uses**
Sex hormones – (sex steroids) Oestrogens	Stilboestrol, Oestradiol benzoate.	Prevent implantation following accidental mating (misalliance). Treat urinary incontinence. Reduce the size of an enlarged prostate gland and anal adenomas.
Progestagens Steroids which mimic the actions of progesterone	Megoestrol acetate, Proligestone	Postpone or suppress oestrus in the bitch and queen. Management of some behavioural problems.
Androgens Esters or analogues of the male sex hormone, testosterone	Methyltestosterone	Hormonal alopecia in dogs and cats. Deficient libido in males.
Anti-androgens Compete with and inhibit the actions of testosterone at its receptor	Delmandione	Treatment of prostatic hypertrophy. Management of aggressive behaviour in male dogs.
Luteolytic agents (Prostaglandins) Cause regression of the corpus luteum	Dinoprost	Management of open pyometra in the bitch (unlicensed use). Synchronisation of oestrus in cattle and sheep. Induction of parturition in pigs.
Myometrial stimulants (Ecbolics) Stimulate the uterus to contract	Oxytocin (extract of posterior pituitary gland)	Dystocia due to weakness of the uterine muscle (uterine inertia).
Drugs used to treat urinary tract disorders **Urinary acidifiers** Lower the pH of the urine	Ethylenediamine hydrochloride	Cystitis (aid action of antibacterials and urinary antiseptics). In the management of urolithiasis (struvite calculi)
Urinary alkalinisers Raise the pH of the urine	Sodium bicarbonate	In the management of urate uroliths.
Urinary antiseptics Hydrolyse in acidic urine to release formaldehyde	Hexamine	Prophylaxis and long term treatment of recurrent urinary tract infections.

Fig. 13.7. Drugs used in the treatment of the reproductive and urinary tracts.

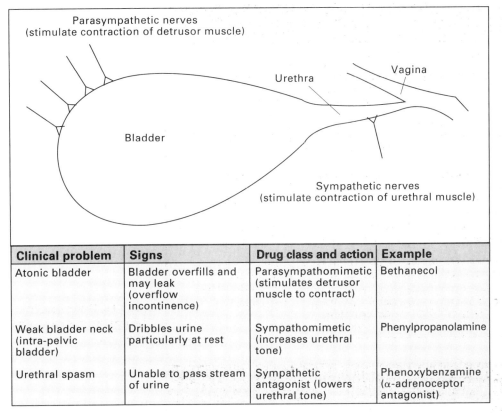

Clinical problem	Signs	Drug class and action	Example
Atonic bladder	Bladder overfills and may leak (overflow incontinence)	Parasympathomimetic (stimulates detrusor muscle to contract)	Bethanecol
Weak bladder neck (intra-pelvic bladder)	Dribbles urine particularly at rest	Sympathomimetic (increases urethral tone)	Phenylpropanolamine
Urethral spasm	Unable to pass stream of urine	Sympathetic antagonist (lowers urethral tone)	Phenoxybenzamine (α-adrenoceptor antagonist)

Fig. 13.8. The bladder and drugs which affect urination. The process of urination is brought about by parasympathetic stimulation of the detrusor muscle and inhibition of sympathetic tone to the urethral smooth muscle, allowing the bladder to contract and empty through the relaxed urethra. When the bladder fills, the sympathetic nervous system is active, maintaining continence by closing the urethra; the parasympathetic system is inactive, allowing the detrusor muscle to relax and the bladder to fill.

Drugs Used to Treat Disorders of the Musculoskeletal System and Joints

Anti-inflammatory drugs

These are considered here although they can be used to reduce or suppress inflammation wherever it occurs in the body. The value of such drugs is to relieve the pain, swelling and fever caused by acute inflammation.

Corticosteroids of the glucocorticoid group will suppress inflammation and, at high doses, can produce **immunosuppression**, which is required in the treatment of immune-mediated diseases that sometimes cause polyarthritis in the dog.

Non-steroidal anti-inflammatory drugs (NSAIDs) inhibit the formation of prostaglandins and related compounds, which are important mediators of acute inflammation. These drugs will reduce pain and swelling following surgery or in a number of acquired inflammatory conditions such as osteoarthritis. Examples: *Phenylbutazone*, *flunixin meglumine*, *aspirin*.

Chondroprotective agents

These prevent further breakdown of cartilage and stimulate the synthesis of new articular cartilage. Example: *Pentosan polysulphate sodium*.

Drugs acting on the eye

Antimicrobial and anti-inflammatory agents can be applied topically to the eye in the form of drops or ointments. Local anaesthetics can also be formulated for topical application to the eye. Other drugs with actions on the eye include:

Mydriatics and cycloplegics

These dilate the pupil (mydriasis) and reduce spasm in the ciliary muscle. Examples: **Antimuscarinic agents**, *atropine, homoatropine*.

Drugs used in the treatment of glaucoma (raised intra-ocular pressure)

Miotics constrict the pupil and thus open the drainage angle for ocular fluid. Drugs which mimic stimulation of the parasympathetic nerve supply to the eye (**parasympathomimetics**) have this effect. Example: *pilocarpine*.

Carbonic anhydrase inhibitors will reduce the formation of aqueous humor. Example: *Dichlorphenamide* (given orally).

Drugs used in keratoconjunctivitis sicca (dry eye)

These replace the tear film, which is deficient in this condition. *Hypromellose* drops are the most commonly used artificial tears. A **mucolytic**, *acetylcysteine*, may be beneficial when the tears are particularly mucoid and viscous. **Parasympathomimetics** (*pilocarpine*) administered by mouth may stimulate lacrimal secretion in some cases.

Drugs Acting on the Ear

Topical preparations containing antimicrobial, ecto-parasiticide and anti-inflammatory agents are all available. **Sebolytics** dissolve wax and cleanse the ear canal. Example: *Squalane*.

Drugs Acting on the Skin

The skin can be treated with drugs given orally or parenterally, which reach the skin via its blood supply, or by topical application of preparations of drugs directly to the affected area. Topical drugs are usually formulated as creams, ointments, lotions, powders, shampoos or sprays. The vehicle or base of these may be selected to suit the type of lesion and location being treated, as described later. The active drugs contained in such preparations may be anti-bacterials, ectoparasiticides or anti-inflammatory agents. Drugs that have not been mentioned else-where which are used for disorders of the skin include the following.

Keratolytics loosen the horny layer of the epidermis, causing it to separate from the deeper epidermis. Examples: *Benzyl peroxide, salicylic acid.*

Astringents precipitate protein on the surface of the skin to produce a protective coating. Examples: *Zinc oxide, calamine.*

Disinfectants in the correct concentration can be used topically to cleanse the skin and chemically destroy surface bacteria. Example: *Chlorhexidine gluconate.*

Essential fatty acids are given orally to animals and have potential *anti-inflammatory* properties with some evidence of beneficial effects in inflammatory skin conditions. Examples: *gammalinoleic acid* (GLA), *eicosapentanoic acid* (EPA).

Drugs Affecting Nutrition and Body Fluids

Electrolyte and water replacement solutions (crystalloid fluids)

These are used to treat animals suffering from dehydration. **Oral rehydration solutions** consist of mixtures of sodium, potassium and chloride ions and an anion which is metabolised by the liver to form bicarbonate (e.g. citrate). In addition, glucose and amino acids such as glycine are included, not for nutritional purposes but because they help the transport of sodium and water across the gut wall and into the blood stream. **Parenteral solutions** are used to replace fluid losses in cases where the oral route is unsuitable and a parenteral route (usually intravenous route) is chosen. The composition of the fluid used depends on the type of losses sustained. For example, *replacement* of extracellular fluid volume requires a fluid with plasma concentration of sodium (about 140 mmol/l). When parenteral fluids are given to *maintain* hydration in an animal that is unable to drink, fluids that are much lower in sodium

are more appropriate. Isotonicity of such fluids is maintained by the addition of glucose (e.g. 4% glucose and 0.18% sodium chloride). **Concentrated additives** such as potassium chloride, glucose (dextrose monohydrate) and sodium bicarbonate are available for addition to commercially available fluids so that the composition of the fluid can be adjusted to suit the requirements of the animal being treated. Nutrient solutions are available to provide nutrition by the intravenous route (*parenteral nutrition*). They consist of concentrated solutions of glucose or emulsions of lipid to provide calories and amino acids. They should only be administered through the jugular vein, as the risk of phlebitis and infection when given through a small peripheral vein is high.

Plasma substitutes

These are large molecular weight **colloids** in solution which are retained in the circulation rather than leaving capillaries and distributing into the whole extracellular fluid volume (as is the case with crystalloid fluids). Thus the volume of such colloid preparations needed to restore the circulating fluid volume in an animal suffering from haemorrhagic shock is small when compared with the volume of replacement crystalloid solutions required. Example: *Gelatin.*

Vitamins and minerals

These can be used as supplements for sick and debilitated animals and, as such, would be regarded as medicines. Nutritional deficiencies may occur but are uncommon in the dog and cat nowadays with the use of commercial pet foods. Specific indications for a mineral would be eclampsia in the bitch where *calcium gluconate* would be given intravenously. *Phytomenadione* (Vitamin K1) is the specific antidote to warfarin poisoning

Vaccines and Immunological Preparations

Vaccines are given to animals to stimulate immunity against an infectious disease (e.g. canine distemper). The body responds to antigens in the vaccine and the immunity produced is termed **active immunity**. **Live vaccines** consist of living organisms of a slightly different strain from that which causes the natural disease making them non-pathogenic (no signs of disease result) but still able to stimulate a protective immune response. The organisms in live vaccines multiply inside the host after administration and stimulate a long-lasting immune response. **Inactivated vaccines** contain sufficient antigen to stimulate an immune response; no multiplication of the organism in question is possible following administration of an inactivated vaccine. **Toxoids** (e.g. *Tetanus toxoid*) are forms of inactivated vaccines where toxins produced by organisms have been extracted and heat-treated to render them harmless. Inactivated vaccines usually contain **adjuvants**, such as aluminium hydroxide or mineral oil, that help to enhance the immune response to the antigens in the vaccine, which is generally not as long-lasting as that obtained with live vaccines. An **autogenous vaccine** is prepared from material collected from an individual animal for administration to the same animal.

Immunoglobulins (antibodies, antisera) can be administered to animals to confer **passive immunity**. Example: *Tetanus antitoxin*. These consist of serum containing antibodies raised in another animal (usually of the same species). They can have a neutralising effect on the organism or toxin in question and therefore give some immediate protection in the face of infection. Passive immunity only persists for about 3 weeks.

Formulation and Administration of Drugs

Systemically Administered Drugs

If a drug cannot be applied locally (topically) to the site at which its action is desired, it must first be administered in such a way that it is **absorbed** into the blood circulation (systemically) from which it **distributes** to the place in the body where it acts. The rate and extent of absorption of the drug from its site of administration will depend upon its route of administration and the physical and chemical form in which it is administered (see below). The body gets rid of (**eliminates**) the drug by converting it into a different chemical compound by a process of **metabolism** followed by excretion of the drug from the body. The liver is the major organ where drug metabolism occurs and excretion of the drug itself or of its metabolites is into the bile or urine. Some volatile agents are excreted from the body via the respiratory tract.

Oral preparations

The oral route is the most convenient route for many drugs used in small animal veterinary practice as owners can dose their own pets at home. However, there are a number of problems with oral dosing:

- The absorption of the drug from the gut into the blood stream is often slower and less complete than when drugs are injected (given by a parenteral route, Fig. 13.9). It may take time for a tablet to dissolve and release its contents: some drugs are absorbed primarily in the small intestine, rather than the stomach, and so their absorption only occurs once the stomach empties.
- If the animal is vomiting the oral route is not reliable.
- Some drugs are unstable in gastric acid or may be destroyed by the enzymes of the gut and so the oral route can not be used (e.g. penicillin G, insulin).
- Some drugs are broken down very rapidly and efficiently in the liver after absorption from the gut and so do not reach the general circulation (e.g. lignocaine, glyceryl trinitrate); or a higher dose is required when the drug is given orally (e.g. propranolol).
- Food in the gastrointestinal tract may affect the absorption of the drug by delaying its entry into the blood stream (e.g. digoxin) or reducing the amount of the drug absorbed (e.g. ampicillin). In other cases, fatty food helps the absorption of some drugs across the gut wall (e.g. griseofulvin, mitotane).
- Some drugs are not absorbed when given orally and remain in the gastrointestinal tract. They can be used as a form of local therapy but will not have systemic effects (e.g. neomycin can be used orally to treat enteric infections but not urinary tract infections).

Tablets. Many oral medications are in the form of **tablets** containing the active drug and some inert ingredients (binder and excipients) that bind the compressed mass together. Tablets may be coated for a number of reasons:

- To protect the tablet from the atmosphere, particularly moisture.
- To delay disintegration of the tablet and so protect the active drug from the acidic environment of the stomach or protect the stomach from irritant effects of the drug (e.g. aspirin).
- To hide the bitter taste of the drug and so facilitate dosing (e.g. bunaminidine).

Grinding up tablets will destroy the properties which the outer layers of the tablet provide. Before this measure is recommended or undertaken, it is important to check with the manufacturer that such action can be taken without altering the properties of the medication. Some tablets are scored to facilitate breaking them in half for dosing.

Capsules. Other oral medications are formulated as *capsules* containing either powder or granules. The outer case of the capsule is made of hard gelatin and comes in two halves which slot together. The outer case prevents the drug (which may have a bitter taste) contacting the oral mucosa. Some capsule formulations of drugs contain granules of differing sizes and composition so that they dissolve at different rates, providing a sustained release of drug from the gastrointestinal tract (e.g. slow release formulations of *theophylline*). This reduces the frequency of dosing required.

Mixtures. Liquid medication (or *mixtures*) can be given by mouth and may contain the drug completely in solution, if it is freely soluble, or in suspension if it is insoluble (e.g. *kaolin* in water). Suspensions require thorough mixing before dosing and should always be labelled with the instruction: 'Shake well before use.'

Parenteral preparations

Strictly speaking, a parenteral route of administration means any route other than the oral route. It is generally taken to mean routes by which drugs are injected into the body of an animal. All preparations for parenteral use must, therefore, be sterile and pyrogen-free. The most common routes of injection of drugs in small animal practice are:

- Intravenous—directly into venous blood.
- Intramuscular—into muscular tissue, usually of the leg or back.
- Subcutaneous—into the tissue beneath the skin.

Occasionally the intraperitoneal route of injection is used, particularly in small rodents. The peritoneal membrane provides a large surface area for drug absorption.

Intravenous route. The **intravenous route** provides the fastest possible distribution of the drug to its site of action, since the drug is placed directly into the blood stream. The peak plasma concentration of the drug is higher than can be achieved by any other route. However, the drug concentration often decreases rapidly (depending on the rate at which the body metabolises and excretes the drug) as absorption of the drug from the site of administration is instantaneous and does not continue over a period of time as it would for the oral route and other parenteral routes (Fig. 13.9).

Preparations for intravenous use must be true solutions, where the drug to be administered is dissolved in sterile water (aqueous solution) or another type of solvent. It is important to make any intravenous injections slowly, because a rapid (bolus) injection can result in a very high concentration of the drug (or solvent) reaching the heart or brain and causing detrimental effects. Suspensions of drugs cannot be administered intravenously as the particles in a suspension may block capillaries in the lungs causing death.

Drugs that may be irritant to the tissues should preferably be administered by the intravenous route, as the drug is rapidly removed and diluted in the circulating blood (if the injection is made slowly). If irritant drugs are given (e.g. sodium thiopentone, vincristine) it is important to ensure that the injection is indeed made into the vein. Accidental injection into the tissues around the vein (perivascular injection) may cause severe damage.

Intramuscular route. **Intramuscular injection** of drugs may be more convenient for less cooperative patients and drugs in suspensions can be given by this route. After inserting the needle into a muscle to make the injection, it is important to draw back on the syringe plunger to ensure that the tip of the needle is not in a blood vessel within the muscle. Intramuscular injections are painful; the severity of the pain depends on the volume of the injection, the viscosity of the material being injected and the chemical nature of the compound (how irritant it is to the tissue). The drug diffuses from the injection site by dissolving in the tissue fluid surrounding the muscle cells and is then absorbed into the blood capillaries and lymphatics supplying the muscle.

Subcutaneous route. **Subcutaneous injections** can be made into any area of the body where there is loose skin—usually over the neck or back. Formulations of drugs for subcutaneous injection should be approximately of blood pH and body fluid tonicity. They should not be irritant, nor should they cause vasoconstriction as this would impede the absorption of the drug into the blood stream. Larger volumes can be administered by the subcutaneous route than by the intramuscular route.

Absorption rates. In general, the rate of absorption of drugs given by the intramuscular route is faster than those given by the subcutaneous route since muscle receives a larger blood supply than subcutaneous tissue (Fig. 13.9). However, the physical and chemical properties of the drug formulation affect the rate of absorption from both of these sites. Formulations of drugs can be produced which contain a combination of different salts of the same drug, one of which is highly soluble (e.g. sodium salt

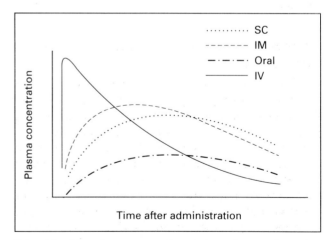

Fig. 13.9. Plasma concentration versus time curve for a 'typical' drug following its administration by: intramuscular injection (IM); intravenous injection (IV); subcutaneous injection (SC); and oral administration.

of penicillin G) and so is rapidly absorbed from the intramuscular injection site, a second which is more slowly absorbed (e.g. procaine salt of penicillin G) and a third which is absorbed very slowly indeed because of its extremely low solubility (e.g. benzathine salt of penicillin G). This principle is used to produce long-acting injections of drugs which are sometimes called *depot preparations.* Insulin is also prepared in different physical forms which give different times to onset of action and durations of effect based on the speed of absorption of insulin form the injection site. Some formulations of insulin (protamine zinc insulin or insulin zinc suspension) may have a duration of action which make them suitable for once daily administration whereas other formulations (Isophane insulin) have a shorter duration of action so that two injections per day may be necessary. *Implants* are an extreme example of a depot preparation: a small disc or cylinder of relatively insoluble drug (often a hormone) is inserted beneath the skin in a sterile manner using a special injection device. The drug can then be released over an extended period, preventing the need for repeated administration.

Other injection sites. Other sites used for injection of drugs include:

- *Intradermal*—into the dermis (allergy testing in dogs).
- *Intra-articular*—into a joint cavity.
- *Intrathecal*—into the cerebrospinal fluid (contrast media for myelography—therapeutic agents are not given by this route in veterinary medicine).
- *Epidural*—into the vertebral canal outside the dura mater (to produce spinal analgesia when local anaesthetics are injected).
- *Subconjunctival*—under the conjunctival membrane of the eye.

These are all forms of local therapy: the injection site is the site at which the drug is desired to produce its effect.

Other ways of administering drugs to produce systemic effects

Inhalation of drugs into the respiratory tract is a means of supplying drugs to this site of the body and for drugs to be absorbed into the blood stream (e.g. gaseous anaesthetics). Formulation of drugs for inhalation is more difficult for administration to domestic animals than to humans, for whom inhalation is a common way of administering drugs such as bronchodilators. In some university hospitals, drugs in solution can be produced in a very fine mist of liquid droplets which are inhaled by the animal. This process is called *nebulisation* and has obvious safety implications for the operators (see below).

Drugs can be absorbed across other mucous membranes of the body and produce systemic effects. For example, desmopressin is supplied in the form of drops, which in humans are instilled into the nose. In dogs, it is more convenient to place these drops into the conjunctival sac. Absorption of the drug from this site into the blood stream occurs and the systemic effects (anti-diuretic action) become evident. This drug cannot be given by the oral route: it is a peptide (small protein) and will be destroyed by enzymes in the gut. This route of administration is more convenient than the frequent injections of the drug which would otherwise be necessary.

Some drugs are able to penetrate intact skin and so be absorbed from the surface of the skin and have systemic effects. An example used in small animal medicine is the nitrovasodilator, glyceryl trinitrate. This drug can not be given by the oral route as it is removed so effectively by the liver. Fenthion, the organophosphate insecticide, is another example of a drug which when applied to a discrete area of skin, is absorbed into the blood stream and distributed systemically.

Topically Administered Drugs

Topical preparations are applied directly to the site at which the drug is required. The most common sites to be treated topically in small animal medicine are the skin, eyes and ears. Enemas could be considered a form of topical therapy where fluids are infused into the rectum to soften the faecal mass. In large animal practice, topical application of drugs are to the mammary gland (*intramammary preparations*) the vagina and uterus (*vaginal suppositories or pessaries*). It is important to remember that drugs can be absorbed across mucous membranes and even intact skin—particularly drugs that are lipid soluble (such as corticosteroids)—and so these drugs should not be assumed to be without systemic effects.

Examples of formulations of topical preparations include:

- *Creams*—semi-solid emulsions of oil or fat, and water (which usually contains the drug). They spread easily without friction and penetrate the outer layers of the skin, particularly if the fat is lanolin. Water-soluble drugs are more active in creams than in ointments.
- *Ointments*—semi-solid and greasy, insoluble in water; the drugs are present in a base of wax or fat (usually petroleum jelly). They are non-penetrating and more occlusive than creams and are most suitable for dry chronic lesions.
- *Dusting powders*—finely divided powders for application to the skin, usually containing ectoparasiticides or antibacterials.
- *Wettable powders*—applied to the skin as a suspension after mixing with a large quantity of water. The animal is then dried by warmth, leaving the powder in the coat (i.e. it is not rinsed off).

- *Lotions*—liquid preparations which consist of solutions of the drugs in water (e.g. calamine lotion).
- *Medicated shampoos*—aqueous solutions or suspensions of drugs that have a detergent base, which gives good penetration of the coat. Shampoos are left in contact with the skin for the recommended period and then rinsed off thoroughly.
- *Aerosol sprays*—a way of applying liquid solutions or suspensions of drugs in fine droplet form. The liquid is packaged in a metal container under pressure. Pressing the nozzle of the container causes the liquid to be expelled.
- *Eye medications* can be in the form of ointments or drops. Ophthalmic ointments tend to be more liquid than the ointments described above, having a soft paraffin base. When applied to the surface of the cornea they melt to form a thin film which covers the whole surface of the eye. Eye drops are aqueous solutions of drugs for instillation to the eye. In general, drops tend to be shorter acting than ointments and require more frequent application. Both forms of medication should be sterile and, once opened, should be stored only for the length of time recommended by the manufacturers.

Calculation of Drug Dosages

The responsibility for ensuring that the correct dosage of drug is administered to an animal under their care lies with the veterinary surgeon in charge of the case. However, veterinary nurses should understand how to calculate dosages.

Weights, Volumes and Concentration

The active ingredient in the preparation of a drug is expressed in terms of its weight. The standard units for weight are kilograms (kg), grams (g), milligrams (mg) and micrograms (no abbreviation used). These weights are related as follows:

> 1 kilogram (kg) = 1000 grams
> 1 gram (g) = 1000 milligrams
> 1 milligram (mg) = 1000 micrograms

If the weight relates to a tablet or capsule, then each tablet or capsule contains the stated weight of active drug. When considering liquid formulations of drugs (solutions or suspensions), the weight of active drug is related to a unit of volume of the suspension or solution. Standard units of volume include litres (l) and millilitres (ml) where 1l = 1000ml. Some drugs are relatively unstable in solution and so are supplied as a solid in a vial; the solvent (often water for injection) is supplied separately. The drug is reconstituted by adding the solvent to the vial.

Unless all the drug is used immediately, it is important to write on the vial the concentration of the solution of the drug you have just made (usually in terms of milligrams of drug per millilitre of solution) and the date on which it was reconstituted. The reconstituted drug may be stable if kept in the refrigerator for several days and so it is important to know the concentration of the solution which has been made.

Percentage solutions

Another way of expressing the concentration of a drug in solution is as a percentage of weight (w) of the drug per volume (v) of solution (w/v). If 1g of the active drug is dissolved in a total volume of 100ml, this produces a **1% solution**. If this fundamental fact is remembered, percentage solutions can be readily converted into concentrations in terms of milligrams per millilitre, which is usually a more convenient form when it comes to calculating dosages.

Exceptions to standard weights and volumes

Some drugs, such as insulin, oxytocin and heparin, are extracted from animal tissues and are not produced in a completely pure form. The concentration of the drug in the product is determined by is effect in a laboratory test system (bioassay) against an International Standard. In most cases, the concentration of such preparations is given in terms of international units (i.u.) or simply units per standard volume (usually per millilitre). For example, all formulations of insulin for human use are produced at a concentration of 100 units per ml. There is now an insulin preparation licensed for veterinary use in the United Kingdom which contains insulin at a concentration of 40 i.u. per ml. Insulin is administered using special syringes which are graduated in units rather than in millilitres. It is important to use a 40 unit syringe for insulin of concentration 40 units per ml, and a 100 unit syringe for insulin preparations of 100 units per ml.

Dosages

Drug dosage rates are usually expressed in terms of weight of drug per weight of the animal to be dosed (most often in milligrams of drug per kg body weight of the animal). Some drugs, particularly those used for cancer chemotherapy, are dosed on a weight of drug per body surface area (milligram per square metre of body surface area). Conversion charts are available which give body surface area from the animal's weight in kilograms. The worked examples given here will illustrate some of the principles in calculation of dosages.

EXAMPLE 1

You are asked to dispense enrofloxacin tablets for a dog weighing 20kg at a dose rate of 2.5mg/kg twice daily for 7 days. The drug comes in tablet sizes of 15, 50 and 150mg. Which tablet size would be most appropriate, how many tablets would you dispense and what instructions for dosing would you give to the owner?

Amount of drug require (mg)
$$= \text{dose (mg/kg)} \times \text{body weight (kg)}$$
$$= 2.5 \text{ (mg/kg)} \times 20 \text{ (kg)}$$
$$= 50 \text{ mg}$$

Thus, the most appropriate tablet size to use would be 50mg and the owners should be instructed to give one tablet twice a day for 7 days. The number of tablets required will be 14 (7x2).

EXAMPLE 2

A 6kg miniature poodle requires digoxin for treatment of congestive heart failure. The dose rate required is 0.01mg/kg each day, which should be divided into two equal doses (0.01mg/kg divided twice daily). The tablet sizes available are 62.5, 125 and 250 micrograms. What tablet size would you use, what would your dosing instructions to the owners be and how many tablets would you dispense for a 30 day course?

Daily dose required (mg)
$$= \text{Dose (mg/kg)} \times \text{body weight (kg)}$$
$$= 0.01 \text{ (mg/kg)} \times 6 \text{ (kg)} = 0.06 \text{mg}$$

To convert milligrams to micrograms multiply by 1000:

$$0.06 \text{mg} = 0.06 \times 1000 \text{ micrograms}$$
$$= 60 \text{ micrograms}$$

This dose should be divided into two equal daily doses, so that each dose should contain:

$$60/2 \text{ micrograms}$$
$$= 30 \text{ micrograms}$$

Thus, the most appropriate size to use would be the 62.5 microgram tablets, and the owners should be instructed to give half a tablet every 12 hours before food. For a course of 30 days, the owners would require 30 tablets.

TIPS
(a) Please note that it is important to be sure of the position of the decimal point in all drug calculations. Always write 0.01 rather than simply .01.
(b) In addition, the dose required in Example 2 was slightly lower than the convenient tablet size. Digoxin is a drug with a low therapeutic index and care should be taken not to overdose an animal. In this case, the inaccuracy was deemed so small as to be of no consequence but such a judgement should always be made by the veterinary surgeon in charge of the case.
(c) In dosing with digoxin, food can interfere with the rate of absorption of digoxin from the gut and so an instruction to give the medication before meals is important.
(d) In Example 2, the total daily dose rate was given and had to be divided into two equal doses. An alternative way of expressing this would be to say that the dose required is 0.005mg/kg to be given twice daily—which was the way the dose rate in Example 1 was expressed.

EXAMPLE 3

For injection, you are given a drug in solution which is 7.5%. The dose required for the dog you are treating is 10mg/kg and the dog weighs 18kg. What volume of the drug should be given to this dog by injection?

Concentration of drug in solution
$$= 7.5 \text{g in 100ml (7.5\% w/v)}$$
$$= (7.5/100) \text{ g in 1ml}$$
$$= 0.075 \text{ g in 1 ml}$$
$$= (0.075 \times 1000) \text{ mg in 1ml}$$
$$= 75 \text{ mg/ml}$$

Amount of drug required
$$= \text{dose (mg/kg)} \times \text{body weight (kg)}$$
$$= 10 \text{ (mg/kg)} \times 18 \text{ (kg)} = 180 \text{mg}$$

Volume of drug require (ml)
$$= \text{amount of drug (mg)/concentration (mg/ml)}$$
$$= 180 \text{ (mg)}/75 \text{ (mg/ml)}$$
$$= 2.4 \text{ml}$$

TIP

To convert the concentration of a solution expressed in percentages into mg/ml, multiply the percentage figure by 10.

Legal Aspects of Medicines and Prescribing

The legislation which governs the storage, handling, use and supply of medicines in veterinary practice includes:

- The Medicines Act 1968
- The Misuse of Drugs Act 1971
- The Misuse of Drugs Regulations 1985
- The Health and Safety at Work Act 1974
- The Control of Substances Hazardous to Health Regulations 1988.

They have also been considered in Chapters 6 (Ethics and Law) and 11 (Occupational Hazards).

The Medicines Act 1968

The Government ensures the quality, safety and efficacy of medicines for human and animal use by a system of licences approved by the Department of Health and the Ministry of Agriculture, respectively. Before a product can be manufactured, imported and distributed widely, the company or person who devises it has to gain a product licence by showing that the drug is safe and efficacious (produces the effects which the data sheet claims) and that the manufacturing process ensures a consistent quality of the product. Manufacturers and wholesale dealers of medicinal products require *manufacturer's* and *wholesale dealer's licences* respectively. As part of the licensing procedure, the company may need to perform a clinical trial of the drug in question and for this purpose they apply for an *animal test certificate*. An exemption to this law is that veterinary surgeons do not require a product licence to prepare a medicinal product themselves (or to request another veterinary surgeon to prepare such a product for them) for a particular animal or herd under their care. The veterinary surgeon is only allowed to stock a very limited supply of a medicine prepared in this way (2.5 kg of solid and 5 l of liquid). It is not permissible for vaccines (other than autogenous vaccines) to be prepared in this way.

Use of unlicensed products in veterinary medicine

The British Veterinary Association has produced a code of practice for the prescribing of medicinal products by veterinary surgeons. In non-food producing animals, the code of practice states that a product which has a veterinary product licence for the species and the condition to be treated, or is licensed for another condition or another veterinary species should, if possible, be chosen before a product which only has a licence for human use. Products licensed only for human use may be used if no veterinary licensed alternative exists. Special products made by the veterinary surgeon or by a pharmacist for the veterinary surgeon, which have no product licence at all, should be used only if a veterinary or human licensed product does not already exist.

Legal categories of medicines

When granting a product licence for a drug the licensing body places the medicine into one of three main categories. In order of decreasing strictness of controls over their supply to the public, these are:

- Prescription only medicines (POMs) including Controlled Drugs (CD).
- Pharmacy only medicines (P) including Merchant's List and Saddler's List medicines (PML).
- General sales list medicines (GSL).

More detailed information about these categories and their subdivisions is given in Fig. 13.10. In

LEGAL CATEGORISATION OF MEDICINAL PRODUCTS			
Legal category	**Sub-category**	**Definition**	**Examples**
Prescription only medicines (POM)	Controlled drugs	A sub-category of POM where the regulations for supply and storage are even more stringent than general POM medicines.	Morphine (S2) Phenobarbitone (S3)
	General POM drugs	Can only be prescribed and dispensed by a veterinary surgeon or dispensed by a pharmacist against a prescription written and signed by a veterinary surgeon.	Many veterinary medicines such as: Antibacterial drugs Vaccines Any drug intended for parenteral administration
Pharmacy only medicines (P)	General P medicines	Any drug in this category may be sold over the counter by a registered pharmacist to the general public. A veterinary surgeon may supply drugs in this category for the treatment of animals under his/her care.	Most P medicines are human products. Veterinary example: Dermisol®
	Pharmacy merchant's list (PML)	Drugs in this sub-category in addition to the general regulations described for P medicines may also be sold by agricultural merchants registered with the Royal Pharmaceutical Society to persons whose business involves animals (e.g. farmers).	Large animal anthelmintics Ectoparasiticides
	Saddler's list (PML)	Saddlers who are registered with the Royal Pharmaceutical Society may sell certain anthelmintics to horse owners.	Anthelmintics for horses
General sale list (GSL)	–	Medicinal products where the hazard to health or the need to take special precautions is sufficiently small that they can be sold without a prescription by pet shops or merchants who are not subject to special regulation. A number of veterinary products are GSL only when produced for external use or, when formulated for oral administration, a maximum strength which may be sold is stipulated.	Piperazine citrate Permethrin flea spray Pipronyl butoxide

Fig. 13.10. Legal categories of medicines.

summary, GSL is the only category of medicine which can be sold direct to the public by a veterinary practice without the owner having consulted with a veterinary surgeon. For all other categories of drugs, the animals for which they are intended should be under the care of a veterinary surgeon, whose authority should be sought before these drugs can be supplied by a trained veterinary nurse.

Storage of medicines

The manufacturer's recommendations should be carefully followed for each medicine in terms of storage temperature and the sensitivity of the compound to light and humidity. The part of the building in which the medicines are stored should not be accessible to the general public. Well designed shelves are essential to allow easy access to the drugs when required and to reduce the possibility of breakage, spillage or misplacement of stock. There should be a work surface, which should be easy to clean, and adequate refrigeration space.

It is convenient to store the medicines on the shelves in their classification groups. Products in large containers should be stocked near ground level for safety. Effective stock control will save time and money, ensuring that old stock is used before new so that medicines in stock do not exceed their expiry date and so that the pharmacy does not run out of a particular medication. In conclusion, a clean and tidy pharmacy makes for efficient and safe dispensing of medications.

Dispensing and labelling of medicines

The containers listed in Fig. 13.11 are recommended by the Council of the Royal Pharmaceutical Society for the dispensing of medicines from bulk packs. Note that paper envelopes and plastic bags are unacceptable forms of container.

PACKAGING OF MEDICINES	
Container	**Medicine**
Coloured flute bottles	Medicines for external application. Examples: shampoos, soaps, lotions. Enemas and eye and ear medications should be similarly dispensed if not already packaged in a suitable plastic container.
Plain glass bottles	Oral liquid medicines.
Wide-mouthed jars	Creams, dusting powders, granules.
Paper board cartons/Wallets	Sachets, manufacturer's strip or blister packed medicines.
Airtight glass, plastic or metal containers (preferably childproof)*	All solid oral medicines (tablets and capsules)

*Discretion can be exercised with childproof containers. Some aged and infirm clients may request plain screw-top containers.

Fig. 13.11. Recommended containers for different medicines.

The Medicines Act and the Medicine Labelling Regulations state the legal requirements for labelling of dispensed medicines. These regulations apply whether the medicines are dispensed in the manufacturer's original container or dispensed from bulk into smaller packages. Labels should be legible and indelible (written in biro or felt pen, not washable ink or pencil). Printed labels can be generated by computers used in modern practices. The specimen shown in Fig. 13.12 indicates essential information which has to be provided on a label by law and also optional (but desirable) information.

If the medication is for external application, the words 'For external use only' should appear on the label. In addition, any safety precautions that the owners should take when handling the drug should be added. When the drug is to be used in food producing animals, the label must also include the withdrawal period (the time between the last dose of the drug and the use of meat, milk or eggs from the animal for human consumption).

MEDICINE LABELLING DETAILS	
Essential	
Owner's name, pet identification and address Date	**For Animal Treatment Only** For Mrs Jones' cat 'Boris' 85, Sister's Avenue, Battersea, London SW11 3SN 18/9/93
Optional	
Quantity and strength of drug Instructions for dosing	21 x 50mg Ampicillin tablets One tablet to be given three times daily before food
Essential	**Keep all medicines out of reach of children**
Name & address of veterinary surgeon	P.J. Barber MRCVS Veterinary Surgeon 12, St John's Hill, London SW18 1JL

Fig. 13.12. Example of label, including information required by law and additional desirable details.

The Misuse of Drugs Act 1971 and The Misuse of Drugs Regulations 1985

This legislation controls the production, supply, possession, storage and dispensing of drugs where the potential exists for abuse by humans. These are the controlled drugs (CD), a special category of POM products, and there are 5 schedules:

- Schedule 1 (S1)—addictive drugs such as *cannabis* and hallucinogens *mescaline* and *LSD*.
- Schedule 2 (S2)—the opiate analgesics *morphine, etorphine, fentanyl* and *pethidine* plus *cocaine* and *amphetamine*.
- Schedule 3 (S3)—the barbiturates *pentobarbitone* and *phenobarbitone* plus the opiate analgesics, *buprenorphine* and *pentazocine*.
- Schedule 4 (S4)—benzodiazepines such as *diazepam* and *chlordiazepoxide*.

- Schedule 5 (S5)—certain preparations of cocaine, codeine and morphine that contain less than a specified amount of the drug. (Examples: *Codeine cough linctus; kaolin and morphine antidiarrhoeal suspension.*)

A veterinary surgeon does not have any general authority to possess or supply drugs from Schedule 1. Some of the other controlled drugs are subject to more stringent regulations than general POM medications, as detailed below.

Purchase. Purchase of S2 and S3 drugs requires a written requisition to a wholesaler, manufacturer or pharmacist. The requisition must include the veterinary surgeon's signature, name, address and profession; the purpose for which the drug is required; and the total quantity of the drug required. If a messenger is sent to collect the drug, written authority has to be given by the veterinary surgeon for the messenger to receive the drug on their behalf.

Storage. S2 drugs and buprenorphine (S3) must be kept in a locked cupboard which is attached to a wall. The key to such a cupboard is the responsibility of the veterinary surgeon, without whose authority the cupboard should not be opened.

Records. A bound register of all transactions involving S2 drugs must be kept. Details of incomings (purchases) of S2 drugs and their outgoings (drugs given to animals on the practice premises or dispensed to an owner to give to their animal) should be recorded in separate parts of the register, with a section for each individual drug in both parts of the register (e.g. the records for pethidine should be separated from those for morphine). Such registers for controlled drugs are available commercially. In addition, any S2 drug which is no longer required by the veterinary practice can only be disposed of in the presence of a Home Office Inspector. A record has to be made in the register which the Inspector is required to sign.

Special prescription requirements for controlled drugs. These apply to drugs that are in S2 and S3. An example of a prescription is shown in Fig. 13.13. The format is the same for any drug which the veterinary surgeon would like a Pharmacist to dispense to a client. In the case of S2 and S3 drugs, the name and address of the client, the date, and the quantity (in numbers and words) and strength of the preparation should be written in the veterinary surgeon's own handwriting.

PRESCRIPTION DETAILS

Mr J. Fishwick, MA, Vet MB MRCVS
50, High Street, Comberton, Cambridge CB4 1RL
Tel: 0223 849623

25th September 1993
Mr J. R. Fox's dog "Smarty"
23, The Green,
Barton, Cambridge.

Rx
Tablets Pethidine 50 mg
Send 10 (ten)

Label: Give half a tablet twice a day for 5 days

For Animal Treatment Only

This animal is under my care

No repeats

Fig. 13.13. Example of prescription form for a controlled drug.

The Health and Safety at Work Act 1974 and The Control of Substances Hazardous to Health (COSHH) Regulations 1988

When common sense is used and a few general ground rules followed, the medicines found in most veterinary practices present a relatively small hazard to the health of employees. All data sheets of licensed medicines will discuss any hazards that the medicine might pose to the operator (the person dispensing and administering the drug). The practice should also have produced a COSHH assessment for the substances (including drugs) which staff come into contact with during the working day (Chapter 11, Occupational Hazards). It is important that these documents are read and the safety measures followed to contain any risk to the absolute minimum.

Drugs can get into the body by accident and have systemic effects in the operator in a number of ways.

Absorption across the skin. This can occur with certain drugs such as prostaglandins (luteolytic agents), insecticides, nitrovasodilators and compounds containing the solvent DMSO (dimethyl sulphoxide), which aids penetration of substances which are dissolved in it across the skin (e.g. the corticosteroid, flumethasone). When handling such substances or when handling any substances when there are cuts or abrasions on the hands, gloves should be worn to prevent absorption across the skin. As a general principle, hands should be washed after handling any veterinary medicine and splashes or spills of medicines should be washed from the skin immediately.

Absorption across mucous membranes. The membranes of the eye (conjunctiva), nose and oral cavities may be reached if aerosols from liquid formulations or dust from powders containing a drug are formed. An aerosol is formed by very fine droplets of liquid which can be accidentally sprayed into the eyes or mouth. They are formed most often when reconstituting (dissolving) drugs for injection in the diluent supplied and when expelling air bubbles from a syringe. Care should be taken not to pressurise the contents of vials when reconstituting drugs. In addition, if the needle cover is kept on the needle when expelling air bubbles from the syringe, potentially dangerous aerosols will be avoided. Cytotoxic drugs should only be reconstituted by trained personnel and in designated areas. Should accidental contamination of the eyes, nose or mouth occur, the initial first aid measure is to wash or flush with copious amounts of water. Further medical help should be sought depending on the drug involved.

Accidental ingestion of drugs. This can occur through aerosols or dust, as described above, or through eating contaminated food. Food and drink must not be consumed or stored in areas where drugs are being handled, including areas where topical sprays (e.g. flea sprays) are applied to animals. Smoking should also be prohibited from these areas.

Inhalation. Inhalation of volatile substances such as gaseous anaesthetics (e.g. halothane), dust from powders and droplets from aerosols may cause irritation of the respiratory tract or the drugs can be absorbed and cause systemic effects. Hazards from inhalational anaesthetics can be minimised by the use of an adequate scavenging circuit attached to the anaesthetic circuit and by providing good ventilation of the operating room. Dust masks and eye protection should be worn when dispensing powders from bulk packs where a large amount of dust is inevitable. Insecticidal sprays should only be used in well-ventilated areas.

Accidental injection. This is the final way in which drugs may get into the body. The risk may be minimised by keeping all needles covered until the injection is made and by disposing of the used needle in a safe way immediately after use. The quantity of drug which enters the body following penetration of the skin with a needle is very small. Oil-based vaccines, however, can produce very severe reactions. Some drugs, such as etorphine, are so toxic to humans that even these minute quantities are hazardous.

Hazardous Drugs Used in Veterinary Practice

The groups of drugs mentioned below carry special risks. It is important to realise that whilst some drugs may produce acute effects on the operator which are obvious shortly after exposure, other drugs can have cumulative effects when exposure to small quantities occurs over a long period, which can be just as detrimental. For this reason it is good practice to keep exposure to all drugs to an absolute minimum by following the ground rules mentioned above.

- **Etorphine**—Highly toxic following accidental injection or exposure of skin or mucous membranes to the drug.
- **Halothane**—Repeated inhalation may damage the liver. Has been incriminated in increasing the risk of miscarriages.
- **Cytotoxic drugs**—Many are mutagenic (they damage genetic material), carcinogenic (they cause cancer) and teratogenic (they damage the unborn foetus).
- **Prostaglandins**—May cause asthma attacks, have serious effects on the cardiovascular system and cause uterine contractions. Should not be handled by asthmatics or women of child-bearing age. The BVA has drawn up a code of practice for using prostaglandins in cattle and pigs.
- **Antimicrobial agents**
  —*Griseofulvin*, the antifungal drug, is teratogenic and should not be handled by women of child-bearing age. Protective clothing, impervious gloves and a dust mask should be worn when handling the powdered form and adding this to feed.
  —*Penicillins* and *cephalosporins* may cause hypersensitivity on exposure in operators who are allergic to these drugs. The reaction can range from mild skin rash to swelling of the eyes, lips and face with difficulty in breathing—symptoms which require immediate medical attention. Those who have a history of allergy to drugs in these two families should not handle them.
  —*Chloramphenicol* can cause a fatal aplastic anaemia in humans, a reaction which is not related to the dose received and occurs in a very small number of people exposed to the drug when prescribed for them by doctors. Nevertheless, it is wise to avoid unnecessary exposure to this drug by taking the precautions mentioned above, including avoiding direct contact of the drug with the skin.

It can be seen from the above discussion that hazards are greatest from drugs which are formulated in a liquid or powder form where aerosols, accidental injection or dust can lead to significant exposure of the operator. Many capsules and tablets can be handled safely with minimal or no contact with the drug, provided that they are not broken or ground up to release the contents in a powdered form. It is still good practice to wear gloves when handling some tablets (e.g. cyclophosphamide, mitotane and griseofulvin). The use of a triangular metal or plastic tablet counter facilitates counting and reduces any contact between the operator and the tablets to a minimum.

Further reading

Brander, G. C., Pugh, D. M., Bywater, R. J. and Jenkins, W. L. (1991) *Veterinary Applied Pharmacology and Therapeutics*, 5th edition. Ballière Tindall, London.

BVA Code of Practice for sale or supply of animal medicines by veterinary surgeons (1990) *Veterinary Record*, **127**, 236–240.

The safe storage and handling of medicines (1990; 2nd edition). National Office of Animal Health.

Debuf, Y. (ed.) (1991) *The Veterinary Formulary.* The Pharmaceutical Press, London.

Wilkins, S. (1991) Hazards of handling veterinary medicines: Part 1. *Veterinary Nursing Journal,* **6,** 15–17.

Wilkins, S. (1991) Hazards of handling veterinary medicines: Part 2. *Veterinary Nursing Journal,* **6,** 53–55.

14
Anatomy and Physiology

A. J. PEARSON

Introduction

This section is concerned with the anatomy and physiology of the species which most concern the veterinary nurse: the dog and the cat.

Definitions

Anatomy describes the actual structure of the body. **Physiology** describes the working of the body.

Histology is the anatomy you can only see down a microscope—the micro-anatomy.

Pathology and **histopathology** describe the diseased states of the body—pathology can be seen with the naked eye, while histopathology (like histology) requires a microscope.

It is important when describing the structure of a body, be it dog, cat or human, to be able to describe where things lie in relation to one another:

Dorsal and **ventral** mean the sides of the body furthest from and nearer to the ground (in the standing quadruped).

Within the limbs, the 'top' is still dorsal, but the underneath—the palm of the hand or sole of the foot—are **palmar** (or **volar**) and **plantar**.

Cranial is towards the head end, and **caudal** is towards the tail—except within the head region, where towards the nose is **rostral**. The terms **anterior** and **posterior** may also be used, particularly within the head.

Within the limbs, **proximal** is the end of the limb nearer to the body, whereas **distal** is towards the toes—further from the body.

Medial means towards the centre midline of the body, whereas **lateral** means towards the sides.

Superficial and **deep** describe relative distances from the surface of the body.

Internal and **external** refer to relative depths within organs and body cavities.

It is sometimes necessary to talk about a section through a body, and these sections are called **planes**.

The **median plane** divides the body longitudinally into two equal halves.

A **sagittal** plane is any plane that lies parallel to the median plane.

A **dorsal plane** is a horizontal section parallel to the back (or dorsum) of the animal.

A **transverse plane** or section runs perpendicular to the long axis of the part to be sectioned. For example, a transverse section of the abdomen runs from the vertebral column to the ventral surface of the abdomen, whereas a transverse section of a limb is a horizontal slice across the limb at one level.

Classification

Classification is the way we organise and systematise the diversity of organisms, living and extinct, according to their degree of relatedness to one another. The dog and cat are **mammals**, which means that they have fur or hair, bear live young, and feed them on milk produced by the mother.

All species in the animal kingdom are divided into those with backbones and those without backbones—the **vertebrates** and the **invertebrates**. Included within the invertebrates are worms and insects (many of them important as parasites of domestic animals), molluscs, crustaceans and protozoans.

The vertebrates are divided into five groups: the fish, the amphibians, the reptiles, the birds and the mammals. Although a veterinary practice will no doubt see examples from all these groups from time to time, the vast majority will be mammals.

The mammals themselves are divided into many orders, including, for example:

- the **carnivores**—the meat eaters
- the **ungulates**—the hoofed animals
- the **rodents**—mice, rats and gerbils
- the **lagomorphs**—rabbits and hares.

All mammalian bodies (indeed all vertebrate bodies) are based on the same basic structural plan. As we start to understand the structure and function of the dog by way of example, we can look at other mammals and see how the same basic body plan has been varied to produce animals that are specialised for running, eating grass, jumping, burrowing etc.

The Systems of the Body

All bodies are made up of a number of systems, each of which has a specific function, for example:

- The **respiratory** system takes oxygen into the body and expels waste gases.
- The **digestive** system takes in and processes food and excretes waste

The systems are divided into three groups: the **structural** systems, the **visceral** systems and the **co-ordinating** systems.

Structural systems

Structural systems make up the basic structure of the body:

- The **skeletal system** consists of the rigid structures that support and protect the soft structures of the body. It is mainly composed of bone and cartilage, plus the tissues that make up the joints.
- The **muscular system** is generally understood to be the skeletal muscle of the body—that which is attached to the skeletal system and under voluntary control. There is muscular tissue elsewhere in the body—for example within the visceral systems—but this is not under voluntary control.
- The **integument** is the skin, the covering of the body.
- the **cardiovascular system** carries blood around the body

Co-ordinating systems

- The **nervous system** carries information to the central nervous system, and instructions away from it. Included in this system are the **special senses**.
- The **endocrine system** is also a communication system, carrying the **hormones**, which are chemical messengers, in the blood.

Visceral systems

The visceral systems are all tubular in design, and have one or two openings onto the surface of the body.

- The **digestive system** takes in food, digests and absorbs it, and excretes waste.
- The **respiratory system** takes in oxygen and excretes carbon dioxide.

- The **urinary system** removes waste from the body.
- **The reproductive system** enables the organism to replicate itself.

Cells, Tissues and Systems

Each of the systems of the body is made up of different types of **tissues**—for example, muscular tissue, nerve tissue, bone. Tissues are made up of three components, which may be present in different amounts in different tissues.

- The **cells** of the tissue.
- **Intercellular materials**—such as fibres and membranes found between the cells.
- **Fluid** bathing the cells or flowing round them.

The smallest unit of a tissue within the mammalian body is the **cell**. Several different types of tissue may be required to construct an organ such as the kidney, and several organs together make up a **system** within the body—for example the urinary system is made up of kidney, ureters, bladder and urethra.

The Structure of the Cell

Each cell in the body of a mammal is in its way as complex a structure as the whole body. Each cell has the ability to take in nutrients, to expel waste, to grow and to repair itself, to respire and to reproduce. All cells within the mammalian body are specialised to some extent, but they still have all the basic cellular structures and functions (Fig. 14.1).

The cell membrane

The cell membrane surrounds the cell. It is made up of a double layer of **phospholipid**, with **protein** molecules interspersed among them. **Transport** of

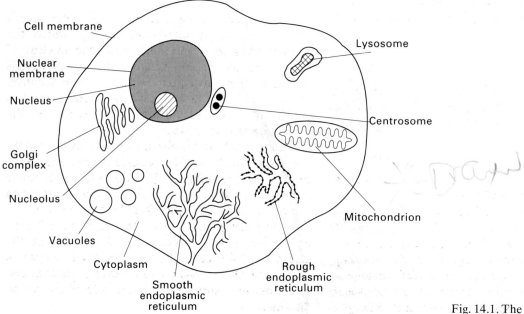

Fig. 14.1. The structure of a cell.

substances across the cell membrane may be by one of a number of methods:

- Small pores in the membrane allow the passage of very small molecules.
- Some molecules cross the cell membrane by being dissolved in the lipid of the membrane and diffusing through.
- Large molecules depend on what are termed **active transport mechanisms**. Proteins in the cell membrane are able to bind to particular molecules and carry them across the cell membrane. This process requires energy expenditure by the cell, but means that molecules can be moved from an area of low to one of high concentration—which is the opposite of what would occur by simple diffusion. Sodium ions are moved by this method.
- Some substances use **carrier molecules**, but are transported from an area of high concentration outside the cell to a lower concentration inside the cell. Glucose is transported into the cell by this method.

Phagocytosis and pinocytosis

Cells may ingest particles of food or fluid by engulfing them in a vesicle of cell membrane. This process is called **phagocytosis** when applied to solid matter, or **pinocytosis** if fluid is taken into the cell.

The nucleus

The nucleus controls the cell and all its activities. A cell without a nucleus cannot reproduce and will eventually die. The nucleus of the cell contains its **chromosomes**, which carry the genetic code for the organism and are responsible for coding for the construction of proteins within the cell. The chromosomes are made of **DNA (deoxyribonucleic acid)**. Except when the cell is dividing, the nucleus is amorphous in appearance except for one or more spherical structures called **nucleoli** (singular: nucleolus) which are responsible for the manufacture of **ribosomes**.

Cytoplasm

The cytoplasm is the semi-fluid substance within the cell, which contains protein, salts, glucose and the nucleus and organelles of the cell.

Organelles

Organelles are the various structures visible within the cell, other than the nucleus:

Mitochondria consist of an inner and an outer membrane, the inner one of which is folded to increase its surface area. The mitochondria convert energy in food to stored energy within the cell. They do this by using a chemical called **ATP (adenosine triphosphate)** which stores energy in the phosphate group linkage to the rest of the molecule. Energy is released when one phosphate group splits from the rest of the molecule, leaving **ADP (adenosine diphosphate)**. The ADP can then be converted back to ATP and more energy is stored.

Lysosomes are membranes within the cytoplasm filled with digestive enzymes. They digest material phagocytosed by the cell, and digest the remains of the cell once it has died. In the case of the phagocytosed matter, the lysosomes are emptied into the **vacuole** containing the engulfed matter.

Endoplasmic reticulum is a network of fine channels running through the cytoplasm. There are two types of endoplasmic reticulum, the rough and the smooth. Rough endoplasmic reticulum has **ribosomes** on it that have been produced in the nucleolus—they give it a rough or knobbly appearance under the microscope. Endoplasmic reticulum and the ribosomes attached to it are responsible for protein synthesis and transport within the cell.

The **Golgi complex** is a series of tubes which store substances such as lysosomal enzymes.

The **centrosome** lies near the nucleus and is made up of two **centrioles** which are important during cell division.

Cell Reproduction—Mitosis and Meiosis

The cells of the body reproduce themselves by a process known as **binary fission** which means that they divide in half. Before this can happen, however, the chromosomes within the nucleus of the cell must replicate themselves, so that there is an identical set of chromosomes for each of the so-called 'daughter cells'. This process of chromosome multiplication and then cell division is called **mitosis** (Fig. 14.2).

Mitosis can be divided into four stages:

- Prophase
- Metaphase
- Anaphase
- Telophase.

What appears to be a resting stage between cell divisions is called **interphase**, during which the chromosomes are duplicated within the nucleus of the cell, so that by the time the process of mitosis begins, each chromosome consists of two identical **chromatids**, joined together at the **centromere**. The individual chromosomes are not visible in the nucleus during interphase.

During **prophase** the chromosomes become visible. The long threads of DNA become shorter and fatter, so that they are visible in the nucleus. Also this stage the centrosome is replicated, and one of the two migrates round to the opposite side of the nucleus.

During **metaphase**, the nuclear membrane breaks down, and all the chromosomes line up along the 'equator' of the cell. The two centrosomes form a **nuclear spindle**, consisting of a series of threads that pass from the centrosome on one side of the cell to the other.

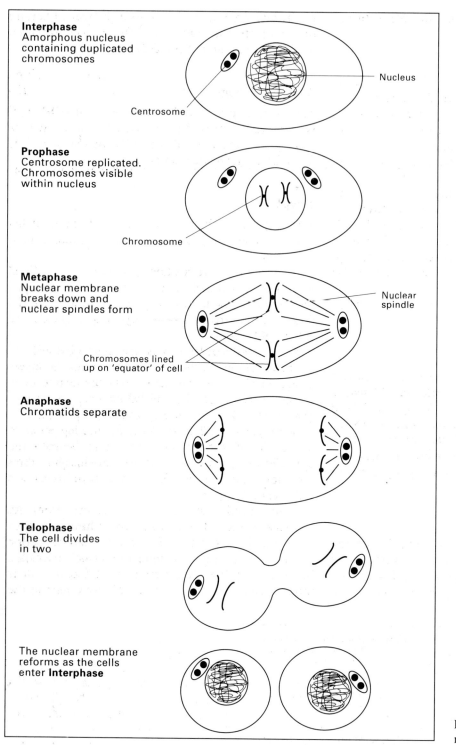

Fig. 14.2. Cell reproduction: mitosis.

During **anaphase**, the chromatids separate from one another, and move towards the opposite sides of the cell along the nuclear spindle.

During **telophase**, the cell membrane starts to form a 'waist', and the cell divides in two, leaving one set of identical chromosomes on either side of the division. The chromosomes then unravel to form a dense nuclear mass, and the nuclear membrane reforms, as the cell enters another **interphase**.

The Tissues of the Body

There are four types of tissue within the body:

- Muscular
- Nervous
- Epithelial
- Connective.

The structure of muscle and of nervous tissue will

be considered under the sections dealing with the muscular and nervous systems.

Epithelial Tissue

Epithelial tissue (Fig. 14.3) covers all the surfaces of the body, both inside and out. The skin is epithelial tissue, but so are the linings of all the body cavities and the hollow organs within the body.

The function of epithelial tissue is to protect, but also, depending on its situation within the body, to allow absorption across its surface. Where filtration or absorption is required across a layer of epithelium, it has to be as thin as possible. **Simple epithelium** is just one cell thick, and the cells may be **squamous** (flattened), **cuboidal** or **columnar** (elongated) in shape. Where a thicker, more protective layer of epithelium is required, there are two or more layers of cells, and the epithelium is known as **stratified** or **compound**.

Mucus and cilia

Many parts of the body are lined with a mucous epithelium or a ciliated mucous epithelium. **Mucus** is a thick proteinaceous fluid secreted by specialised epithelial cells to protect the tissue beneath. (Note: 'mucus' is the noun: 'mucous' is the adjective.) **Cilia** are very small hair-like projections on the surface of epithelial cells that move mucus along by constant waves of movement.

Keratinisation

Keratin is a tough protein that is found in the top layers of a stratified squamous epithelium in positions where a great deal of protection is required, such as the skin. The cells in the outer layers of the epithelium dry out and form a tough layer of keratin that protects the underlying tissue from bacterial invasion, drying and physical damage.

Transitional epithelium

Transitional epithelium is a stratified epithelium that is very elastic. It can be stretched to many times its resting size, and then return to its original size. It is found lining the bladder and ureters.

Glands

All the glands in the body are derived from epithelial tissue. Glands may be unicellular or multicellular, (Fig. 14.4).

An example of **unicellular glands** is the modified epithelial cells found in the linings of, for example, the digestive tract, secreting mucus to protect the lining of the tract. These very simple glands are called **goblet cells**.

Some **multicellular glands** are quite obviously of epithelial origin, as they lie mainly within the layers of epithelial tissue, and have ducts connecting them to the surface of the epithelium—e.g. sebaceous glands in the skin, and sweat glands in the paw pads.

Some glands still have ducts connecting them to the epithelial surface, but are found beneath the epithelium—e.g. salivary glands, discharging their secretion into the mouth. Glands with ducts are called **exocrine glands**.

Some glands are not only remote from an epithelial surface, but also no longer have a duct to discharge their secretion. These are called **endocrine glands**. The secretions of **endocrine** glands are called **hormones**, and they are carried in the blood to their target organ, which may be in a different part of the

Cells Basement membrane	**Simple squamous epithelium** found lining blood vessels and body cavities
	Simple cuboidal epithelium found lining the renal nephron
	Simple columnar epithelium found lining the gastro-intestinal tract
	Ciliated columnar epithelium lines the respiratory tract. The goblet cells produce mucus
	Stratified squamous epithelium found in the epidermis of the skin
	Transitional epithelium is a stratified (layered) epithelium, but the cells do not become flattened at the surface. Transitional epithelium can be stretched and return to its original shape. It is found lining the bladder.

Fig. 14.3. Epithelial tissues.

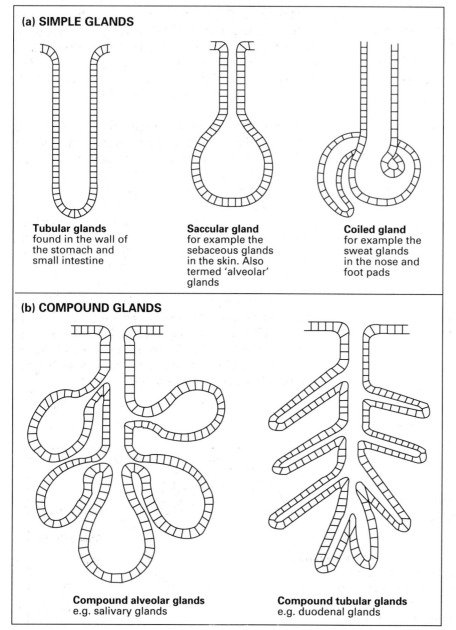

(a) SIMPLE GLANDS

Tubular glands
found in the wall of
the stomach and
small intestine

Saccular gland
for example the
sebaceous glands
in the skin. Also
termed 'alveolar'
glands

Coiled gland
for example the
sweat glands
in the nose and
foot pads

(b) COMPOUND GLANDS

Compound alveolar glands
e.g. salivary glands

Compound tubular glands
e.g. duodenal glands

Fig. 14.4. Glands.

body to the gland. Examples of endocrine glands are the thyroid gland and the gonads (testes and ovaries).

Connective Tissue

Connective tissue (Fig. 14.5) binds all the other body tissues together. It supports them and acts as a transport system.

Connective tissues often have a lot of intercellular material among the actual cells—this material is called the **ground substance**.

The types of connective tissue are:

- Loose connective tissue
- Dense connective tissue
- Bone
- Cartilage
- Blood.

Details of the structure of bone will be dealt with in the section on the skeletal system, and that of

blood in the section on blood and the circulatory system.

Loose connective tissue

Loose connective tissue is sometimes called **areolar tissue**. It is found between and surrounding organs within the body, and forms the layer between the skin and the tissues beneath.

It consists of a loose network of **collagen fibres** and **elastic fibres** with a few cells such as fibroblasts (which produce the fibrous collagen fibres) and **fat cells**. There are usually blood vessels and nerves within the tissue

Adipose tissue

Adipose or **fatty tissue** is essentially the same as areolar tissue, but the spaces between the collagen and elastic fibre network are filled up with fat cells. It forms a food reserve and an insulating layer, and in

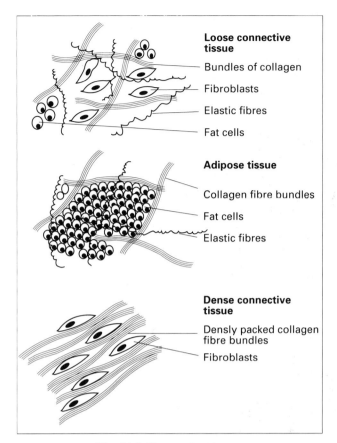

Fig. 14.5. Connective tissue.

some cases pads of fat support and protect vulnerable organs such as the kidney and the eye.

Dense connective tissue

Dense connective tissue is also known as **fibrous tissue**. It consists of large numbers of collagen fibre bundles with fibroblasts between them. The fibres may be arranged at random, with the fibres all running in different directions, or they may be arranged in parallel, as in tendons or ligaments. This latter arrangement gives the tissue great strength. The sheaths of **fascia** that support and bind together muscles throughout the body are also made up of dense connective tissue, but this time arranged to form flat sheets of tissue.

Cartilage

Cartilage (Fig. 14.6) is a dense, clear, blue–white substance which is tough and (with the exception of elastic cartilage) quite rigid. It is found principally at joints and between bones. It does not contain blood vessels (unlike bone) but is covered by a membrane called **perichondrium**, from which it derives its blood supply.

There are three different types of cartilage:

- Hyaline cartilage
- Fibrocartilage
- Elastic cartilage.

Hyaline cartilage. The cartilage—producing cell is called a **chondrocyte**. Hyaline cartilage consists of chondrocytes lying within a **hyaline matrix**, with a few very fine collagen fibres running through it. It is a very smooth tissue, and forms the rings of the trachea and the articular surfaces of joints.

Fibrocartilage. Fibrocartilage is stronger than hyaline cartilage. It has a similar basic structure, but has more collagen fibres in it, and is therefore stronger. Fibrocartilage surrounds and so deepens the articular sockets of some bones (e.g. the acetabulum of the pelvis and the glenoid fossa of the scapula). It also forms the intra-articular cartilages (**menisci**) of the stifle, and contributes to the structure of the intervertebral discs of the vertebral column.

Elastic cartilage. Elastic cartilage has a hyaline matrix and chrondrocytes, but also numerous elastic fibres within the matrix, which give the tissue its elastic properties. It is found in the pinna of the ear and in the epiglottis of the larynx. It is very flexible, and readily springs back into shape.

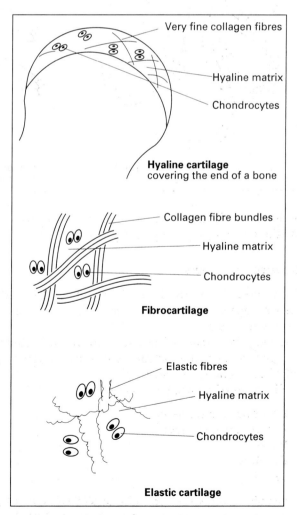

Fig. 14.6. Types of cartilage.

The Body Cavities

There are three body cavities: the **thorax**, the **abdomen** and the **pericardium**. (Sometimes the abdominal cavity is divided into abdominal and pelvic cavities, but this is an unnatural division as there is no physical barrier between them.)

All the body cavities are lined with **serous endothelium**. A serous membrane is a shiny, smooth membrane that produces a watery fluid to act as a lubricant between two surfaces (as opposed to the mucous membrane that produces the thick protein-aceous mucus as a protective layer). Examples of serous membranes are the pleura that lines the thoracic cavity and the peritoneum that lines the abdominal cavity. **Endothelium** is simply the term used for an epithelium lining a body cavity.

The boundaries of the thoracic cavity are:

- anteriorly, the thoracic inlet;
- dorsally, the thoracic vertebrae and hypaxial muscles;
- ventrally, the sternum;
- laterally, the ribs and intercostal muscles;
- posteriorly, the diaphragm.

The boundaries of the abdominal/pelvic cavity are:

- anteriorly, the diaphragm;
- dorsally, the sub-lumbar hypaxial muscles;
- ventrally, the abdominal muscles and the floor of the pelvis;
- laterally, the abdominal muscles and the lateral walls of the pelvis;
- posteriorly, the pelvic diaphragm.

The thoracic cavity

The serous lining of the thoracic cavity is called **pleura**. The thoracic cavity is divided into two pleural cavities (Fig. 14.7), between which lies the potential space of the **mediastinum** (a double layer of pleura that separates the two pleural cavities from one another). The lungs lie in out-pouchings of the pleura. The pleural cavities themselves are empty except for a small amount of the lubricating pleural fluid. Different parts of the pleura are given different names according to their position: so the diaphrag-matic pleura covers the diaphragm, the costal pleura covers the ribs, etc.

The mediastinum varies from species to species in its toughness. In humans, and to a lesser degree in the dog and cat, it is quite strong—it is possible for one lung to collapse yet leave the other functioning efficiently. However in the ruminants, and particu-larly the horse, the mediastinum is weak and damage to the chest wall may lead to the collapse of both lungs.

The abdominal cavity

The serous membrane lining the abdominal cavity is called the **peritoneum**. All the viscera within the abdominal cavity lie either behind the peritoneum (for example the kidney lies against the dorsal body wall in its kidney capsule), or in a fold of **mesentery**, which is a continuation of the peritoneum. So, although the abdominal cavity is full of viscera, the peritoneal cavity, like the pleural cavity, simply contains a little serous fluid.

The **pelvic diaphragm** consists of the structures that close the posterior part of the pelvis—mainly the muscles that surround the muscular anal sphincter. The pelvic diaphragm is important as it has to hold its shape against the regular muscular straining involved in defecation. Weakness in this area can lead to 'perineal rupture', with the breakdown of the muscles of the pelvic diaphragm.

The pericardial cavity

The pericardial cavity lies within the mediastinum in the thoracic cavity.

The pericardium

The pericardium, which contains the heart, consists of a double layer of membrane. The inner layer, a serous membrane closely attached to the heart, is called the **serous pericardium**. The outer layer, a thicker fibrous membrane with serous endothelium on its inner side, is called the **fibrous pericardium**. With this arrangement, the heart lies within a double sac of pericardium with serous fluid between the two layers. This fluid acts as a lubricant, allowing the heart to move freely.

The Chemistry of the Cell

Although cells may be specialised to perform different tasks, they all share some basic biochemical processes.

Before considering gross anatomical structure, it is useful to consider some of the basic chemical processes within the cell, and in the generalised multi-cellular animal. We need to consider respiration, digestion, temperature regulation and water balance at a simple, cellular level, before we can understand how these functions are performed in a complicated mammal.

Inorganic Content of the Body

The body is made up of organic materials (carbon-based molecules) and inorganic materials.

The **inorganic** content of the body is made up of water, and minerals such as calcium, phosphorus, magnesium, chlorine, iron, copper, manganese and iodine. None of these minerals exists in the body in the form of the pure element (copper in its pure form

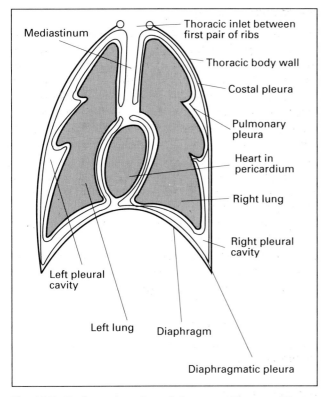

Fig. 14.7. Horizontal section of thorax, to illustrate pleurae and pleural cavities.

is a brown metal, and chlorine is a gas); they are instead in the form of **ions**.

Ions are positively or negatively charged particles which may be made up of one element, for example H^+ the hydrogen ion, or of two or more in combination, for example OH^- the hydroxyl ion, or HCO_3^- the bicarbonate ion.

An **electrolyte** is a substance that will split up into ions when it is dissolved in water. Sodium chloride (salt) is an electrolyte; in solution it splits up into Na^+ and Cl^-.

Ions that carry one or more positive charges are called **cations**, ions that carry one or more negative charges are called **anions**.

Water

About 60–70% of the body's weight is water. This is divided between the **intracellular water** and the **extracellular water**.

The intracellular water can be further divided into that in the intracellular fluid in the blood cells, and that in the cells in the rest of the body. The extracellular water can be divided into **plasma** (the fluid part of the blood) and the **interstitial fluid** that surrounds the cells of the body outside the blood vascular system.

Diffussion and osmosis. A **semipermeable membrane** is one that allows the passage through it of small molecules, but not large ones.

Diffusion is the movement of substances from a fluid of high concentration to a fluid of lower concentration, across a semipermeable membrane, in an effort to equalise the two concentrations (Fig. 14.8). Diffusion can only occur if the molecules are small enough to pass through the holes in the semipermeable membrane.

Osmosis is the movement of water through a semipermeable membrane from a weak (low concentration) solution to a stronger (higher concentration) solution.

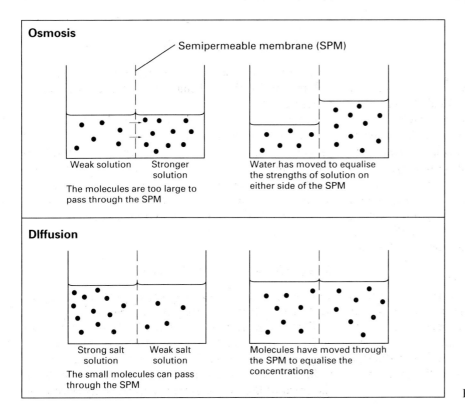

Fig. 14.8. Osmosis and diffusion.

If the actual molecules in the solution on either side of the membrane are too large to pass through the holes, the water will tend to move instead, in order to equalise the concentration on both sides of the membrane (Fig. 14.8).

Osmotic pressure is the pressure difference that would be required to stem the flow of water across the membrane.

Osmotic pressures within the body are described relative to the osmotic pressure of plasma. A fluid, relative to plasma, is either: **isotonic** (the same osmotic pressure); **hypertonic** (a greater osmotic pressure); or **hypotonic** (a lower osmotic pressure).

The osmotic pressure of plasma is maintained largely by the plasma proteins.

Fluid balance. The water in the body is constantly moving. It is taken in through food and drink, and is lost not just through the obvious means, in the urine and faeces, but also through tears, sweat, vaginal secretions and the moisture in expired air. It may also be lost to the body in increased amounts if an animal vomits, has diarrhoea, or loses blood after an accident.

It is very important to the body to maintain the correct fluid balance between input and output.

The proportional water content of the body varies with age and obesity—it is slightly higher in young animals, and slightly lower in obese ones.

Typical water loses from the body per 24 hours are:

20 ml/kg through respiratory system and sweat
20 ml/kg in urine
10–20 ml/kg as faecal losses.

Thus a healthy animal, eating, drinking and producing urine and faeces, needs between 50–60 ml of water/kg body weight per day. A vomiting animal, or one with, say, a copious vaginal discharge or diarrhoea, will need much more.

Acidity and alkalinity. It is also important for the body to maintain the correct degree of acidity or alkalinity.

An acid is a substance that liberates hydrogen ions in solution, and an alkali or base is one that accepts hydrogen ions.

For example the following equation:

$$H_2CO_3 \rightleftharpoons H^+ + HCO_3^-$$

means that carbonic acid (H_2CO_3) in solution gives hydrogen ions and bicarbonate ions. Carbonic acid is an acid because it gives up or produces a hydrogen ion in solution. The bicarbonate is an alkali or base, because, if the chemical reaction is reversed, the bicarbonate will accept the hydrogen ion to form carbonic acid.

The acidity of a solution is measured by its hydrogen ion concentration, on a scale of 1 to 14, and is called the pH ('per Hydrogen') value. A neutral pH is 7; acidity increases as the numbers decrease, and alkalinity or basicity increases as the number increases.

Body fluids are at pH 7.4, and it is very important that they are kept stable at this level.

Because the pH scale is logarithmic, an increase or decrease of 1 means a 10-fold increase in acidity or alkalinity.

Other inorganic substances within the body

The most important inorganic substances after water are the minerals **calcium**, **phosphorus** and **magnesium**. These are stored in the body within the bones and teeth, and give rigidity and strength to these structures. They are also essential for muscle and nerve function, and play a part in blood clotting and in milk production.

It is important not only to have sufficient of these minerals but also, particularly in the case of phosphorus and calcium, to have them in the correct proportions.

Sodium, **potassium** and **chlorine** are important in the regulation of fluid balance between the intracellular and extracellular fluid. Sodium and chlorine are found mainly in the extracellular fluid, whereas potassium is mainly found within cells.

Iron and **copper** are found in all tissues but are particularly important in the production of **haemoglobin**, the oxygen-carrying compound within the blood.

Organic Compounds within the Body

Organic compounds are chemicals built on a carbon base.

Three types of organic compound are important to the body:

- **Amino acids and proteins**
- **Sugars and carbohydrates**
- **Fatty acids and lipids**.

These are the main classes of foodstuffs.

Amino acids and proteins.

Amino acids are the building blocks of proteins. Two amino acids join together to form a **peptide**; when a larger number join together the new unit is called a **polypeptide**; and when there are several hundred it is called a **protein**. This process of joining together simple units to make complex ones is called **polymerisation**.

Amino acids contain carbon, hydrogen, oxygen and nitrogen, and may also contain sulphur and iodine. There are twenty different amino acids, which are constant throughout nature.

Proteins within the body may be either **structural** (such as collagen and keratin) or **functional** (such as enzymes and hormones).

Dietary proteins must be broken down to amino acids before they can be absorbed by the body.

Sugars and carbohydrates

Sugars are made up of carbon, hydrogen and oxygen. Simple sugars join together in chains to form the **polysaccharides** or **carbohydrates**. Sugars are important as a source of energy for the animal and are stored in the body as **glycogen**, a polysaccharide. Carbohydrates must be broken down to simple sugars before they can be absorbed by the body.

Fatty acids and lipids

Fatty acids are also made up of carbon, hydrogen and oxygen. **Lipids** are important in the formation of cell membranes and steroids, in the insulation of nerves and, in the form of fat, as a food store and insulation against cold. Lipids must be broken down to fatty acids before they can be absorbed by the body.

Enzymes

Enzymes are organic catalysts. A catalyst is a substance that assists or accelerates a chemical reaction without itself taking part in the reaction or being changed by it in any way.

Enzymes are involved in chemical reactions throughout the body—they assist in the breakdown of food in the gut and regulate the chemical reactions going on all the time in every cell. It has been estimated that there are 200 or more enzymes within each cell.

Chemical Reactions within the Body.

The **Law of Conservation of Energy** states that energy cannot be created or destroyed, but it can be stored as potential energy, or dissipated as heat or electrical energy.

Some chemical reactions need or use up energy, others release it. A chemical reaction requiring energy is called an **anabolic reaction**, whereas one releasing energy is called a **catabolic reaction**.

The body is in a constant state of degradation and repair and all the time, throughout the body, there are catabolic and anabolic reactions releasing and using energy. The sum total of all this energy use, be it gain or loss, is the **total metabolism** of the body.

The **basal metabolic rate**, (BMR) is defined as the rate at which a resting animal produces heat.

All animals require energy. Plants use solar energy and carbon dioxide to produce sugars and carbohydrates. Animals eat plants, or they eat other animals that have eaten plants, and so they in turn have access to the stored solar energy.

The Skeletal System

The skeletal system consists of the hard structures that protect and support the soft parts of the body. Usually included in this are the bones, and also the cartilage and the joints that connect the bones and provide for movement between them.

The functions of the skeleton are:

- To support the body.
- To provide leverage for voluntary muscles, and surfaces for their attachment.
- To protect the soft internal organs of the body, especially those inside the chest (the heart and lungs).
- To provide a store of minerals, particularly calcium and phosphorus, for use in the body.

The Structure of Bone

There are two types of **bone tissue**:

- **Compact bone**
- **Spongy bone**.

Compact bone (Fig. 14.9) is the hard whiteish substance we think of as bone. It is a complex tissue, in the form of a series of canals running along the length of the bone, surrounded by layers of bone tissue. The canal in the centre of each of these **Haversian systems** carries the blood vessels, nerves and lymphatics that serve the bone.

The bone tissue itself consists of:

- calcium-containing minerals, chiefly calcium phosphate
- collagen fibres
- mucopolysaccharide polymer, forming the ground substance
- **osteocytes** (bone cells) within **lacunae** or spaces within the bone lamellae.

Compact bone is found in the cortices (the outer layer) of all bones.

In **spongy** or **cancellous bone** the Haversian canal systems are spread widely apart, and the spaces between them are filled with red bone marrow, which is made up of fat and blood cells. This type of bone tissue is found in the ends of long bones, and forms the core in both short and flat bones.

All bones are covered by a tough fibrous membrane called the **periosteum**.

Bones can be classified as one of three types by shape and composition:

- long bones
- flat bones
- irregular bones.

Long bones have a shaft and two ends (Fig. 14.9), the proximal end is often called the 'head' of the bone. They have an outer layer of compact bone (a cortex), with spongy bone at the extremities, forming

266

A. J. Pearson

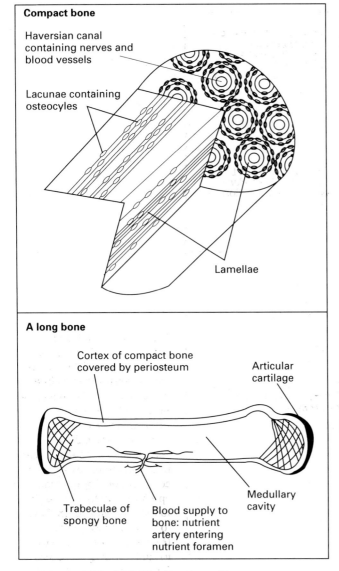

Fig. 14.9. The structure of bone.

lines of **trabeculae**, which give strength to the bone without adding too much to its weight.

Long bones have a medullary cavity, which is filled with marrow. However, most of the blood cell formation takes place at the ends of the bone, among the spongy tissue.

Flat bones consist of two layers of compact bone with a layer of spongy bone between them. Examples of flat bones are the those of the vault of the skull, the scapula and the pelvis.

Irregular bones are also made up of two layers of compact bone with spongy bone between them. Examples of irregular bones are those of the vertebral column, and the carpal and tarsal bones. The carpal and tarsal bones are sometimes put in a separate category as 'short' bones.

Sesamoid bones (e.g. patella) develop within the tendon and occasionally a ligament, particulary where a tendon operates over a ridge of underlying bone.

Development of Bone

Bones form by one of two methods:

- intramembranous ossification
- interchondral ossification.

Ossification is the term used for the development of bone.

Membrane bones—those that form by intra-membranous **ossification** are formed between two layers of membrane which are the layers of periosteum. An example of membrane bones is the flat bones of the skull.

In the case of **interchondral ossification**, the bone develops from a cartilage model of the bone formed within the embryo (Fig. 14.10).

Centres of ossification appear within the cartilage; there may be as few as two or as many as seven. Centres of ossification start as groups of bone-producing cells called **osteoblasts**, that break down the cartilage and lay down bone instead. The bone tissue gradually extends towards the ends of the bone, and a little later from the extremities towards the shaft.

The area of bone development within the shaft of the bone is called the **diaphysis**, and the areas of bone at the ends of the bone are called the **epiphyses**. Between the developing diaphysis and the epiphyses is a strip of cartilage called the **epiphseal plate** or **growth plate**, which is where growth continues until the plate is overtaken by bone growth, at which point the bone ceases to grow.

The **medullary cavity** of the bone develops by the activity of **osteoclasts**, or bone-destroying cells, which remove bone from the centre of the diaphysis, and the continuing activity of osteoblasts laying down bone on the outside of the shaft as the animal grows.

Bone is a living tissue, and has the potential to remodel and change its shape throughout life. The bone of a young animal is relatively smooth, but that of an old one shows roughened areas where periosteum has been pulled away from bone, and remodeling at the site of damaged tendons, as well as possibly arthritic change.

Joints

Joints are formed wherever two or more bones meet—but not all joints allow movement. Other terms for a joint are an **arthrosis** or an **articulation**.

Joints can be classified in three groups:

- **Synovial joints**
- **Cartilagenous joints**
- **Fibrous joints**.

Synovial joints

Synovial joints (Fig. 14.11) occur where the articular or joint surfaces of the bones involved are covered with hyaline cartilage. The whole joint is surrounded by a **joint capsule** consisting of an outer layer, which

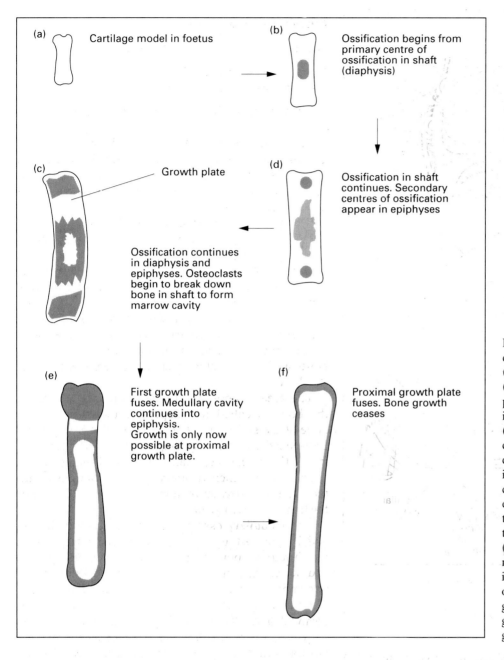

(a) Cartilage model in foetus

(b) Ossification begins from primary centre of ossification in shaft (diaphysis)

(c) Growth plate

(d) Ossification in shaft continues. Secondary centres of ossification appear in epiphyses

Ossification continues in diaphysis and epiphyses. Osteoclasts begin to break down bone in shaft to form marrow cavity

(e) First growth plate fuses. Medullary cavity continues into epiphysis. Growth is only now possible at proximal growth plate.

(f) Proximal growth plate fuses. Bone growth ceases

Fig. 14.10. Growth and development of a long bone: (a) cartilage model in foetus; (b) ossification begins from primary centre of ossification in shaft (diaphysis); (c) ossification in shaft continues—secondary centres of ossification appear in epiphyses; (d) ossification continues in diaphysis and epiphyses, osteoclasts begin to break down bone in shaft to form marrow cavity; (e) first growth plate fuses, medullary cavity continues into epiphysis, growth is now only possible at proximal growth plate; (f) proximal growth plate fuses, bone growth ceases.

is the continuation of the periosteum, and an inner layer of **synovial membrane** which lines the joint cavity and secretes **synovial fluid**. This fluid lubricates the joint surfaces and provides nutrients for the articular cartilage; it varies in consistency, being more viscous and plentiful in fit and athletic animals but more sparse and watery in the unathletic.

Synovial joints may have stabilising ligaments associated with them, either on the outside or the inside of the joint capsule. Most commonly the ligamentary support is in the form of 'collateral ligaments' that lie on either side of the joint.

Synovial joints may also have one or more fibro-cartilage **menisci** (singular meniscus) within them, which increase the range of movement of the joint and reduce wear and tear on the articular surfaces. Examples of joints containing menisci are the stifle (Fig. 14.12) and the tempero-mandibular (jaw) joint.

Cartilagenous joints

In cartilagenous joints the bones are connected by cartilage, and may or may not allow a degree of movement:

- Synarthroses are cartilagenous joints allowing little or no movement. An example is the pelvic symphysis between the two pelvic bones.
- Amphiarthroses are cartilagenous joints that allow a reasonable degree of movement between the bones. An example of this type is the inter-vertebral joints.

The intervertebral disc that separates two adjacent vertebrae consists of two parts: a fibrous outer shell called the annulus fibrosus and a jelly-like inner substance called the nucleus pulposus. These discs form a cushion between the vertebrae that absorbs sudden jarring movements and helps prevent damage to the spinal cord (Fig. 14.13).

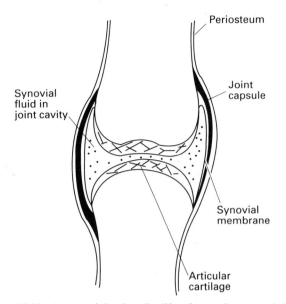

Fig. 14.11. A synovial joint. In life, the periosteum, joint capsule and synovial membrane are fused to form one sheet of tissue.

Fibrous joints

In fibrous joints the bones are joined together by dense fibrous connective tissue and there is very little or no movement between the bones. An example of fibrous joints is the sutures between the flat bones of the skull.

Both fibrous and cartilagenous joints may eventually become ossified, or may develop pockets of synovial fluid. The latter commonly occurs in the sacro-iliac joint, which tends to relax during parturition.

Movement of joints

The movement of joints can usually be described as being one or more of the following:

- Flexion and extension—flexion decreases the angle between two bones: extension increases it.
- Abduction and adduction—abduction moves the limb away from the body (as when the male dog lifts his leg): adduction moves it towards or beneath it
- Inward and outward rotation—one end of the bone swivels round in the joint, allowing the other to move in a circle towards or away from the body.
- Gliding or sliding—when one articular surface slides over the other.

Anatomists have devised many ways to categorise joints. Here is one relatively simple method:

- **Hinge joints** allow movement in one direction only—for example the elbow joint, which flexes and extends again to a (more or less) straight line.
- **Condylar joints** allow flexion, extension to the straight line, then over-extension. An example is the carpal joint.

- **Pivot joints** allow rotation. An example is the radio-humeral joint in the cat.
- **Ball and socket joints** are the most freely moveable of joints. An example the hip joint.
- **Plane joints** allow a restricted amount of gliding movement of one bone over another—for example the small bones in the carpus and tarsus.

The Skeleton

Skeletons of any vertebrate animal—be they mammal, bird, reptile, amphibian or fish—are really very similar. They all have a skull and a vertebral column. They nearly all have four limbs, and each limb has the potential for up to five digits.

They may have different numbers of toes or different numbers of ribs but the basic structure is the same; and the bones have the same names, though they may differ in shape from species to species.

The skeleton is divided into three parts:

- **The axial skeleton**—the skull, vertebral column, ribs and sternum.
- The **appendicular skeleton**—the limbs.
- The **splanchnic skeleton**—bony elements that develop in tissue unattached to the rest of the skeleton; for example, the os penis of the dog and cat.

It is useful when studying the skeleton to have access not only to a skeleton but also to a tolerant living dog, so that each bone can be considered in place, held against the living animal (Fig. 14.14).

The Axial Skeleton

The bones of the head consist of the skull, the mandible or lower jaw, and the hyoid apparatus.

The skull

Different breeds of dog have very different head shapes, which can generally be placed into one of three categories:

- The long, thin **doliocephalic** head—for example the borzoi.
- The short, broad **brachiocephalic** head—for example the bulldog.
- The 'normal' **mesocephalic** head.

Although the shapes of the skulls may differ, they all contain the same bones. The skull consists of two parts:

- **The cranium**, which encloses the brain.
- **The maxilla**, which forms the upper jaw and contains the nasal chambers.

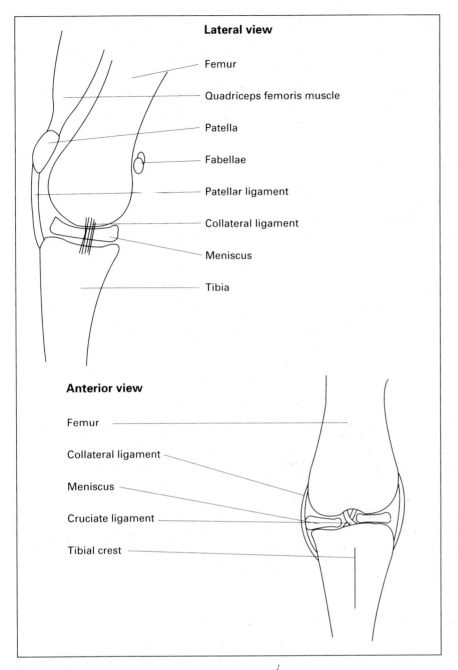

Lateral view

- Femur
- Quadriceps femoris muscle
- Patella
- Fabellae
- Patellar ligament
- Collateral ligament
- Meniscus
- Tibia

Anterior view

- Femur
- Collateral ligament
- Meniscus
- Cruciate ligament
- Tibial crest

Fig. 14.12. The stifle joint.

The only way to become thoroughly familiar with the skull is to handle one, noting the following points (Figs 14.15 and 14.16):

- At the back and towards the base of the cranium is the **foramen magnum**—the large hole through which the spinal cord enters the cranial cavity.
- The back of the skull, above the foramen magnum, consists of a flat area—the **occipital region**. Muscles that support the head on the neck attach over this area.
- At the base of the skull, on either side of the foramen magnum, are the **occipital condyles**, where the first cervical vertebra articulates with the skull.
- On either side of these are two prominences, the **jugular processes**—again for muscle attachment.

- Just in front of each jugular process is a round protruberance—the **tympanic bulla**—which houses the structures of the middle ear. On the lateral aspect of each tympanic bulla is the **external acoustic meatus**—the opening where the external ear canal attaches to the skull.
- Continuing forward up the ventral midline of the skull, the flat bone enters a canal with walls of bone on either side. This bone forms the roof of the pharynx, and the soft palate is attached between the 'walls' on either side.
- Imagine the soft palate in place, and go up a step on to the **hard palate**, which forms the roof of the mouth. In life, the hard palate is covered with tough, ridged mucous membrane. It is possible to see on the skull the suture lines between the three bones contributing to the hard palate. These are

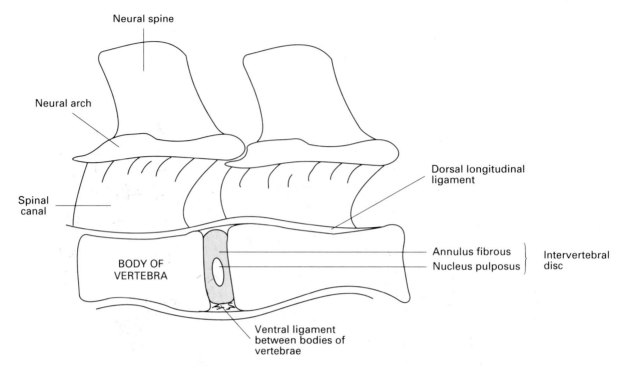

Fig. 14.13. Position of the intervertebral disc.

(from the back) the **palatine**, the **maxilla** and the **premaxilla** (or incisive).

- Now turn the skull on its side, and follow the maxillary bone and the premaxilla on to the side and top of the nasal cavity. One other pair of bones contributes to the maxillary region: the nasals, which run down the top of the nose. Notice that the bones stop well short of where the nose of the dog actually is. This is because the pad of the nose is supported by cartilage, not bone.
- Two bones make up the bulk of the vault or top of the cranium. At the front, occupying the 'forehead', is the **frontal bone**, which contains the **frontal sinus**. (A sinus is an air-filled cavity within a bone.) Behind the frontal bones are the **parietal bones**, with the little **interparietal bone** between them.
- Now look at the orbit, which in life contains the eye and eye muscles. See how it is protected on the lateral side by the bony **zygomatic arch**.
- Other bones that lie within the orbit are the little **lacrimal bone**, which carries the lacrimal drainage to the nasal chamber, and the **sphenoid**, a bone near the base of the orbit with many holes, or **foramina**, in it. Foramina are found throughout the skull, particularly on its base. They provide an exit from the cranial cavity for the cranial nerves, and allow blood vessels to enter the cranium to supply the brain.
- The nasal chamber is divided into two longitudinally by a cartilagenous **nasal septum**. In each chamber there are two **nasal turbinates**, which are much-branched, thin, scroll-like bones covered with ciliated mucous epithelium.

- On the front of the **mesethmoid bone**, which separates the cranial from the nasal cavities, are some more delicate turbinate bones, the **ethmoturbinates**, which carry smell receptors in their covering mucous membrane.

The mandible

The lower jaw of mammals is made up of two bones, the **dentaries** (Fig. 14.17). They join together at the chin in the **mandibular symphysis**. This is always a point of weakness in the jaw, and a common site for fractures following road traffic accidents, especially in cats.

The lower jaw is divided into two parts, the **horizontal** and the **vertical rami** (singular ramus).

The **coronoid process** provides an area for muscle attachment of the temporal muscle, and the **masseteric fossa** for the masseter.

Teeth

The mammals are unique among the vertebrates in having teeth in different parts of jaw specialised to perform different functions (Figs 14.15 and 14.17). Mammalian teeth can be divided into four groups: **canines (C), incisors (I), premolars (P)** and **molars (M)**. For each species there is a 'dental formula' for the temporary and for the permanent teeth.

The dental formulae for the dog are:

$$\frac{\text{I3 C1 P4 M2}}{\text{I3 C1 P4 M3}} \quad \text{and} \quad \frac{3.1.3}{3.1.3}$$

for the milk teeth. There are never any temporary molars.

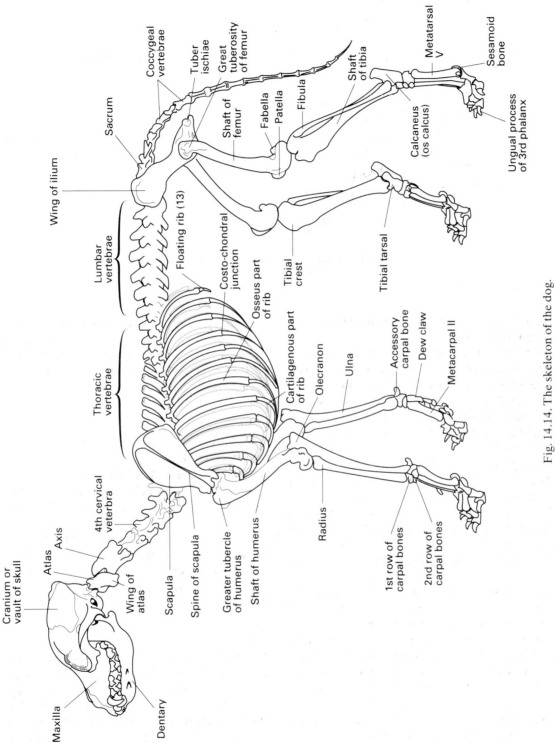

Fig. 14.14. The skeleton of the dog.

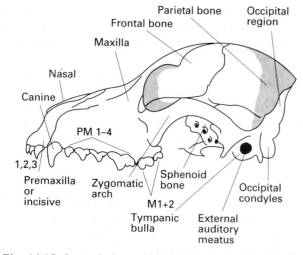

Fig. 14.15. Lateral view of the skull of the dog, showing main bones and permanent dentition.

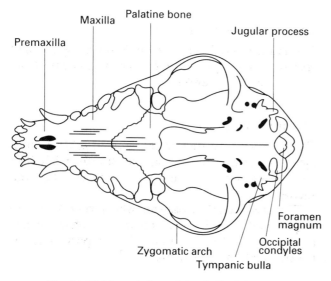

Fig. 14.16. Ventral view of the skull of the dog.

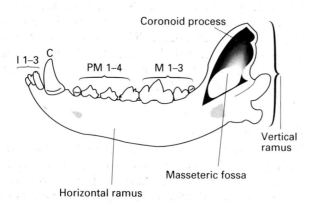

Fig. 14.17. Permanent dentition of the dog.

The dental fomulae for the cat are 3/3, 1/1, 3/2, 1/1, for the permanent teeth and 3/3, 1/1, 3/2 for the deciduous teeth.

Both of the above are acceptable methods of writing dental formulae. In the example given for the dog, the characters above the line identify the top teeth, and those below are the teeth in the lower jaw. For the cat, the formulae have a 'slash' separating top and bottom teeth.

Both pups and kittens lose their deciduous teeth and start to gain their permanent set between (usually) 4 and 5 months old. The process is complete by about 7 months old.

The structure of teeth

- The tooth can be divided into a **crown** and a **root**, the division being at the line of the gum (Fig. 14.18).
- The crown is covered with **enamel**, a very hard, white, calcified substance.
- Beneath the enamel, making up the bulk of root and crown, is **dentine**. Within the dentine is a **pulp cavity** containing the nerves and blood vessels supplying the tooth.
- The root is covered with **cement**, which may overlap with the enamel at the gum margin, and which fixes the tooth firmly in the socket in the bone, via the fibrous **periodontal ligament**.

The different teeth have different functions.

- The incisors (I) are relatively unimportant in carnivores. They help the canine teeth to hold prey, particularly in the dog.

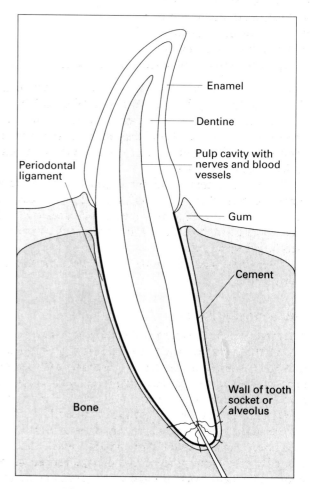

Fig. 14.18. The structure of a tooth.

- The canines (C) are long and sharp, and are the main implement for catching and holding prey.
- The premolars (P) and molars (M) of carnivores are not designed for grinding and crushing (as in the case of human cheek teeth) but for shearing chunks of meat off bone. Dogs and cats do not chew their food: they swallow pieces, and leave the rest to the digestive juices.

The carnassial tooth

The carnassial tooth is the last premolar in the upper jaw. It is a very large tooth, with three roots, that shears against the first lower molar to form a very efficient scissor-like cutting action.

The hyoid apparatus

The hyoid apparatus is a series of small bones and cartilages that hang down from the tympanic bone of the skull and suspend the larynx below the pharynx. The two arms of the hyoid apparatus move backwards and forwards, allowing the larynx to move back and forth as if on a swing.

The vertebrae

The vertebrae are divided into regions:

- Seven **cervical** vertebrae
- Thirteen **thoracic** vertebrae
- Seven **lumbar** vertebrae
- Three fused **sacral** vertebrae
- Up to twenty or more **coccygeal** vertebrae.

The vertebrae of each region are distinctive in shape and slightly different in function (Fig. 14.19).

The basic plan of a vertebra is of a **body** or **centrum**, with a **neural arch** above it, topped with a **neural spine**. The spinal cord runs through the neural arch in the **spinal canal**.

There are lateral **transverse processes**. (Where there are ribs, they are called transverse processes, but where there are no ribs they are properly called costo-transverse, to indicate that the rib is incorporated into the process.)

There may also be other processes for muscle attachment.

The cervical vertebrae

The first cervical vertebra is the **atlas**. It has no body, and consists mainly of a canal and a large wing-like pair of transverse processes. In common with all the cervical vertebrae, it has intervertebral foramina running through it, to allow the passage of blood vessels. It articulates with the base of the skull.

The second cervical vertebra is the **axis**. It is elongated, has a blade-like neural spine, and a cranially projecting process, the **dens**, attached to its body. The dens was originally the centrum of the atlas.

Attached to the neural spine of the axis is the **nuchal ligament**, a thick fibrous band that attaches to the neural spine of the first thoracic vertebra, and so helps support the head.

There are synovial joints between the skull, the atlas and the axis, allowing an enormous range of movement. The remaining five vertebrae are similar however, they have poorly developed spinous processes and have fibrous joints between them.

The thoracic vertebrae

The thoracic vertebrae have short bodies, and tall neural spines that gradually decrease in height throughout the series. They also have articular depressions, or **foveae**, (singular fovea) on the centra, where they form a synovial joint with the head of the rib, which has a further articulation with the transverse process.

The lumbar vertebrae

The lumbar vertebrae have bulky neural spines and costo-transverse processes for the attachment of the powerful lumbar muscles.

The sacral vertebrae

The three sacral vertebrae are fused together to form the sacrum, which forms a support for the pelvis. The joint between the sacrum and pelvis is called the sacro-iliac joint.

The **sacro-sciatic ligament**, which runs from the sacrum to the sciatic tuberosity on the pelvic bone, is a strong band of fibrous tissue that supports much of the musculature of the rump.

The coccygeal vertebrae

The coccygeal vertebrae in the dog vary in number from breed to breed, and depending on whether the dog has had its tail docked. They decrease in size as they go down the tail. The first few have a neural arch and costo-transverse processes, but the last few are merely small rods of bone.

The ribs and sternum.

The dog and cat both have 13 sets of ribs, which are made partly of bone (the osseus part) and partly of cartilage (the costal cartilage). They have two articulations proximally with the thoracic vertebrae: the **capitulum** articulates with the body of the vertebra, and the **tuberculum** with the transverse process.

The distal ends of the first eight ribs join on to the **sternum**, which is composed of eight **sternebrae**. The first sternebra is called the **manubrium**, and the last has a flap of cartilage attached to it called the **xiphisternum**, or **xiphoid cartilage**.

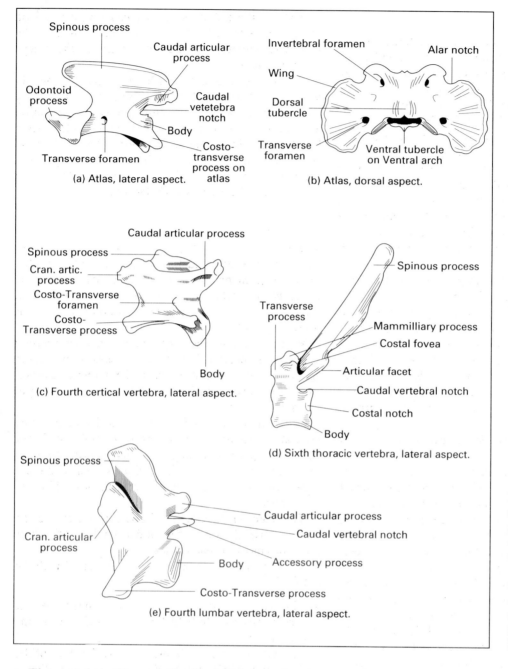

Fig. 14.19. Regional differences in vertebral structure: (a) lateral view of 1st cervical vertebra (atlas); (b) dorsal view of 1st cervical vertebra (atlas); (c) lateral view of 4th cervical vertebra; (d) lateral view of thoracic vertebra; (e) lateral view of lumbar vertebra.

The costal cartilage of ribs 9 to 12 join on to the cartilage in front of them, and form the costal arch. The 13th rib is called the 'floating' rib: it is very short and the end lies free within the muscle of the body wall.

The Appendicular Skeleton

The forelimb and hindlimb are joined to the body in different ways. The forelimb of the running animal has no pectoral girdle—it is joined to the trunk by muscles. This allows a degree of shock absorption as the limb hits the ground, because the muscular attachment allows the weight of the body to drop between the two forelimbs, instead of jarring as it would with a rigid bony attachment. The hindlimb, however, has a rigid girdle, because the hindlimb produces the main propulsive force for the body.

It is important to be familiar with the shapes of the bones of the limbs, and to be able to identify them. Most of the long names given to the different features seen on bones are not that complicated once you know the meaning of just a few of the words.

- A tuberosity, a trochanter or a tubercle are all bumps on the bone; they are usually sites for muscle attachment.
- The greater tuberosity is a big bump or protruberance and is usually on the lateral aspect of the bone.
- Most long bones have a head, sometimes a neck, and always a shaft.
- A trochlea is a groove for a pulley (usually a tendon).
- Condyles are rounded articular surfaces. Epicondyles are the bits of the bone lateral to the condyles.
- A fossa is a hole or depression in a bone.

The Forelimb

The scapula is a flat, roughly triangular bone with an obvious **spine** on the lateral side, that divides the lateral surface into a **supraspinous fossa** and an **infraspinous fossa**. There is a neck, an articular surface called the **glenoid cavity**, and an **acromion**, which projects from the distal end of the spine.

The humerus is a classic long bone with a head and a neck, a shaft and greater and lesser tubercles—it forms the shoulder joint with the scapula. Distally it forms the elbow joint with the radius and ulna.

The radius and ulna lie side by side and are the bones of the forearm. The ulna has the **olecranon** at its proximal end, and just in front of it the **anconeal process**. It has a deep **articular notch** that holds it close to the humerus.

The radius is a relatively simple rod-like bone that lies on top of the ulna at the elbow joint.

At the carpus, the ulna lies laterally and the radius medially, and the **styloid processes** at the end of each lie on either side of the first row of carpal bones.

The **carpus**, or wrist, consists of two rows of small bones held together by numerous ligaments. The **accessory carpal bone** projects from the ventral aspect of the carpus, and provides a point for muscle attachment.

The **metacarpus** of the dog consists of four long metacarpal bones.

There are five digits in the forelimb of the dog and cat, the innermost (digit I) being the dew claw, which attaches to the carpus, not to a metacarpal bone.

Each digit (toe) consists of three phalanges (Fig. 14.26): the proximal (or first) phalanx, middle (or second) and distal (third). The toes are numbered from the medial side in Roman numerals.

The first and second phalanges are relatively simple long bones, but the third phalanx carries the ungual process that forms the core of the nail.

Behind the metacarpo-phalangeal joint and the distal inter-phalangeal joint are pairs of small sesamoid bones. These are bones that form within a tendon to ease the passage of that tendon over a joint.

The Hindlimb

The pelvis

The two pelvic bones are in fact each formed from three large and one very small bone. The three large bones are the **ilium**, the **ischium** and the **pubis**, and the small bone the **acetabular** bone.

The two pelvic bones are attached to the sacrum, and join each other in the midline at the **pubic symphysis**, so forming the floor of the pelvic cavity.

Lateral to the pubic symphysis on each side is a large hole, the **obturator foramen**, which allows blood vessels and nerves to pass out of the pelvic cavity into the hindlimb.

Parts of the pelvic bone that can be palpated on the live dog include the wing of the ilium and the **ischial tuberosity**, which is the origin of the biceps femoris muscle.

The pelvis articulates with the femur at the **hip joint**, a ball-and-socket joint and therefore very mobile—it allows flexion and extension, adduction and abduction and rotation of the femur. The socket for the hip joint is the **acetabulum**. The head of the femur is held in the socket by the **round ligament**, which attaches to the non-articular area in the centre of the acetabulum, the **acetabular fossa**.

The femur

The femur has a head, a neck, greater and lesser tubercles, a shaft, and lateral and medial condyles. (The hip joint has been discussed above.) **The stifle joint**, at the articulation of femur with tibia and fibula, has been called the most complex joint in the body (Fig. 14.12).

When studying the dry bones, this articulation looks most unstable, but the soft tissues round and in the joint make it very stable, and relatively resistant to injury (considering its position and the stresses put upon it.)

The stifle joint is stabilised by four ligaments. The **cruciate ligaments** run across from tibia to femur within the joint, and stop the bones sliding forward and back on one another. The strong collateral ligaments on either side of the joint prevent sideways movement.

Two **menisci** cushion the bones, and increase the area for articulation as they move back and forth as the bones move on each other.

Three **sesamoid bones** are also associated with the stifle joint:

- The **patella**, which lies in the tendon of the quadriceps muscle (which inserts on the top of the tibial crest).
- Two **fabellae**, which lie on the caudal aspect of the distal femur, within the origins of the two bellies of gastrocnemius.

The tibia and fibula

The tibia and fibula lie together. The tibia is much the larger bone and has a flat articular surface proximally, for articulation with the femur at the stifle joint. The fibula lies lateral to the tibia throughout its length.

On the front of the tibia is the **tibial crest**, which provides a broad area for muscle attachment.

The tarsus

Like the carpus, the tarsus is made up of a number of small bones closely attached to one another. Two of special significance are the tibial tarsal and the fibular tarsal bones. These two bones form the articular surface for the tibia and fibula at the hock joint. The fibular tarsal bone, or **calcaneus**, is enlarged to form the point of the hock—the point of attachment for the Achilles tendon.

The metatarsus and digits

The metatarsus and digits of the hindlimb are very similar to those of the forelimb, except that the dew claw is often absent, leaving only digits II to V.

The splanchnic skeleton

The os penis, the bone of the penis, has a groove in it that surrounds the urethra within the penis. In the dog, the groove is on the ventral side of the bone, whereas in the cat (owing to the different position of the penis) the groove is dorsal.

The Muscular System

Muscle tissue

There are three types of muscle tissue (Fig. 14.20):

- Skeletal (striated or voluntary) muscle
- Smooth (unstriated or involuntary) muscle
- Cardiac muscle.

Skeletal muscle is found attached to the bones of the body. It is under the control of the animal, and so is also called voluntary muscle.

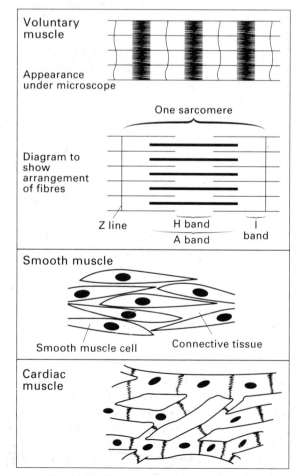

Fig. 14.20. The structure of muscle tissue.

The cells of striated muscle are called muscle fibres, and they lie parallel to one another in bundles, bound together by connective tissue. Groups of bundles together then make up the whole muscle, which is surrounded by a muscle sheath

Smooth muscle is found throughout the body. It is found, for example, in the bowel, in the walls of blood vessels, in the walls of the bladder and uterus and in the respiratory tract. Smooth muscle is not under voluntary or conscious control.

The cells of smooth muscle are spindle-shaped, and have less connective tissue associated with them than does striated muscle.

Cardiac muscle, as its name implies, is found only within the heart. The cells are short and cylindrical, and are bound together by connective tissue. The cells are arranged longitudinally, as in voluntary muscle, and contract automatically and rhythmically throughout life—they are not under voluntary control.

Muscle Contraction

Muscle contraction occurs as a result of the stimulation of a fibre by a nerve impulse. Muscle fibres are made of thick and thin fibres: the thick fibres are of the protein **myosin**, and the thin ones of **actin**.

In striated muscle the different types of fibres are arranged so that they overlap. Where there are thick myosin fibres, or where the actin and myosin fibres overlap, the tissue looks dark, but where there are just actin fibres the tissue appears lighter in colour. The alternating light and dark bands give rise to the name striated or striped muscle.

There are numerous attachments between the actin and myosin, and when the muscle contracts the attachments break and reform as the myosin and actin fibrils slide along one another, so shortening the muscle fibre.

All the muscle fibres that are activated by a single nerve fibre are termed a **motor unit**. The size of the motor unit varies throughout the body: a muscle that makes small, intricate movements will consist of very small motor units, whereas a muscle performing only large movements may have 200 or more fibres innervated by a single nerve fibre.

Muscles are nearly always in a state of slight tension, which is called **muscle tone**:

- **Isometric** contraction inceases muscle tone without shortening the muscle.
- **Isotonic** contraction shortens a muscle without changing its tension.

To retain its tone a muscle must be used constantly. Muscles that are not used tend to get weak and lose muscle fibres (**atrophy**), whereas a muscle that is constantly and vigorously exercised will hypertrophy (get bigger).

Muscles, Tendons, Bursae and Sesamoid Bones

Muscles may be the classic 'muscle shape' or they may be in the form of flat sheets. They may have one origin or starting point and one insertion on bone; or there may be several muscle bellies (the thick, fleshy, central part of a muscle) inserting together at one point, in which case the muscle is said to have two or more heads.

The muscle sheath which surrounds each muscle may be quite delicate, or it may be thick and fibrous. The muscle sheath continues at each end of the muscles into the dense fibrous tissue of the tendons of origin and insertion of the muscle. (To avoid confusion: a ligament runs from bone to bone, whereas a tendon runs from muscle to bone.)

Muscles may have very short tendons, and appear to start or end with the fleshy part of the muscle, or they may have long tendons attaching the belly to the bone. Examples of the latter are the long muscles of the limbs of the dog, where the tendon of insertion may be longer than the muscle belly itself.

Where the muscle is in the form of a flat sheet, the tendon is drawn out into a fibrous sheet as well—this is then called an **aponeurosis**.

A **bursa** is a cavity lined with synovial membrane, and filled with synovial fluid, that lies between tendons and bone, or between tendon and tendon, to minimise friction between the structures as they move backwards and forwards. If a bursa wraps itself completely round a tendon, it is called a **synovial sheath**.

'**Acquired**' **bursae** may form on, for example, the point of the elbow or hock in large dogs, particularly those that habitually lie on hard surfaces. A bursa forms to protect the bony prominence from the constant friction with the ground.

Sesamoid bones are small bones that form within a tendon, to ease the passage of that tendon over a joint. Examples are the **patella**, and the **proximal and distal sesamoids** in the paws.

Skeletal Muscle Groups

This section deals only briefly with the most important muscle groups in the body. Wherever possible, the text should be related to a skeleton to help understand the muscles' positions, and palpation of the muscles of a good-natured dog will help in appreciating their positions and actions in the live animal.

Intrinsic and extrinsic muscles

Intrinsic muscles lie completely within one region of the body (the head, the trunk or a limb) and alter the position of parts of that region of the body—for example they close an eye, bend the spine or curl a toe.

Extrinsic muscles run from one region of the body to another, and alter the position of one region in relation to another—for example they turn the head on the neck or pull a limb forward in relation to the trunk.

Muscles of the Head

The muscles of the head can be categorised as follows:

- the muscles of facial expression
- the muscles of mastication
- the eye muscles
- muscles of the tongue, pharynx, larynx and soft palate
- extrinsic muscles of the head.

The **muscles of facial expression** are formed from a single sheet of muscle. There are muscles that raise the lips (to snarl), move the ears, move the eyelids and nostrils. All these muscles are innervated by the facial nerve (cranial nerve VII), and damage to this nerve will result in flaccid paralysis of these muscles.

The main **muscles of mastication** are:

- **Digastricus**, the jaw-opening muscle which runs from the mandible to the base of the skull.
- **Temporalis**, one of the jaw closing muscles, which fills the temporal fossa of the skull and inserts on the medial side of the vertical ramus of the mandible.
- **Masseter**, the other jaw-closing muscle, which runs from the zygomatic arch to the lateral side of the vertical ramus of the mandible.
- **Medial and lateral pterygoids**, which produce side-to-side movement of the lower jaw. This is important in the carnivores for pushing the carnassial teeth against the lower molars so that they can have an effective scissor action. In herbivores these muscles are much larger and produce the grinding action of the molars against one another.

The **eye muscles** enable the eye to be moved up and down or from side to side, and to be drawn back into the socket (which allows the third eyelid to move across the eye). There is also a small amount of rotatory movement. The eye muscles are:

- medial, lateral, dorsal and ventral rectus
- retractor oculi
- dorsal and ventral oblique.

Muscles of the tongue may be intrinsic or extrinsic. The intrinsic muscles of the tongue allow it to curl up, flatten out or move from side to side, while the extrinsic muscles draw it forwards or backwards or lift it towards the roof of the mouth.

Muscles of the pharynx, larynx and soft palate allow the movements needed for voice production, respiration and swallowing.

The extrinsic muscles of the head move the head on the neck.

Vertebral Column Muscles

The vertebral column muscles are divided into:

- **Epaxial muscles** above the vertebral column
- **Hypaxial muscles** below the vertebral column.

The **epaxial** muscles attach to the pelvis, the sacrum, the vertebrae and the ribs. Some of these muscles are long, running a good proportion of the length of the spine, and some are short, spanning only two or four vertebrae. They support the spine, help to move the spine as the animal runs, support the weight of the head and neck and tail, and allow a certain amount of rotation between the vertebrae.

The **hypaxial** muscles are less bulky than the epaxials—they do not have to support the vertebral column, head and neck. They act to flex the lumbar spine as the animal runs, and to bend the neck downwards.

Muscles of the thorax

The most important muscles of the thorax are the **internal and external intercostals**. These run from rib to rib, and are important muscles of respiration.

The diaphragm

The **diaphragm** (Fig. 14.21) separates the thoracic from the abdominal cavity. It is made up as follows:

- A peripheral muscle that occupies the outer part of the diaphragm
- A central tendon

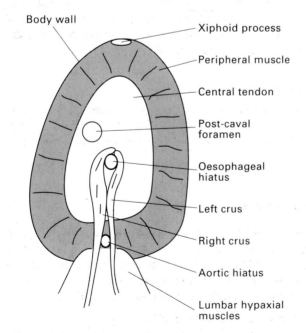

Fig. 14.21. The structure of the diaphragm and the structures that pass through it (viewed as if from the abdomen, with the dog lying on its back).

- Two muscular crura—the right crus being larger than the left.

There are three holes where structures pass through the diaphragm:

- the **post-caval foramen**, carrying the posterior vena cava.
- **the oesophageal hiatus**, carrying the oesophagus and the vagal nerves
- the **aortic hiatus**, carrying the aorta, the azygos vein and the thoracic duct.

Abdominal muscles

There are four muscles on each side of the body that together make up the abdominal wall:

- **External abdominal oblique**
- **Internal abdominal oblique**
- **Transversus abdominis**
- **Rectus abdominis**.

The main function of the abdominal wall is to enclose and protect the abdominal viscera. The four abdominal muscles are so arranged that all their fibres run in different directions, so giving the abdominal wall great strength.

Each abdominal muscle (except rectus abdominis) ends in a sheet of aponeurosis, and all the sheets join in the ventral midline to form the **linea alba** (white line).

Because of the different origins of the muscles there is a small area in the groin where there is no muscle in the wall, merely a sheet of fascia (part of the aponeurosis of external abdominal oblique). In this area there is a small hole or slit known as the **inguinal ring**, which carries the structures in the spermatic cord to and from the scrotum, and allows blood vessels out of the abdomen to supply the mammary glands and external genitalia. **Hernias** are quite common in this region, as the inguinal ring may enlarge, producing a hole that will let other structures such as bladder and uterus out of the abdomen, to lie subcutaneously in the groin or on the medial aspect of the thigh.

The **rectus abdominis** muscle has its origin on the first rib, and inserts on what is called the pre-pubic tendon on the front of the pubis, next to the pubic symphysis. It supports the abdominal cavity and also helps to flex the lumbar spine.

Muscles of the forelimb

The extrinsic muscles of the forelimb attach the forelimb to the trunk. Among them are:

- **trapezii** (singular trapezius) which run from the spine of the scapula to the dorsal midline, and support the limb on the body
- **brachiocephalicus**, which runs from the anterior aspect of the humerus to the base of the skull, and either bends the neck, or brings forward or

protracts the forelimb (depending on the action of other muscles and whether the forelimb is on the ground)

- **latissimus dorsi**, which runs from the humerus to form a large fan of muscle attached to the dorsal midline—it retracts the forelimb (pulls it backwards)
- **pectorals**, which run from the humerus round the front of the thorax to the sternum and ribs. The pectorals are adductors: they hold the forelimb in close to the body.

Muscles of the shoulder

- **supraspinatus** runs from the supraspinous fossa of the scapula to the greater tuberosity of the humerus and extends the shoulder
- **infraspinatus** runs from the infraspinous fossa of the scapula to the lesser tuberosity of the humerus, and helps support the shoulder joint.

Muscles of the elbow

- **triceps** is a four-headed muscle that originates from the scapula and humerus, and inserts on the olecranon of the ulna. It extends the elbow joint
- **biceps brachii** runs from the bicipital or scapular tuberosity, and inserts on the ulna. It flexes the elbow
- **brachialis** originates just beneath the head of the humerus and inserts with biceps brachii. It too flexes the elbow.

Muscles of the carpus and digits

Although there are many small muscles within the paw, most of the action of flexing and extending the carpus and digits is performed by eight muscles:

- two carpal flexors
- two carpal extensors
- two digital flexors
- two digital extensors.

To help understand these muscles, look at a forearm (either of a dog or your own) and locate the proximal and distal ends of the radius and ulna. The ulna (starting at the olecranon) starts ventral and ends up lateral, and the radius starts dorsal and ends up medial.

You will notice that there are two masses of muscle—one dorso-lateral, and one ventro-medial.

The dorso-lateral muscle mass consists of the two carpal extensors (originating on the humerus and inserting in the carpal region) and two digital extensors (originating on the humerus and inserting on the third phalanx).

The ventro-medial muscle mass contains the two carpal flexors and two digital flexors. The superficial digital flexor inserts in the second phalanx, and the deep digital flexor on the third phalanx.

Muscles of the Hindlimb

The very mobile ball-and-socket joint of the hip is moved by a number of relatively short muscles at the top of the leg, among them the gluteal muscles that make up the muscle mass of the curve of the rump.

The hamstring group consists of three muscles that lie on the caudal aspect of the thigh, but act together on the hip, stifle and hock joints to extend the whole limb backwards, providing the main propulsive force in the running animal.

The hamstring group consists of:

- **Biceps femoris**, the most lateral of the group
- **Semitendinosis**
- **Semimembranosus**, the most medial of the group.

Other important muscles of the upper part of the hindlimb are:

- **Quadriceps femoris**, the bulky muscle that runs down the front of the thigh. It extends the stifle.
- **The Adductor group**, on the inside of the thigh, that hold the limb in towards the body.

The **Achilles tendon** runs down the back of the shank to the point of the hock (the tuber calcis). It includes the tendons of **superficial digital flexor**, which runs over the point of the hock and then on down towards the digits, and also the tendons of **gastrocnemius**, **biceps femoris** and **semitendinosis**, which all insert on the tubor calcis.

Muscles of the hock

- **Anterior tibial** is the main flexor of the hock—it arises from the proximal end of the tibia, on the side of the tibial crest, and inserts on the tarsus.
- **Gastrocnemius** is the main extensor of the hock (along with the hamstrings). It arises from the ventral aspect of the distal part of the femur, and inserts on the tuber calcis. It forms the muscular bulge at the top of the calf.

Muscles of the digits

The muscles of the digits of the hindlimb are very similar to those of the digits of the forelimb, except that there are three digital extensors and two digital flexors.

The Integument

The integument is the covering of the body. It includes the skin, hair or feathers, and the claws or nails. It blends with the mucous membrane at the various natural openings of the body.

In mammals, the skin has several functions:

- It protects the surface of the body.
- It protects the body against invasion by micro-organisms.
- It plays a part in temperature control.

- It helps prevent excessive water loss (or, in the case of aquatic mammals, water uptake) by the body.
- It manufactures vitamin D.
- The hair and the pigment in the skin protect the body from the harmful effects of ultraviolet radiation.
- It contains pressure, temperature and pain receptors and so can be thought of a sense organ.
- It contains glands (sebaceous and sweat glands) and so has a secretory function.

Epidermis, Dermis and Hypodermis

There are three distinct layers to the skin:

- The **epidermis**
- The **dermis**
- The **hypodermis**.

The epidermis

The epidermis (Fig. 14.22) is the most superficial layer of the skin, and is made of **stratified squamous epithelium**. It consists of four layers, or strata:

- stratum germinativum;
- stratum granulosum;
- stratum lucidum;
- stratum corneum.

   The whole of the epidermis is avascular (i.e. contains no blood vessels at all).

   The deepest layer of the epidermis is the basal cell layer, or **stratum basale**, also known as the **stratum germinativum**. In this layer the cells divide rapidly. Between the basal skin cells are the **melanocytes** that give colour to skin. This deep layer of the epidermis rests on the **dermal papillae**, which are deeper and more numerous where the skin is thickest and most liable to trauma (e.g. in the pads).

   The next layer of epidermal cells is the **stratum granulosum**, where the cells are starting to flatten and become infiltrated with the protein keratin.

   Above this is the **stratum lucidum**, where the skin cells start to lose their nuclei. The top layer is the

stratum corneum, where the process of keratinisation is complete, and the cellular outlines have disappeared.

The Dermis

The dermis, deep to the epidermis and firmly attached to it, consists of vascular dense connective tissue. It also contains elastic fibres, nerve fibres and the sensory nerve endings of the skin. It is invaded by hair follicles, sweat and sebaceous glands, which grow downwards from the epidermis.

The Hypodermis

The hypodermis, beneath the dermis, is not truly part of the skin: it consists of loose connective tissue, often infiltrated by fat.

Hair

Hair is formed from epidermis that firstly extends down into dermal tissue to form a 'hair cone' over a piece of dermis called the **dermal** or **hair papilla** (Fig. 14.23). As the hair starts to grow from the hair cone, the epidermal cells around and above it are destroyed, so leaving an open channel or hair follicle for the hair. The hair then grows continuously until it dies and becomes detached from its hair cone. The hair may be shed then, or may stay attached to the skin, supported by hairs around it, until it is combed out.

   Associated with each hair follicle is a **sebaceous gland**. This is a coiled gland that opens off the side of the follicle and secretes sebum. The functions of sebum are:

- to lubricate and waterproof the hairs
- to produce a smell that is thought to act as a territorial marker (the distinctive smell of a wet dog is due to sebum.).
- to produce pheromones, which play a part in attracting the opposite sex.

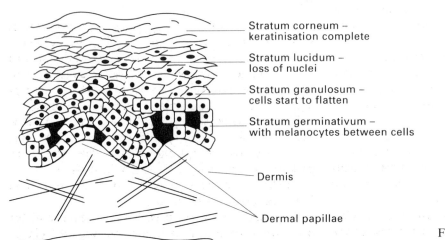

Stratum corneum – keratinisation complete

Stratum lucidum – loss of nuclei

Stratum granulosum – cells start to flatten

Stratum germinativum – with melanocytes between cells

Dermis

Dermal papillae

Hypodermis

Fig. 14.22. The structure of the epidermis.

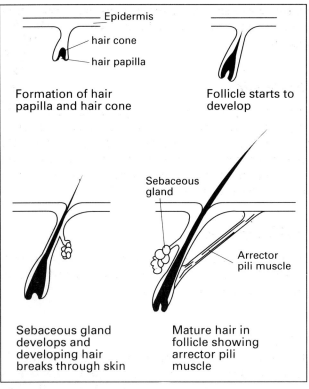

Epidermis
hair cone
hair papilla

Formation of hair papilla and hair cone

Follicle starts to develop

Sebaceous gland

Arrector pili muscle

Sebaceous gland develops and developing hair breaks through skin

Mature hair in follicle showing arrector pili muscle

Fig. 14.23. The formation of hair.

There are three types of hair:

- Guard hairs
- Undercoat (wool hairs)
- Vibrissae.

The **guard hairs** are the long hairs of the topcoat and provide the waterproof layer of the coat. Only one guard hair grows from each follicle. Associated with each guard hair is an involuntary **arrector pili** muscle, which raises the hair from its resting position. This happens as a result of exposure to cold or, in the case of the dog, when the hackles are raised. It may also be seen when a cat goes into a threat stance with a 'bottlebrush' tail.

The **wool hairs**, or undercoat, provide an insulating layer of shorter, softer hairs beneath the topcoat. They trap air between them, and so keep the body warm. Wool hairs make up the main part of the 'puppy' coat, and in the adult there are more of them in the winter than in the summer coat.

There may be many wool hairs growing from a single follicle with its guard hair. The chinchilla, which has no guard hairs except on its tail, has the densest coat known, with up to seventy wool hairs growing from each hair follicle.

Density of coat varies over the body and with the individual and breed. Generally, hair is more sparse on the underside of the body, and what there is tends to be mainly guard hairs, with less undercoat than on the top of the body.

The **vibrissae**, or tactile hairs, are even thicker than guard hairs, and project beyond the rest of the coat (Fig. 14.24). They grow from specialised

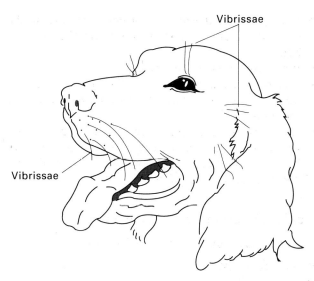

Fig. 14.24. Vibrissae.

follicles that project deep into the hypodermis. At their base they have nerve endings that respond to the movements of the hair. In this way the vibrissae are important sensory organs, particularly in the cat, but also in the dog, and should never be cut without good reason.

Most vibrissae are found round the head—on the upper lip and above the eyes. Dogs also have a substantial tuft on the cheek, and cats have a tuft on the carpus as well.

Moulting

Moulting is the seasonal shedding of hair. Most dogs shed during spring and autumn, although many household pets shed to some extent all the year round. This is due to the effect of household living, with central heating and possibly electric lighting upsetting the normal stimuli of seasonal temperature change and increase or decrease of photoperiod (day length). Cats moult most heavily in the spring, then less heavily throughout summer and autumn.

Pads

The epidermis of the footpads of dogs and cats is very thick and hairless (Fig. 14.25). The dermis is similarly thickened, is very vascular and contains adipose tissue. This forms a '**digital cushion**' that supports the foot and provides some shock absorption as the feet of the running animal hit the ground.

The **rhinarium** or nosepad is also thick, keratinised and hairless. Like the fingerprints of people, each dog's nose gives a unique print that reflects the pattern of dermal papillae beneath the surface.

Unlike the hairy skin of the dog, the nose and footpads contain sweat glands.

Dogs and cats have on each foot a main pad (or metacarpal/metatarsal pad) and four digital pads. In addition, there is on the forelimb a digital pad on the dew claw (digit I), and a carpal pad covering the accessory carpal bone.

Claws

The horny part of a nail is modified epidermis, and grows from a specialised part of the epidermis called the **coronary border** or **coronary band**, which lies underneath a fold of skin, the **claw fold**.

The claw grows in two sheets which form the walls of the claw, and cover the **ungual process** of the third phalanx.

The **sole**, in the groove between the two walls of the claw, is made of softer horn.

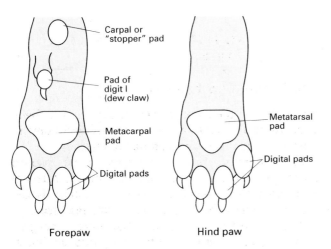

Fig. 14.25. Ventral view of dog's (a) forepaw and (b) hind paw, showing footpads.

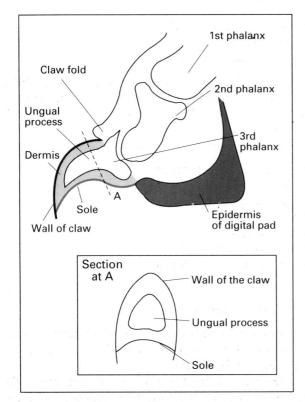

Fig. 14.26. Longitudinal section of dog's toe, showing claw.

The dermis lies between the horn and the third phalanx, and provides the blood and nerve supply to the claw. Trimming of claws should be done with great care so as not to cut into the sensitive dermis.

The claws of the cat are held retracted and are only extended by the action of the digital flexor muscles, which pull the claw forwards against the pull of two little **elastic ligaments** that run from the third to the second phalanx and hold the claws off the ground.

Sweat Glands

Sweat glands, or sudiferous glands, are epidermal structures but lie deep within the dermis, not alongside the hair follicle. They are coiled glands, and in the dog and cat they are only found on the hairless epidermal areas, i.e. the nose and footpads.

Mammary Glands

Mammary glands (mammae) (Fig. 14.27) are really modified sweat glands. Bitches usually have five pairs of glands and queens have four pairs, though the number is variable.

Mammary glands develop in the embryo from **mammary ridges** that run from the axilla to the groin. A **teat papilla** develops on the surface of the body, then solid epidermal buds or 'sprouts' grow downwards into the hypodermis and branch. When the branching system has been well established, the epidermal tissue hollows to produce the duct system of the gland. Rudimentary teats are found in the males of most but not all mammal species.

Mammary tissue consists of glandular tissue surrounded by fibrous connective tissue and fat. During pregnancy it becomes active and hypertrophies, and towards the end of the pregnancy it starts to produce mammary secretion. The teats hypertrophy as well, so they stand up proud from the skin that by the time the young are born, and are easily found by the pups or kittens.

There are two ways of naming the mammary glands, particularly of bitches, where mastectomy for neoplasia is a common operation. The anatomist's terminology describes two thoracic pairs, two abdominal pairs and one inguinal pair. Some clinicians name them as three thoracic and two either abdominal or inguinal and this terminology relates to the lymphatic drainage of the glands. The front three pairs drain into the axillary lymph node, and the posterior two pairs into the superficial inguinal lymph node.

Milk

The first milk produced is the colostrum, which is important in many species as a source of antibodies for the young (Chapter 19).

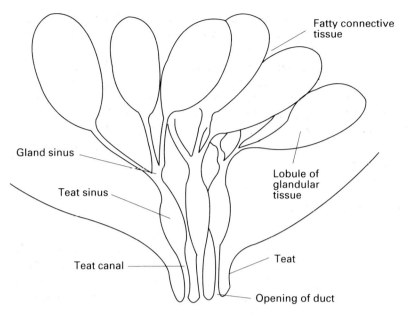

Fatty connective tissue

Gland sinus

Teat sinus

Lobule of glandular tissue

Teat canal

Teat

Opening of duct

Fig. 14.27. Section through a mammary gland.

In the bitch and queen, antibodies are produced over a period of days, but the bowel ceases to absorb various antibodies at different times. As a general rule, all pups and kittens should have sucked within eight hours—and preferably four hours—of birth. Ideally, the young should find themselves a teat as soon as the mother has finished cleaning them.

Milk contains fats, protein, and carbohydrate as the milk sugar lactose. Solids may make up less than 20% or more than 70% of the content of the milk, depending on species. Milk also contains calcium, phosphate, magnesium, sodium and chloride, vitamins A, E and K, and the B vitamins.

Specialised sebaceous glands

These epidermal structures include:

- tail glands
- circum-anal glands
- glands of the anal sacs.

The **tail glands** are a group of sebaceous glands that lie on the dorsal surface of the tail in the dog. Particularly in middle-aged and elderly dogs, the hair may get very sparse in this area and hypertrophy of the glandular area may occur until the tail looks swollen. The glandular secretion lying on the surface may smell, and cause irritation to the dog.

The **circum-anal glands** are sebaceous glands that form a ring around the anus, where their ducts drain into the ducts of modified sweat glands. It is thought that it is the secretion from these glands that dogs smell when they sniff each other's anal areas.

The **anal sacs** are small sacs with ducts leading to the exterior. They lie beneath the skin on either side and just below the anus. The lining of these sacs contains numerous modified sebaceous glands that produce the foul-smelling anal sac secretion, which in the normal animal is squeezed out a little at a time on to the surface of faeces as the animal defecates, and so acts as a territorial marker.

The Respiratory System

Respiration is the gaseous exchange between a living structure (be it plant or animal) and its environment. Respiration may be either external or internal.

External respiration in an animal is the gaseous exchange between the air and the blood. **Internal respiration**, also known as tissue respiration, is the gaseous exchange between the blood and the tissues.

The respiratory system transports oxygen-containing air from outside the body into the lungs, where it can be absorbed into the bloodstream.

The composition of inspired air is:

- Nitrogen: 79%
- Oxygen: 21%
- Carbon dioxide: 0.04%
- Water vapour
- Other gases: traces only.

In expired air the oxygen is down to about 16%, the carbon dioxide has risen to about 4–5%, and the water vapour may have increased. The other gases are unchanged.

The respiratory system consists of:

- the nose and nasal chamber
- the pharynx
- the larynx
- the trachea
- the bronchi
- the bronchioles
- the alveolar ducts and alveoli.

The Nasal Chamber

The nasal chamber extends from the **external nares**, or nostrils, to the **internal nares** where the air enters the pharynx (Fig. 14.28).

The nasal chamber is divided into left and right chambers by a cartilagenous **nasal septum**, and these are partly filled by the dorsal and ventral **naso**

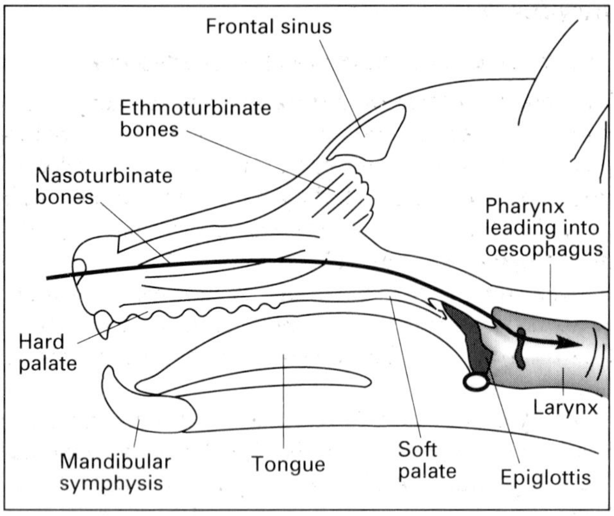

Fig. 14.28. Midline section through dog's head, to show the respiratory passage.

turbinate bones, which arise from the dorsolateral wall of the chamber and are covered with ciliated mucous membrane. The function of the nasal turbinates and their coverings is to moisten, warm and filter the air that passes over them, so that it is warm, moist and clean before passing into the lower respiratory tract.

From the nasal chamber the air passes across the pharynx and into the larynx at the top of the trachea. The **pharynx** is the name given to the area at the back of the mouth used by both the respiratory and digestive tracts. The openings into the pharynx are:

- the nasal chamber
- the mouth
- the two **Eustachian tubes** from the middle ear
- the oesophagus
- the larynx.

Paranasal Sinuses

Sinuses are air-filled cavities within a bone, lined with ciliated mucous epithelium and having drainage, usually into the nasal chamber.

The dog has only one true sinus—the **frontal sinus**—within the frontal bone of the skull. The **maxillary sinus** in the dog is not a true sinus, as it is not enclosed within a single bone—it is merely a recess at the caudal end of each nasal chamber, between the maxillary and palatine bones. Other species, particularly the large herbivores (horses and cattle), have many paranasal sinuses that lighten an otherwise heavy and massive skull.

The Larynx

The larynx is a rigid, hollow structure made up of a number of cartilages. It forms the opening to the lower part of the respiratory tract, and is also the 'voice box' for the production of sound. It is attached

to the skull by the **hyoid apparatus** (see Fig. 14.39), which allows it to move backwards and forwards between its two arms like the seat of a swing.

The opening at the front of the larynx is called the **glottis**. When the larynx moves forwards (during swallowing) this opening is closed by the elastic cartilage of the **epiglottis**. When the larynx moves backwards to its resting position, the epiglottis falls forward and the glottis is open again.

In its resting position the tip of the broadly triangular epiglottis lies above the **soft palate**, so that there is a continuous open passage for air from the nasal chambers to the larynx.

The vocal folds

Inside the larynx there is a pair of folds of mucous membrane that can lie against the walls of the larynx, or contract and partially obstruct the larynx. These are the **vocal folds**. The leading edge of these folds contains a muscle, and this leading edge is sometimes termed the **vocal cord**. The vocal folds project into the larynx at an angle so that there is a cavity behind them, which is known as the **lateral ventricle**. It is this mechanism that is responsible for the production of sound.

The Trachea

The trachea is a permanently open tube that runs from the laryngeal cartilages through the thoracic inlet into the thorax, where just above the heart it divides into the right and left bronchi.

It is made up of a series of incomplete rings of hyaline cartilage separated by fibrous connective tissue and smooth muscle fibres, and lined with ciliated mucous epithelium.

The open part of each tracheal ring is on the dorsal aspect and it has been suggested that this enable the oesophagus, lying above it, to expand without hindrance when a large bolus of food passes along it.

The Bronchi and Bronchioles

The bronchi are similar in structure to the trachea. Each bronchus divides to enter one of the lobes of the lungs, and then the air passages continue to divide throughout the lung substance, getting smaller with each division. In the very small bronchioles the cartilage gets very sparse, and eventually disappears altogether. The structure of air passages formed by this division is called the bronchial tree.

The Lungs

The lungs are two large spongy organs that lie in the thorax on either side of the **mediastinum**. Each lung is divided into lobes—the left into three and the right into four lobes (Fig. 14.29). On the right lung these are called:

- the apical (or **cranial**) lobe
- the cardiac (or **middle**) lobe
- the diaphragmatic (or **caudal**) lobe
- the **accessory** lobe.

The left lung does not have an accessory lobe.

The Terminal Air Passages

The smallest of the bronchioles are called the **respiratory** or **terminal bronchioles** (Fig. 14.30). They have no cartilage in their walls, and no cilia on their epithelium. Each of them gives rise to two or three **alveolar ducts** and each duct terminates in an **alveolar sac**. Each alveolar sac is divided into **alveoli**, which make up the soft tissue of the lung. The alveoli are where the gaseous exchange takes place, and are very well supplied with blood.

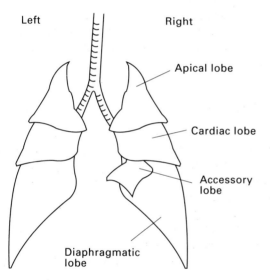

Fig. 14.29. The lobes of the lungs.

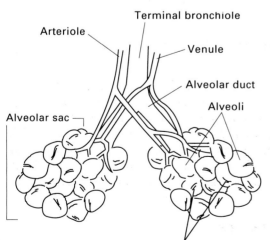

Fig. 14.30. The terminal air passages.

Respiration

The muscles and movements of respiration

The main muscles of inspiration are the diaphragm and the external intercostals. Expiration is mainly passive, caused by the relaxation of the muscles of inspiration, but is assisted by the internal intercostals and, in the case of forced expiration, by the abdominal muscles as well.

The lung tissue contains no muscle: it cannot expand on its own. It is, however, very elastic tissue that returns to a collapsed state when there is nothing to expand it forcibly.

The lungs lie within and nearly fill the thoracic cavity. The pleural cavity that lies between them and the body wall contains nothing but a little pleural fluid.

When an animal breathes in, it increases the volume of the thoracic cavity by flattening the diaphragm, increasing the length of the thorax, and by swinging the ribs out so as to increase the diameter of the thorax. Because of the vacuum between the lungs and the chest wall, the lungs are forced to expand to fill the enlarged thoracic cavity and so air is drawn into the bronchial tree and so into the lung tissue.

When the animal breathes out, the diaphragm is relaxed (decreasing the length of the chest) and the ribs fall back to their resting position (reducing the diameter of the ribcage). As the lungs collapse to their resting volume, air is expelled from the respiratory tract.

The control of respiration

The **respiratory centres** are in the hindbrain, in the pons and the medulla. One centre is responsible for inspiration (the apneustic centre), one for expiration, and one prevents over-inflation of the lungs. **Stretch receptors** in the walls of the bronchioles feed information to these centres on the degree of inflation of the bronchial tree (the **Hering–Breuer reflex**).

The rate of respiration is also controlled by centres in the medulla that monitor the pH of the blood. If respiration is too slow or too shallow, carbon dioxide builds up in the blood and in the form of carbonic acid decreases the pH of the blood (and of the cerebrospinal fluid, which is what is directly monitored). The respiratory pacemaker is then stimulated to increase the rate and depth of respiration to blow off the surplus carbon dioxide and restore the pH of the blood to its correct level.

There are also chemoreceptors in the walls of arteries (the **aortic** and **carotid bodies**) that respond to changing levels of oxygen and carbon dioxide in the blood and influence the medullary respiratory centre accordingly.

Respiratory rate and lung capacity

When animals are at rest and breathing quietly, they are only using a small fraction of their total lung capacity. The **resting respiratory rate** in the dog varies between about 10 and 30 breaths per minute (depending on the size of the dog). In the cat it is between 20 and 30 breaths per minute.

The amount of air breathed in and out during quiet respiration is called the **tidal volume**. If there is a forced intake of breath, the extra air drawn into the lungs in addition to the normal tidal volume is called the **inspiratory reserve volume**. The tidal volume plus the inspiratory reserve volume is called the **inspiratory capacity**.

A forced exhalation after quiet respiration will give the **expiratory reserve volume**, and this plus the normal tidal volume will give the **expiratory capacity**. However, even after the hardest possible expiration, there is still some air left in the lungs—this is the **residual volume**. The **functional residual capacity** is the air left in the lungs after quiet expiration, which allows gaseous diffusion to carry on during expiration.

Dead space is the volume of air drawn in at each respiration that never reaches the alveoli—i.e. it is the volume of the trachea, the bronchi and the bronchioles.

Blood and the Circulatory System.

The **blood-vascular** or **circulatory system** is a system of tubes distributed throughout the body to allow the circulation of blood. The **lymphatic system** is closely allied to the blood vascular system and carries lymph, which is essentially excess tissue fluid, from the periphery back to the circulation.

The **heart** is part of the blood vascular system. It is a folded and elaborate piece of muscular tubing that is modified to form a four-chambered pump.

The blood circulation can be divided into **pulmonary** and **systemic** parts. The pulmonary circulation takes deoxygenated blood from the heart through the lungs, where it is oxygenated, and returns it to the heart. The systemic circulation takes oxygenated blood from the heart to the rest of the body, where the oxygen is used by the tissues. It then returns the deoxygenated blood to the heart.

An **artery** is a relatively large vessel carrying blood away from the heart, whether it is in the pulmonary or the systemic circulation (Fig. 14.31). Arteries have relatively thick walls, which contain smooth muscle, and can constrict or dilate to allow a greater or lesser flow of blood to a particular organ.

As the arteries divide they get smaller in diameter. These smaller arteries, called **arterioles**, lie within the organs they are supplying with blood.

Within the tissues themselves the blood vessels become very small and very thin-walled, so as to allow oxygen exchange—these are the **capillaries**.

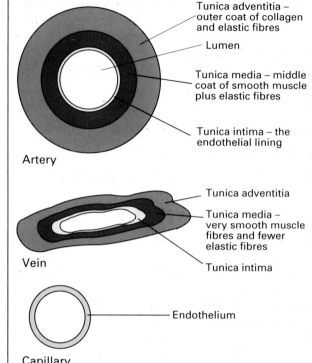

Fig. 14.31. The structures of an artery, a vein and a capillary.

The capillaries form a network (the **capillary bed**) within the tissue.

A **vein** is a relatively large, thin-walled vessel, carrying blood towards the heart. A **venule** is a small vein within an organ, receiving blood from the capillary bed.

As well as being thinner walled than arteries, veins also have valves, which offer no resistance to the flow of blood towards the heart but prevent any back flow. These valves are most numerous in the veins of the limbs, and quite sparse in the veins of the internal organs.

Veins and arteries have a similar structure. Both have an outer fibrous coat, a middle layer composed of muscular and elastic fibres, and an inner lining membrane of elastic fibres and flattened epithelial cells.

Although most tissues are supplied by a network of capillaries, there are three organs within the body that have a system of end arteries instead. End arteries are capillaries that branch like the branches and twigs of a tree, getting smaller all the time but never joining up with one another. The organs that have end arteries rather than a capillary bed are the brain, the heart and the kidneys.

The reason for end arteries in these organs is thought to be protection against sudden drops in blood pressure, for example after blood loss. All the other organs of the body can survive a period of vasoconstriction and poor blood supply, while the available oxygenated blood is diverted to these three vital organs.

This system does have a disadvantage as well, in that obstruction of a vessel (for example with a blood clot) will cause the death of the tissue supplied by that vessel, whereas in a network capillary bed there are many routes for blood to reach each section of tissue.

The Functions of Blood

The functions of blood are:

- to carry oxygen to and carbon dioxide away from the tissues.
- to carry digested food products to the tissues
- to supply water to the tissues
- to carry waste away from the tissues to the kidneys for excretion.
- to help regulate body temperature by distributing heat throughout the body.
- to stop haemorrhage when it occurs, through the blood clotting mechanism
- to act as a transport system throughout the body for hormones and enzymes.
- to protect the body against infection by the blood borne cells of the immune system. The transport of antitoxins and antibodies in the blood.
- to assist in the maintenance of the correct pH of the tissues.

The Composition of Blood

Blood is a red fluid—it is brighter red in the systemic arteries, where it is rich in oxygen, and darker in the veins after it has given up some of its oxygen to the tissues.

It has a pH of approximately 7.4, and forms about 7% of the total weight of the body.

Blood consists of a fluid part and a solid part. The solids are cells and cellular fragments; the straw-coloured fluid is called plasma.

The Composition of Plasma

The composition of plasma reflects the different functions of blood:

- **Water**.
- **Mineral salts**. Sodium is the main extracellular cation and chloride the main anion. There are also significant amounts of potassium, calcium, phosphate and carbonate. The mineral salts in plasma act as buffers, maintaining the correct pH of the body fluids.
- **Plasma proteins**. These include albumin, globulin, fibrinogen and prothrombin. They are large molecules that cannot pass out of the circulation to the tissues, and so they help to maintain the osmotic pressure of the blood, stopping too much fluid leaking out of the circulation into the tissue spaces. Most of the plasma proteins are produced by the liver, with the exception of the immuno-globulins (part of the immune system) which are produced by plasma cells.
- **Foodstuffs**. The amino acids, fatty acids and glucose that are the end products of food break-down are carried in the plasma.
- **Gases** in solution. Most of the oxygen for the tissues is carried in the red blood calls as oxyhaemoglobin, and only a very little is dissolved in the plasma. However, a significant amount of carbon dioxide is carried in the plasma as bicarbonate.
- **Waste products**. Urea and creatinine are carried to the kidneys for excretion.
- **Hormones** and **enzymes**
- **Antibodies** and **antitoxins**.

Blood Cells

Blood cells are divided into three types: two are true cells, the third are cell fragments:

- **Erythrocytes** red blood cells
- **Leucocytes** white blood cells
- **Thrombocytes** platelets.

Red blood cells

Red blood cells are very small (in diameter 7 μm micrometres or 0.007 cm) biconcave discs without nuclei. A biconcave disc is like a ring doughnut where the hole has not gone all the way through—a disc with a dent top and bottom. They contain an iron-containing protein called haemoglobin, which is what gives the cells their red colour, and enables them to carry oxygen.

Before birth, red blood cells are produced in the bone marrow, the liver and the spleen, but after birth they are only produced in the bone marrow. They are formed from cells called **erythroblasts**, which have nuclei. These develop into **normoblasts** as they take up haemoglobin and the nucleus shrinks. The nucleus then disappears completely, leaving only a network of fine threads in the cytoplasm. At this stage the cell is called a **reticulocyte**. Finally the network disappears and the mature erythrocyte passes into the bloodstream. It has a lifespan of about 120 days, after which it is broken down in the spleen or lymph nodes. The haemoglobin in spent cells is broken down—the 'haem' part into iron (which is re-used) and waste pigment (which is converted by the liver into bile pigments). The 'globin' part may be re-used or further broken down.

The level of red cell production is regulated by the amount of oxygen reaching the tissues. When there is a low oxygen level the kidney secretes **erythropoietin factor** (or **erythrogenin**), a substance that converts an inactive plasma protein to **erythropoietin**, which stimulates the bone marrow to produce more erythrocytes. In some circumstances—for example after anaemia, when there is a significant deficit to be made up—immature reticulocytes will be seen in the blood alongside mature red blood cells.

White blood cells

The white blood cells, or leucocytes, are larger than red blood cells and can be divided into two groups:

- **Granulocytes**, which can be subdivided into:
  —neutrophils
  —basophils
  —eosinophils.
- **Agranulocytes**, which can be subdivided into:
  —lymphocytes
  —monocytes.

Granulocytes

Granulocytes, also known as **polymorphonuclear leucocytes**, have a granular cytoplasm and a multi-lobed nucleus. They make up about 70% of all the leucocytes in the body, and have a lifespan of about 21 days.

The three types of polymorphonuclear leucocytes are classified according to their ability to take up different dyes, which gives them different appearances in a stained blood film:

Neutrophils, which account for over 90% of the granulocytes, take up both acid and alkaline dyes, and the cytoplasm remains clear after staining. They are **phagocytes**, which means that they can move about and ingest small particles such as bacteria and cell debris. Neutrophils increase in number in the presence of bacterial infection, when immature forms, with a banded instead of a segmented nucleus, are seen in the blood. Hence the terms 'bands' and 'segs' in blood counts. An increase in the 'bands' indicating recent bacterial infection.

Basophils absorb alkaline dyes and stain blue. They produce heparin and histamine.

Eosinophils take up acidic dyes and stain red. They increase in number with parasitic infestation.

Agranulocytes

The agranulocytes have clear cytoplasm:

Lymphocytes make up over 80% of the agranulocytes in the body. There are two types of lymphocytes: T-lymphocytes and B-lymphocytes. They are both produced in the foetus, but those destined to become T-lymphocytes pass to the thymus, and the others to the spleen where they mature into B-lymphocytes.

Monocytes are the largest of the leucocytes and are phagocytic.

Platelets

Platelets (or thrombocytes) are cell fragments that are an essential part of the body's blood-clotting mechanism. They are formed in the bone marrow with the other blood cells from cells called **mega-karyocytes**

Blood Clotting

When a blood vessel is damaged, a series of reactions take place which result in the vessel being sealed with a 'clot' of blood:

(1) platelets stick to the damaged walls of the vessel, and broken platelets release an enzyme, **thromboplastin**.
(2) The protein **prothrombin** (normally present in plasma), in the presence of thromboplastin and calcium, is converted to **thrombin**.
(3) Thrombin is an active enzyme, which acts on the plasma protein **fibrinogen** to produce insoluble fibres of **fibrin**.
(4) The fibrin sticks to the platelets to form a firm clot.

After some time, the clot shrinks, and serum is released (i.e. serum is plasma minus the clotting factors.)

Vitamin K is required for the manufacture of prothrombin, and the tendency to bleed is increased if this vitamin is destroyed (as in the case of Warfarin poisoning).

The anticoagulant **heparin** is normally present in the blood, and prevents unwanted clots forming in the body.

Blood clotting does not only occur when there is major damage to the body; it deals all the time with minor damage to vessels throughout the body—particularly in areas that are constantly moving or subject to minor trauma, such as the lungs, the lining of the gut and the joints.

The Immune System

The **immune system** is the body's mechanism to deal with invasion by foreign matter (most commonly infectious agents such as bacteria or viruses).

The **humoral immune response** relies on the production of antibodies by the **B-lymphocytes**. (An antibody is a substance that reacts with a particular foreign body or antigen to render it harmless.) When an antigen enters the body, the particular B-lymphocyte that can produce the appropriate antibody multiplies to produce many **plasma cells**, which then produce antibodies against the invader.

The **cellular immune response** relies on the ability of **T-lymphocytes** to recognise any cell that does not belong to the body, including cells that have been invaded and altered by viruses. T-lymphocytes act within the blood, but also elsewhere in the tissues, such as on mucous surfaces.

The Reticuloendothelial

The **reticuloendothelial system** is the system of phagocytic cells that move about through the body and consume foreign matter such as bacteria. These cells are given different names when they occur in different parts of the body. In the blood they are the **monocytes**; in connective tissue they are **macrophages** or **histiocytes**. They are also found in the lymph nodes, the bone marrow, the spleen and the liver.

The Heart

The function of the heart is to pump blood round the body under pressure. It is supplied with blood by the coronary arteries, which are the first two branches of the aorta.

The heart lies within the pericardium, which in turn lies within the mediastinum in the thorax, between the lungs. It is more or less conical in shape. The point, or apex, points downwards, and lies to the left of the thorax, near the sternum, at the level of rib 7. The heart lies at a slight angle, pointing forward.

When the heart within the thorax is viewed from the side, as in a lateral radiograph, the right side of the heart is more anterior, while the left ventricle is more posterior.

The epithelial inner lining of the heart is the **endocardium**, and is continuous with the endothelium of the blood vessels. The muscle of the heart is called the **myocardium**. The outer layer of the heart is the **serous pericardium**, also known as the **epicardium**.

The heart has right and left sides, and each side is divided into an **atrium**, a thinner walled chamber, and a thicker walled **ventricle** (Fig. 14.32). In the adult animal there is no connection between the cavities of the left and right sides of the heart.

On each side of the heart, blood enters the atrium, then is forced by the contraction of the wall of that chamber through a valve and into the ventricle, the valve preventing backflow of blood. Contraction of the ventricle then pushes the blood through a second valve and out of the heart into the circulation.

The valves, which consist of fibrous **cusps** or flaps, are as follows:

- The **right atrio-ventricular** or tricuspid valve lies between the right atrium and the right ventricle; it has three cusps.
- The **left atrio-ventricular** or mitral valve lies between the left atrium and left ventricle; it has two cusps.
- The **aortic valve** lies between the left ventricle and the aorta; it has three cusps
- The **pulmonary valve** lies between the right ventricle and the pulmonary artery; it has three cusps.
- The **atrio-ventricular valves** are restricted in their movement by 'guy-ropes' called chordae tendinae, which are in turn attached to papillary muscles.

The conducting mechanism of the heart.

Cardiac muscle is able to contract rhythmically without a constant nerve supply (the autonomic nerves to the heart serve only to control heart rate). Co-ordination of the contraction of heart muscle is

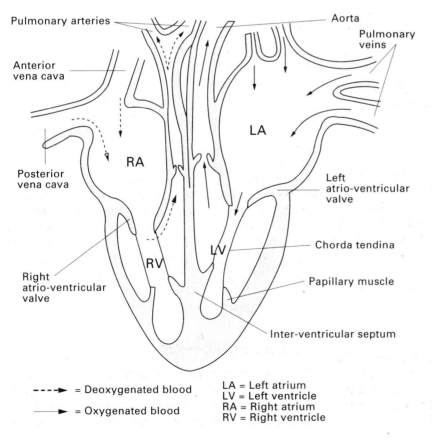

Pulmonary arteries

Aorta

Pulmonary veins

Anterior vena cava

LA

Posterior vena cava

RA

Left atrio-ventricular valve

Chorda tendina

Papillary muscle

Right atrio-ventricular valve

RV

LV

Inter-ventricular septum

- - - ▶ = Deoxygenated blood

—— ▶ = Oxygenated blood

LA = Left atrium
LV = Left ventricle
RA = Right atrium
RV = Right ventricle

Fig. 14.32. The flow of blood through the heart.

carried out by a conducting mechanism that involves the following structures:

- the **sinu-atrial** (or sinoatrial) **node** (SA node)
- the **atrioventricular node** (AV node)
- the **atrioventricular bundle**, or bundle of His
- the **fibrous plate**
- the **Purkinje fibres**

Before considering the conduction system of the heart (Fig. 14.33), it is important to understand that the exit for blood from the ventricles is at the top of the ventricles, towards the base, not the apex of the heart. The aorta and the pulmonary artery twist round each other as they leave the heart in the centre of the heart tissue.

The **SA node** is an area of specialised heart muscle situated in the wall of the right atrium, near where the anterior vena cava enters the heart. It is from the SA node that the impulse for a wave of muscle contraction starts and spreads across the atria.

The cardiac muscle of the atria and ventricles is not continuous, but is separated by a fibrous plate, so that the only electrical connection between the atria and ventricles is at the top of the inter-ventricular septum.

The impulse activates the AV node, which lies at the top of the inter-ventricular septum, and passes the impulse down the bundle of His to the apex of the heart, where it spreads out over the ventricles in the network of Purkinje fibres.

In this way the wave of contraction of the ventricles starts at the apex of the heart, and the blood is pushed upwards towards the aortic and pulmonary valves.

The whole cycle of contraction then relaxation of atria then ventricles is called the **cardiac cycle**. Within the cardiac cycle, the period of contraction is called **systole**, and the period of relaxation is termed **diastole**.

The Circulation of the Blood

Deoxygenated blood returning from the body to the heart enters the right atrium (Fig. 14.34). It is then pumped through the right ventricle and enters the pulmonary circulation via the pulmonary artery. It then enters the lungs, where it is oxygenated, before returning to the left atrium in the pulmonary vein.

This oxygenated blood is then pumped through the left atrium and ventricle and enters the systemic circulation through the aorta, branches of which supply the trunk, the limbs and the thoracic, abdominal and pelvic viscera. The deoxygenated blood returns to the right atrium via the veins, culminating in the anterior and posterior vena cavae.

The Hepatic Portal System

The hepatic portal system lies within the systemic circulation.

The function of the hepatic portal system is to enable the products of digestion absorbed by the gut to be transported directly to the liver for storage or use.

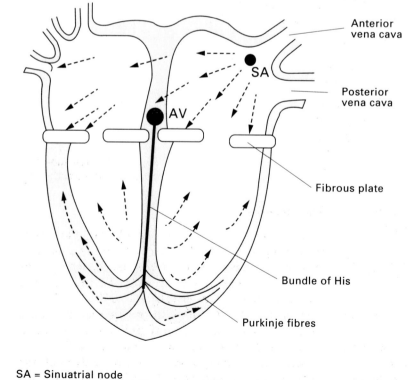

SA = Sinuatrial node
AV = Atrioventricular node
-----► Spread of contraction across the heart

Fig. 14.33. The conduction system of the heart (aorta and pulmonary arteries omitted for the sake of clarity).

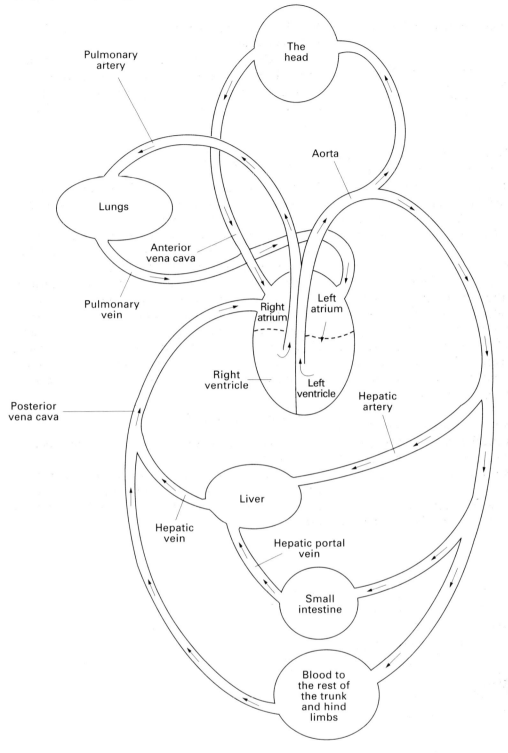

Fig. 14.34. Circulation of blood round the body.

The general rule throughout most of the body is that blood passes from the heart through arteries to a capillary bed and, then returns to the heart via veins.

In the case of the hepatic portal system, however, the blood passes through two sets of capillaries before returning to the heart:

(1) The blood moves from the heart to the capillaries of the stomach and intestine.
(2) It then moves into the **hepatic portal vein** to the liver, where it enters another capillary bed.
(3) Blood from the liver then drains into the **hepatic vein**, which joins the posterior vena cava.

The Arteries

Apart from the pulmonary circulation, the major vessels supplying blood to the body of the animal all arise as branches of the **dorsal aorta**, which runs from above the heart through the thorax and abdomen and into the pelvis (Fig. 14.35).

From the thorax down to the sacrum the aorta gives off pairs of arteries that supply the bones and muscles of the vertebral column and body wall.

After the coronary arteries have been given off the aorta, there are two large branches that come off what is termed the **aortic arch**. The first of these is

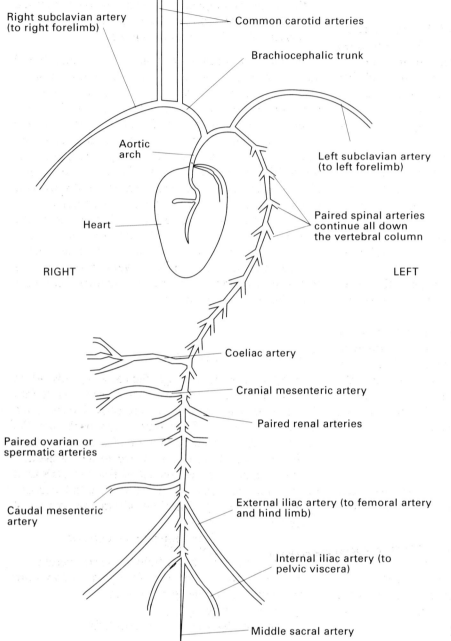

Right subclavian artery
(to right forelimb)

Common carotid arteries

Brachiocephalic trunk

Aortic
arch

Left subclavian artery
(to left forelimb)

Paired spinal arteries
continue all down
the vertebral column

Heart

RIGHT

LEFT

Coeliac artery

Cranial mesenteric artery

Paired renal arteries

Paired ovarian or
spermatic arteries

External iliac artery (to femoral artery
and hind limb)

Caudal mesenteric
artery

Internal iliac artery (to
pelvic viscera)

Middle sacral artery

Fig. 14.35. The main branches of
the aorta.

the **brachiocephalic trunk**, which gives rise to the two **common carotid arteries** that travel up the neck to supply the head with blood. The **brachiocephalic trunk** then becomes the **right subclavian artery**, which continues as the **right axillary**, and then the **right brachial artery** as it supplies the right forelimb with blood. The second large branch off the aorta is the left subclavian, which becomes the **left axillary** and then the **left brachial artery** as it supplies the left forelimb.

In the abdomen, several important pairs of arteries are given off the aorta, including the **renal arteries** and the **spermatic or ovarian arteries**. There are also three large unpaired arteries in the abdomen:

• The **coeliac artery** supplies the stomach, the liver and the spleen with oxygenated blood.

• The **cranial mesenteric artery**, supplies the small intestine, and it anastomoses (joins up with) branches of the third unpaired artery.

• The **caudal mesenteric artery** supplies the large intestine.

In the lower abdomen and pelvis there are aortic branches to supply the hindlimb, in particular the **femoral artery**, and branches to the various pelvic viscera and much of the external genitalia.

The aorta, by now a very slender artery, ends as the **median sacral artery**, running along the ventral aspect of the coccygeal vertebrae.

The pulse in the brachial artery can be felt on the medial aspect of the humerus, distally, just above the elbow. The pulse of the femoral artery can be felt on the medial aspect of the thigh.

The Veins

The head is drained by branches of the **jugular veins**, which run down the neck. The forelimbs are drained by a double system: the brachial veins which run with the brachial artery; and the **cephalic vein** which lies on the anterior aspect of the antebrachium (forearm). All the veins draining the head and forelimbs join the **anterior vena cava**, which in turn empties into the right atrium

Another vein which may cither join the anterior vena cava or empty independently into the right atrium is the **azygos vein**, which runs along the right side of the aorta and collects the venous blood from the intercostal spaces.

The **posterior vena cava** collects all the venous blood from the abdomen, pelvis and hindlimbs, returning it to the right atrium. The hindlimb, like the forelimb, has a double venous system—the veins that run with the arteries and a more superficial system.

The cephalic vein is more superficial than the brachial and therefore more useful for **venepuncture**. One vein in the hindlimb that is occasionally used for venepuncture is the **saphenous**, which crosses the lateral aspect of the limb just above the hock—however, the vein is very mobile under the skin and is therefore rarely a first choice of vein.

The Foetal Circulation

There are significant differences between the foetal circulation and that of the mammal after birth. These differences are because:

- there is a single umbilical vein that brings blood to the foetus from the placenta, and two umbilical arteries that carry blood back to the placenta.
- the lungs of the foetus are collapsed and not in use (all the oxygen the foetus uses comes to it in the umbilical vein);

- the nutrients supplied to the foetus come from the mother via the umbilical vein, having been already processed by the liver of the mother.

Because the lungs only require a very small blood supply prior to being inflated at birth, the pulmonary circulation does not need to be separate from the systemic circulation. There is therefore in the inter-atrial septum a hole, the **foramen ovale**, allowing mixing of blood from both sides of the heart, and also a link between the pulmonary artery and the aorta (**the ductus arteriosus**). Both of these close shortly after birth as the lungs expand and start their job of oxygenating the blood for the whole body.

The **umbilical vein**, bringing blood from the placenta, runs into the **ductus venosus**, which bypasses most of the liver tissue. In the adult animal the remains of the umbilical vein persist in the **falciform ligament**, a fat-filled structure that runs from the umbilicus to the liver.

The Lymphatic System

As the blood passes through the capillary network in the tissues, some fluid leaks out of the vessels into the interstitial spaces between the cells. This is called **tissue fluid**. Some of the fluid seeps back into the capillaries under osmotic pressure, but much remains in the tissues and must be returned to the circulation by the lymphatic system—a set of fine vessels found throughout the body except in the central nervous system (Fig. 14.36). The fluid within this system of vessels is called **lymph**.

The functions of the lymphatic system are:

- to return excessive tissue fluid to the circulation;
- to filter bacteria and other foreign substances out of the fluid within the lymph nodes;
- to produce lymphocytes;
- to transport digested food, particularly fat.

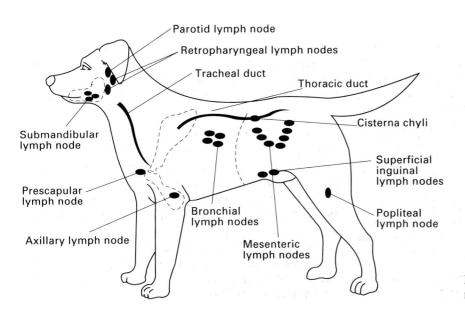

Fig. 14.36. The lymphatic system: major nodes and ducts.

The lymphatic system consists of

- **lymphatic capillaries**
- **lymphatic vessels**
- **lymphatic tissues** (the **lymph nodes** and **spleen**)
- **lymphatic ducts**.

Lymphatic capilliaries

The **lymphatic capillaries** are very fine channels that collect up the surplus tissue fluid. They join to form larger lymphatic vessels. The lymphatic capillaries found in the small intestine, in the intestinal villi, are called **lacteals**; they have a role in collecting fat from the small intestine after a meal, at which time the lymph in all the vessels proximal to the small intestine can appear milky as a result of the fat in it.

Lymphatic vessels

The **lymphatic vessels** are thin-walled structures rather like veins. However, they are more numerous within tissues than veins, and have valves throughout their length. There is no smooth muscle in their walls: they rely on the movement of their surrounding tissues to 'milk' the lymph along the vessels past the non-return valves.

Lymphatic nodes

As they travel back towards the circulation, lymph vessels pass through one or more **lymph nodes**, which consist of lymphocytes joined together by a network of connective tissue.

They enter the node through **afferent vessels**, which may enter the node from all sides, and leave it through the efferent vessels, which are all clustered together at one point.

The functions of the **lymph nodes** are:

- to filter bacteria and other foreign matter from the lymph;
- to manufacture lymphocytes.

Lymph nodes are found mainly at the tops of the limbs, and at what can be called the portals of the body (where the inside meets the outside) in the neck and pharynx, in the mediastinum, on the bronchi, and in the abdomen—particularly in the mesentery of the small intestine.

Some lymph nodes are palpable in the healthy animal, while others are only palpable if they are enlarged as a result of local infection or infiltration by tumour cells.

Lymphatic ducts

After passing through the lymph nodes, the lymphatic vessels enter one of the two large **lymphatic ducts**. The smaller right lymphatic duct drains the right forelimb and the right side of the head and neck. The larger duct drains the whole of the rest of the body; in the abdomen it is called the **cisterna chyli** but once it has crossed the diaphragm it is called the **thoracic duct**. Both lymphatic ducts empty into either the right jugular vein or the anterior vena cava.

Lymphatic tissues

Other structures that contain lymphatic tissue are the tonsils, the spleen and the thymus.

The spleen is made up of lymphatic tissue and lies within the layers of the great omentum, next to the greater curvature of the stomach. It is not essential to life and can be surgically removed. Its functions are:

- the storage of red blood cells;
- the destruction of worn-out red blood cells;
- the production of lymphocytes;
- the removal, by phagocytosis, of bacteria and other foreign matter from the circulation.

The **tonsils** are masses of lymphoid tissue within the pharynx. They are situated in the **tonsillar fossae**, on either side of the pharynx near the root of the tongue, and when enlarged are easily visible when a compliant animal opens its mouth.

The **thymus** is a lymphoid organ situated in the anterior part of the thoracic cavity. In the first few months of life it is an important site of lymphocyte production, but after this it reduces in size and the lymphoid tissue is replaced by fat.

The Digestive System

The digestive system is one of the visceral systems of the body. Its function is to take and break down complex foodstuffs into simple compounds that the body can absorb. The waste is then excreted.

The digestive system starts with the mouth. The teeth, used to prehend (take hold of) food, have been discussed as part of the skeletal system.

The Tongue

The **tongue** (see Fig. 14.28) is a muscular organ attached to the base of the pharynx. Its functions are:

- the manipulation of food;
- tasting food, by means of the taste buds on its surface
- grooming.

In cats, the tongue is covered by many backward-facing papillae, which 'comb' the coat as the animal grooms itself. This also means that the hair which is groomed out by the tongue must be swallowed, as the papillae will not let it be passed forward out of the mouth.

Dogs and cats do not chew their food in the same way that humans do. The food (in the wild, mainly animal prey) is cut up by the shearing action of the carnassial teeth against the lower molars, and is swallowed in lumps.

The Salivary Glands

While it is in the mouth, the food is moistened by saliva from the salivary glands (Fig. 14.37). There are four pairs of salivary glands in both the dog and the cat:

- the **zygomatic**
- the **sublingual**
- the **mandibular**
- the **parotid**.

All the salivary glands have ducts that open into the mouth. The secretion of saliva is stimulated by the sight of food, the smell of food, or even just the anticipation of food (for example, the sight of an owner wielding a tin opener). The production of saliva is continuous, but may increase or decrease in response to the above stimuli. The salivary glands are innervated by both sympathetic and parasympathetic nerves, which act on the glandular tissue and also on the blood vessels to increase or decrease the flow of blood to the glands.

Saliva has a number of functions:

- it moistens and softens the food, helping to break it up physically, so that the digestive enzymes can then break it up chemically.
- it lubricates the food to ease its passage down the oesophagus.
- it moistens the mouth, helping prevent drying of mucous membranes.
- The smaller salivary glands (zygomatic, sublingual and mandibular) produce mucus to help keep the mouth moist.
- The parotid gland produces a serous fluid which contains the enzyme **ptyalin**, or α (alpha)-amylase, which starts to digest carbohydrate.

Swallowing

When food is swallowed, the following sequence is performed:

- A bolus (lump) of food is positioned on the tongue and pushed to the back of the mouth.

- The soft palate is raised, blocking off the naso-pharynx.
- The hyoid apparatus (Fig. 14.38) moves forward and the epiglottis is pushed backwards to close off the larynx, preventing the entry of food.
- The pharynx is opened.
- The tongue pushes the bolus of food into the top of the pharynx, which closes behind it.
- Waves of muscular contraction (peristalsis) then carry the food from the pharynx to the stomach.
- The soft palate is lowered.
- The hyoid apparatus moves backwards and the epiglottis falls forward, leaving the larynx open again.

The Abdominal Part of the Digestive System

The digestive system within the abdomen can be divided into four parts (Fig. 14.39).

- The stomach, where storage and mixing of the food takes place.
- The small intestine, the main site of digestion and absorption of nutrients. The small intestine is further divided into duodenum, jejunum and ileum.
- The colon, where water absorption takes place.
- The rectum, where faeces are stored before excretion.

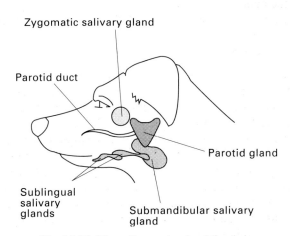

Fig. 14.37. The salivary glands of the dog.

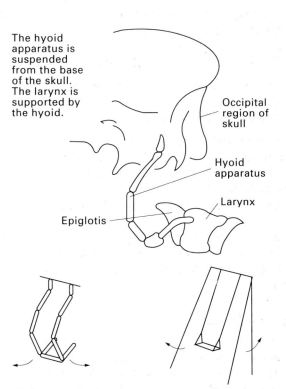

Fig. 14.38. The hyoid apparatus.

A. J. Pearson

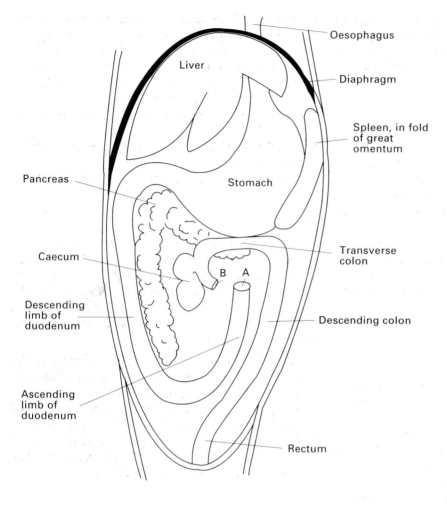

A. Junction of duodenum and jejunum
B. Junction of ileum and ascending colon (ileo-caeco-colic junction)

Fig. 14.39. Position of the gastrointestinal tract within the abdomen. (The view is from the ventral aspect. The jejunum and ileum have been removed.)

The Stomach

The stomach lies on the left side of the abdomen. It is divided into three areas:

- The **cardia**, the area where the oesophagus enters the stomach.
- The **fundus**, or body of the stomach.
- The **pylorus**, where the stomach narrows, and where the food passes into the small intestine.

The stomach is capable of considerable distension. It varies in size a good deal, as the carnivores, (particularly the dogs) are able to gorge very large amounts of food at one time. In the wild, the stomach is the storage organ for perhaps several days' supply of food, and the means by which food is carried home to a den full of puppies. This explains the 'bottomless pit' nature of the average dog's appetite.

All of the gastrointestinal tract is attached, either firmly or loosely, to the dorsal body wall by a dorsal mesentery. The dorsal mesentery of the stomach is massively expanded to form a double sheet of doubled mesentery which is the great omentum.

The spleen lies within the layers of the **great omentum** which lies over the ventral surface of the small intestine as a covering, and is the first organ to be seen when the abdomen is opened along the mid-ventral line.

Gastric Secretions

A number of different secretions are produced by cells in the stomach wall.

- **Mucus** is produced in all parts of the stomach. It protects the lining of the stomach.
- **Hydrochloric acid (HCl)** is produced in the fundus by goblet or parietal cells. A low (acid) pH is required for the enzyme pepsin to act.
- **Pepsinogen** is produced in the fundus, and is acted on by the hydrochloric acid to produce pepsin, an active enzyme that breaks down protein.
- **Gastrin** is a hormone produced by what are termed 'G cells' in the fundus. The gastrin is carried in the bloodstream to the goblet cells in the stomach wall, and stimulates them to produce hydrochloric acid.
- **Lipase**, an enzyme that breaks down fat, is also produced, but only in small amounts.

The food in the stomach is mixed with the various gastric secretions, then the resulting fluid is passed out of the stomach and into the small intestine. The mixture of food, saliva and gastric secretions that leaves the stomach is called **chyme**.

Vomiting

The entry into the stomach, known as the cardiac sphincter, normally remains closed unless food reaches it from the oesophagus. However, vomiting (the forceful expulsion of gastrointestinal contents through the mouth) does occur as a response to over distension of the stomach or irritation of the stomach lining (gastritis). The smooth muscle of the stomach wall relaxes, the cardiac sphincter opens and the stomach contents are forced up the oesophagus by the forceful contraction of abdominal muscles.

The Small Intestine

The small intestine is the site for further digestion and also the main site for absorption of the products of digestion.

The first part of the small intestine is the **duodenum**. It lies on the right side of the abdomen and forms a U-shape. It has three ducts leading into it—**two pancreatic ducts** and a **bile duct**.

The second and third parts of the small intestine—the **jejunum** and **ileum**—are indistinguishable to the naked eye and can be considered together. This is the very long section of the gut that lies loose in the abdominal cavity within a loop of what is called the great mesentery, and is not firmly attached to the dorsal body wall.

There are three secretions into the small intestine:

- **Pancreatic juice**
- **Bile**
- **Intestinal juice**.

Pancreatic Juice

The pancreas is a mixed gland, containing both exocrine and endocrine tissue. It lies between the two arms of the duodenum.

The exocrine secretion of the pancreas is involved in digestion, and enters the duodenum through two pancreatic ducts.

Pancreatic juice contains bicarbonate (HCO_3^-), which is alkaline, and so helps to neutralise the acid within the chyme and produce a suitable pH for the pancreatic enzymes that are released by the action of cholecystokinin (produced by the stomach) on the intestinal lining. The pancreatic enzymes are:

- **Amylase**, which continues the breakdown of carbohydrate started by the salivary amylase.

- **Trypsin**, which acts on proteins and on the products of protein breakdown started by the pepsin in the stomach. It is secreted as trypsinogen, which is converted to the active enzyme trypsin by the action of **enterokinase**, secreted in the intestinal juice.
- **Lipase**, which breaks down fats to fatty acids and glycerol.
- **Peptidases**, which break down polypeptide chains to free amino acids.
- **Nucleotidases**, which break down RNA and DNA.

Bile

Bile enters the duodenum down the bile duct. It is produced in the liver and then stored in the gall bladder, which is attached to the liver, until it is required for digestion. Bile is essential for the breakdown of fats. If too little bile is produced, then there will be fat in the faeces. The two main constituents of bile are:

- **Bile salts**, which act as detergents: they break the surface tension between fats and water so that the fats are broken into small droplets, forming an emulsion. It is easier for the lipase to act on small droplets in an emulsion than on large drops of fat.
- **Bile pigments**, which are waste produced in the liver from the breakdown of blood pigments. They give the faeces their distinctive colour.

Intestinal Juice

Intestinal juice is the third secretion into the small intestine. It is produced by cells in the wall of the small intestine. Like the pancreatic juice, it contains bicarbonate, and also the following enzymes (some of which are also pancreatic):

- **Disaccharidases**, which break down the disaccharides (e.g. maltose, sucrose and lactose) into simple sugars that can be absorbed.
- **Peptidases** to break down peptides into amino acids.
- **Nucleotidase**.
- **Enterokinase**.

Absorption

Absorption of the products of digestion—the amino acids, the fatty acids and the sugars—takes place almost entirely through the villi of the wall of the small intestine (Fig. 14.40). Amino acids and simple sugars are absorbed into the blood capillaries, and are carried in the blood to the liver, via the hepatic portal system.

The fatty acids and glycerol are absorbed into the lacteals (lymph vessels within the villi), where in the form of minute fat droplets they are carried to the cisterna chyli then into the thoracic duct and back into the bloodstream.

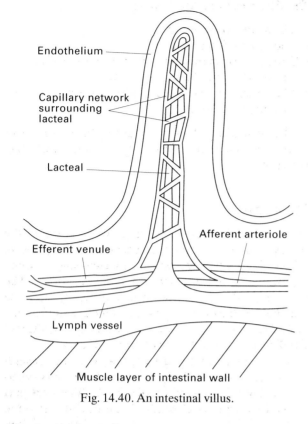

Fig. 14.40. An intestinal villus.

The Large Intestine

The large intestine is composed of the caecum, the colon and the rectum.

The **caecum** is a small blind-ended sac that has no significant function in the carnivores. In herbivores such as the rabbit and guinea pig it is much larger and is a site where bacteria are used to break down coarse vegetable matter so that it can be used by the animal.

The **colon** is attached to the dorsal body wall and has three parts: the ascending, transverse and descending colon.

Water, electrolytes and water-soluble vitamins are absorbed in the large bowel, and the waste products are then passed down towards the rectum, where they are held before being excreted.

Defecation

Defecation is a combination of voluntary and involuntary acts. The involuntary movement of the large bowel moving faeces into the rectum produces the wish to defecate. However, the relaxation of the external anal sphincter, which allows faeces to be passed, is a voluntary act.

The Liver

Closely associated with the digestive system is the liver, sometimes termed 'the largest gland in the body'. It lies against the diaphragm, in front and to the right of the stomach, and is divided into a number of lobes.

The liver receives blood from two sources: about 20% is normal arterial blood from a branch of the aorta, and the rest comes from the veins carrying venous blood away from the intestine, in the hepatic portal system. This blood, of course, carries many of the products of digestion.

The liver performs many chemical functions for the body:

- **Protein metabolism**. Many of the plasma proteins are synthesized in the liver, as are fibrinogen and other proteins involved in blood clotting.
- **Urea formation**. Ammonia, the toxic waste product of protein breakdown, is converted to the less toxic urea.
- **Carbohydrate metabolism**. Blood sugar levels are kept within narrow limits as surplus is stored in the liver as glycogen, and then released into the circulation as energy is required by the body.
- **Fat metabolism**. Some lipids required by the body are synthesised in the liver, and fatty acids are metabolised to produce energy.
- **Formation of bile**.
- **Detoxification and conjugation of steroid hormones**.
- **Vitamin storage**. The liver is the main store of the fat-soluble vitamins (A, D, E and K). Some of the water-soluble vitamins, particularly B12, are also stored.
- **Production of heat** and regulation of body temperature.
- **Iron storage**.

The Urinary System

The urinary system is responsible for removing waste products—including surplus water—from the body (Fig. 14.41). The system consists of:

- the two **kidneys**, which filter the blood
- the **ureters** that carry the urine from the kidneys
- the **bladder**, the storage organ
- the **urethra**.

The Kidneys

The two kidneys lie against the dorsal wall of the abdomen, attached to it by a covering or 'capsule' of fibrous tissue. They are, needless to say, kidney shaped (although this is not the case in all species). The right kidney is about half a kidney's length in front of the left.

The indented part of the kidney is called the **hilus**, and is the point at which blood vessels and nerves and also the ureters enter or leave the kidney.

A cross-section of a kidney (Fig. 14.42) shows that the organ can be divided into three main areas: a **cortex**, which is darker in colour; the paler **medulla**; and the hollow collecting area of the **renal pelvis**.

(a)

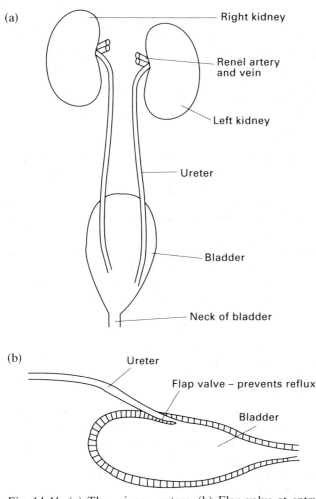

(b)

Fig. 14.41. (a) The urinary system. (b) Flap-valve at entry of ureter into bladder—it prevents urine flow back up the ureter.

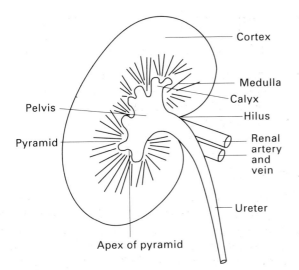

Fig. 14.42. The kidney.

The blood supply to the kidneys comes from the renal arteries, which leave the aorta close to the kidneys.

The Functions of the Kidney

- The formation of urine.
- The production of renin.
- The conversion of vitamin D to an active form.
- The production of erythropoietin.
- The maintenance (with other organs) of the correct pH of the body.

The formation of urine involves the excretion of excess and waste materials from the body (including excess water).

The Nephron

The **nephron** (Fig. 14.43) is the functional unit of the kidney. There are many thousands of nephrons in kidney tissue and they are the mechanism by which the blood is filtered and urine is produced. The nephron starts in the cortex of the kidney with the cup-shaped **Bowman's capsule**, which contains the **glomerulus**, a knot of capillaries fed by an **afferent arteriole** and drained by an **efferent arteriole**.

As the tubule leaves the capsule, it makes several twists and turns and this part of the nephron is called the **proximal convoluted tubule (PCT)**. The next part forms the long **loop of Henle** that dips down into the medulla then returns to the cortex. There is then another series of convolutions—the **distal convoluted tubule (DCT)**—before the nephron empties into a **collecting duct** that serves a number of nephrons, and carries the urine through the medulla to the renal pelvis. The collecting ducts all discharge their contents into the renal pelvis at the apices (singular apex) of the **pyramids** of the medulla.

The indentations of the renal pelvis that lie between the pyramids of the medulla are called **calyces** (singular calyx).

The Ureters

The **ureters** (one from each kidney) are thick-walled, narrow tubes that carry urine from the renal pelvis to the **bladder**. They are lined with mucous membrane and have smooth muscle in their walls which undergo peristaltic movements to move the urine on down towards the bladder. The ureters enter the bladder close to its neck, on its dorsal aspect, and there is a simple flap valve that prevents the return of urine up the ureter under the high pressure of a full bladder

The Bladder

The bladder is capable of considerable distension. It is covered with peritoneum, it has a double layer of smooth muscle fibres in its wall, and a lining of **transitional epithelium** which continues into the urethra. The lining of the empty bladder is thrown into folds, which allows for tremendous expansion when it is full.

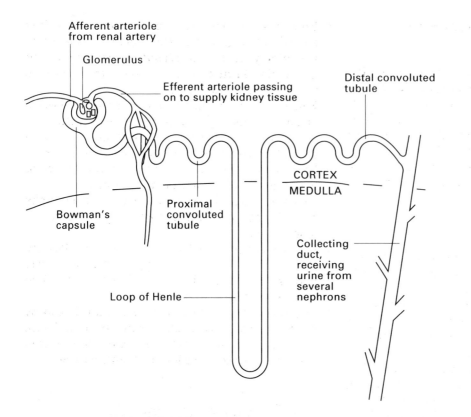

Fig. 14.43. A kidney nephron.

The area between the ureteral openings and the neck of the bladder is known as the **trigone** of the bladder.

The Urethra

In the male, the urethra carries urine from the bladder to outside the body. In the female, it carries the urine from the bladder to the **urethral orifice**, which opens into the genital tract at the junction of vagina and vestibule.

The urethra has two sphincters near to where it leaves the bladder. The **internal sphincter** is involuntary, but the **external sphincter** is under voluntary control.

Renal Filtration and Absorption

The blood in the glomerulus is under high pressure, and the low pressure in the hollow Bowman's capsule allows some of the constituents of blood to enter the glomerulus. This is known as the **glomerular filtrate**. It can be described as an ultrafiltrate of plasma, as it is very similar to plasma except that the larger protein molecules have remained, with the blood cells, in the circulation.

The difference in pressure between the blood in the glomerulus and the pressure of the fluid in the Bowman's capsule is known as the filtration pressure. Over 100 litres of glomerular filtrate may be produced in a day by a large dog—and as only a fraction of this ends up as urine (1–2 litres), there must be considerable reabsorption down the length

of the nephron. Urine volume may be from 0.5% to 15% of the original glomerular filtrate.

Reabsorption and secretion in the renal tubule

Most of the substances in the glomerular filtrate are reabsorbed lower down the nephron either by active transport across the lining membrane or by passive diffusion.

- **Water** is actively absorbed, mainly in the Proximal convoluted tubule PCT but also in the Distal convoluted tubule DCT.
- **Sodium** is actively absorbed in the PCT, with chloride following by passive diffusion.
- **Glucose** is very efficiently absorbed in the first part of the PCT unless the plasma concentration is very high and overtakes what is called the **renal threshold**, when glucose starts to appear in the urine (for example in diabetes mellitus).
- **Amino acids** are reabsorbed completely in the convoluted tubules.
- In the healthy animal, any **protein** that is filtered is reabsorbed in the PCT.
- The waste product **urea** is reabsorbed in the PCT, then re-secreted into the tubule in the loop of Henle.
- **Acids and bases** in the filtrate are selectively absorbed, and **hydrogen ions**, **bicarbonate** and **ammonia** may be secreted into the tubule to help maintain the correct pH within the body.
- There are some other substances, for example **penicillin**, which are also actively secreted into the PCT.

Control of Filtration and Reabsorption

Water

The reabsorption of water is controlled by the hormone **ADH** (**anti-diuretic hormone**), secreted by the posterior pituitary gland. When the body needs to decrease the volume of urine to conserve fluid within the body, ADH acts on the DCT to increase water reabsorption. Conversely, a fall in secreted ADH will decrease water reabsorption in the DCT and allow more urine to enter the collecting ducts.

Sodium

The reabsorption of sodium is controlled by **aldosterone**, which is secreted by the adrenal cortex. When the plasma sodium level falls, the kidney firstly produces the enzyme **renin**, which acts on **angiotensinogen** in the plasma to convert it to angiotensin I. The **angiotensin I** is then converted to **angiotensin II** which stimulates the adrenal cortex to release aldosterone. Aldosterone acts on the DCT to increase reabsorption of sodium and chloride. The angiotensin also increases blood pressure by causing vasoconstriction, and so increases the glomerular filtration rate as the filtration pressure is increased.

Vitamin D

The kidney also converts the fat-soluble form of vitamin D to the more active water-soluble form.

Erythropoietin

Active **erythropoietin**, the substance that stimulates the production of red blood cells in the bone marrow, is produced from an inactive plasma protein by 'erythropoietin factor', which is produced by the kidney in response to low oxygen levels in the blood.

Urine and Micturation (Urination)

As the bladder fills with urine, stretch receptors in its wall send messages to the brain giving the animal the wish to pass urine. These stimuli can be suppressed for a certain time, but then when the situation is right or the bladder is very distended, voluntary motor nerves will cause relaxation of the external sphincter and shortening and so dilation of the urethra, allowing urine to be passed.

A dog passes between 20–80 ml of urine per kg body weight per day, while a cat passes rather less, at 10–15 ml per kg. Analysis of urine is very useful as a diagnostic aid in veterinary medicine, as many disease conditions may be reflected in abnormal urine contents:

- pH and specific gravity: The urine of a carnivorous animal when it is fed on a meat-based diet, is normally slightly acid, in the range pH 5–7, with a specific gravity of between 1.016 and 1.060 in the dog and 1.020–1.040 in the cat.

- **Protein** should not appear in the urine of a healthy animal, although it may do if there is damage to the urinary tract or increased permeability of the glomerulus. Protein appears in the urine in chronic renal disease and in cystitis.
- **Blood** may appear in urine as a result of physical damage to the urinary tract, or as contaminant from, say, the prostate in the male, or blood-stained discharge from an in-season bitch.
- **Bile** will show up in the urine in certain types of liver disease or blockage of the bile duct.
- **Glucose** in the urine usually reflects an abnormally high plasma glucose, most frequently as a result of diabetes mellitus.
- **Ketones** are produced by the body when fats are being oxidised as an energy source, and may appear in the urine in diabetes mellitus, or when there is insufficient calorie intake.
- **Deposits** in urine may also be useful for diagnostic purposes and may include **cells** from different parts of the urinary tract, **crystals** or larger stones (**calculi**), or **casts** of the inside of renal tubules.

The Male Reproductive System

The reproductive or genital system of the male is responsible for the production, storage and nourishment of sperm, and for their transport into the genital tract of the female so that the ova of the female may be fertilised (Figs 14.44 and 14.45).

The male reproductive system consists of:

- the testes
- the epididymides (singular epididymis)
- the vasa deferentia (singular vas deferens) or deferent ducts
- the prostate gland
- the urethra
- the penis
- the prepuce.

The urethra and penis are common to both the reproductive and urinary tracts, and indeed the systems are often considered together as the urogenital tract.

The Testes

The testes of the dog lie in the scrotum, a sac of skin between the hind legs. In the cat the scrotum lies on the perineum, below the anus.

In the foetus, the testes develop from undifferentiated gonads—glands with the potential to be either ovary or testis. These gonads start life in the abdomen, just behind the kidneys. As they develop into testes, they start to move down through the abdomen, out through the inguinal ring in the abdominal wall, and so come to lie in the scrotum, surrounded by a double fold of peritoneum—the internal and external tunic (**tunica vaginalis**). Because

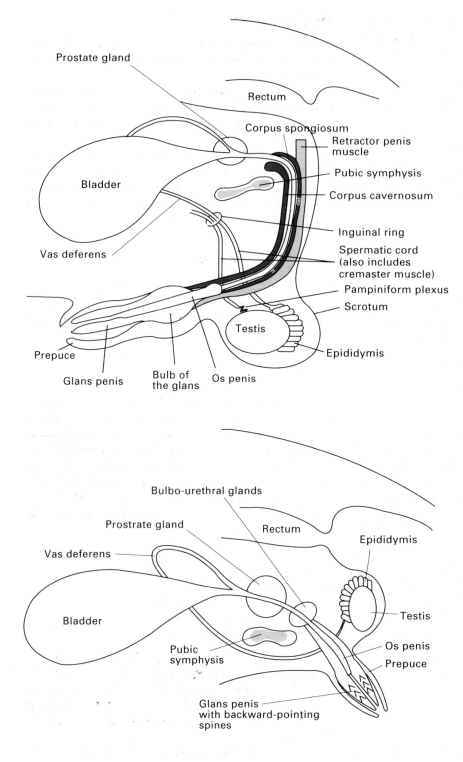

Fig. 14.44. Reproductive tract of the dog.

Fig. 14.45. Reproductive tract of the tom cat.

the blood supply, nerve supply and ducts that run to and from the testis originate from when the testis was an intra-abdominal organ, they run from the abdomen out through the inguinal ring, taking the same route as the migrating testes.

In some cases the testes do not complete their journey, and may end up either lying just subcutaneously in the inguinal region, or still within the abdomen. A dog with both testes undescended is termed a **cryptorchid**, and a dog with only one is termed **monorchid**. In the normal puppy the testes are palpable in the groin by 8 to 10 weeks of age, though the scrotum may not be fully formed by then,

and of course the testes are still small in the pre-pubertal dog.

The group of blood vessels, nerves and ducts that run from the scrotum through the inguinal ring into the abdomen is called the **spermatic cord**. It also has a thin strip of muscle running with it, called the **cremaster muscle**, which originates from the internal abdominal oblique muscle of the abdominal wall and allows the raising or lowering of the testes within the scrotum, to bring them closer to or further from the body wall.

Surgical removal of the testes is termed castration or neutering. Early castration (before the onset of puberty) can affect the development of the secondary sexual characteristics—the heavier musculature (particularly in the neck) and the development of erectile tissue in the penis in the dog; and the heavier shape, and distinctive smell and voice of the tom cat.

The blood supply to the testis is from the testicular artery, which originates from the abdominal aorta. As it enters the scrotum and runs alongside the epididymus it becomes massively convoluted, forming the **pampiniform plexus**. The reason for these convolutions is said to be to allow blood to cool and to smooth out the pulsations in the vessel before the blood reaches the gonad.

Structure of the Testis

The internal structure of the testis is made up of several hundred convoluted **seminiferous tubules** with supportive connective tissue and cells between them. They are lined with two different types of cell:

- **Spermatogenic** cells, which divide by meiosis to produce spermatozoa.
- **Sertoli cells**, which produce oestrogens, and also nutritive fluid for the sperm.

The cells among the supportive connective tissue are called the **interstitial cells**, or the **cells of Leydig**, and they produce the male hormone **testosterone**, which is responsible for spermatogenesis and the development and maintenance of secondary male sexual characteristics.

Testosterone is also responsible for the descent of the testes into the scrotum, and in the young animal it has an inhibitory effect on the hypothalamus in the brain. At puberty, however, it stops being inhibitory, and the hypothalamus stimulates the anterior pituitary gland to produce **interstitial cell stimulating hormone (ICSH)** and **luteinising hormone (LH)**, which stimulate the development of the seminiferous tubules and so sperm production, and also increase testosterone production by the cells of Leydig.

The Epididymus

Sperm leave the testis in a series of small ducts, **the vasa efferentia** or **efferent ducts**, which carry them to the **epididymus**, a larger, much coiled duct that lies alongside the testis in the scrotum and is where the sperm are stored.

The Vas Deferens

The **deferent duct** or **vas deferens** lies within the spermatic cord. It carries the sperm from the epididymus, through the inguinal ring, to the urethra. It empties into the urethra through the tissue of the prostate gland.

The Prostate Gland

The prostate gland of the dog lies just below the neck of the bladder. In the cat it lies a little further down the urethra.

The prostate produces a large part of the **seminal fluid** that makes up the volume of ejaculate in the dog. It is a bilobed structure about the size and shape of a peeled walnut, and surrounds the urethra at the level of the pelvic brim. Enlargement of the prostate can cause obstruction to the passage of faeces through the pelvis, or when very large it may move into the abdomen, where it can often be palpated as a mass posterior to the bladder.

The Bulbo-urethral Glands

The bulbo-urethral glands are found in the cat but not in the dog. They, like the prostate, make a contribution to the seminal fluid. They lie further down the urethra, near to the perineum.

The Penis

The penis runs from the ischial arch of the pelvis, down the perineum and between the hind legs of the dog. The distal part is contained within the **prepuce**, a sheath or fold of abdominal skin suspended from the midline of the ventral abdominal wall. The prepuce is lined with mucous epithelium. It covers and protects the distal part of the penis, but is pushed back during coitus (mating) to expose the erect glans penis.

The penis itself consists of:

- the urethra
- the os penis
- the corpus cavernosum penis
- the corpus spongiosum penis
- the retractor penis muscle.

The **corpus cavernosum penis** consists of two **crura** or strips of erectile tissue that originate at the **root of the penis** on the ischial arch of the pelvis, and continue down into the body of the penis, although not as far as its tip. The **urethra** runs in a groove between the two crura.

The **corpus spongiosum penis** runs beneath the corpus cavernosum and the urethra, and is expanded proximally into the bulb of the penis and at its tip into the glans, where it completely surrounds the urethra and forms the apex of the organ.

The penis of the cat differs from that of the dog in that it does not lie along the ventral abdomen, but points backwards. It also differs in having a number of backward-facing spines on the glans.

The **os penis** in the dog lies dorsal to the urethra, but in the cat, owing to the different orientation of the penis, it lies ventral to the urethra. In both species the os penis is v-shaped, with the urethra lying along the groove in the bone.

The **retractor penis** muscle originates from the first few coccygeal vertebrae, and its action is to pull the penis back into the prepuce.

The Female Reproductive System (Cat/Dog)

The female reproductive system (Fig. 14.46) consists of:

- The two ovaries
- The Fallopian tubes or oviducts
- The uterus—horns, body and cervix
- The vagina
- The vestibule
- The clitoris
- The vulva.

The genital system of the female produces eggs, or ova, which are fertilised in the Fallopian tubes, then carried to the uterine horns, where they are implanted. It is here that the foetus grows throughout the gestation period.

The Ovaries

The ovaries are situated in the abdomen, behind the kidneys. Each one is attached to the dorsal body wall via the kidney capsule by an ovarian ligament, which may also be called the suspensory ligament. The blood supply comes from the ovarian artery, which comes off the aorta and is very convoluted as it follows the ovarian ligament to the gonad.

Like all structures within the abdominal cavity, the ovaries lie within a fold of mesentery, in this case called the mesovarium, but in this case there is an opening into the fold to allow the ova to escape. This opening is the opening to the **ovarian bursa**.

Within the ovary are many **primary ovarian follicles**, each of which can develop into a ripe ovarian follicle (**Graafian follicle**). Some species release just one egg at a time; others, including the dog and cat, release groups of follicles together. Each ripe follicle contains a large amount of fluid, and one ovum.

At ovulation, the follicle ruptures at the surface of the ovary, releasing the ovum, which is usually taken up by the **fimbria** of the **infundibulum** at the head of the oviduct.

After ovulation there may be some bleeding into the ruptured follicle, but then the cells of the follicular wall proliferate to form a solid corpus luteum.

The Oviduct

The oviduct is a narrow tube that runs from the horn of the uterus to the trumpet-like infundibulum that encloses the ovary and captures the released ova.

The Uterus

In the cat and the dog the uterus consists of two long horns, and then a body leading to a single cervix. It lies within the mesometrium (or broad ligament) of the uterus, and is dorsal within the abdomen, except when it is enlarged, when it may hang down under its own weight and lie more ventral.

The wall of the uterus is made up of layers of smooth muscle which together are called the myometrium, and a mucous epithelial lining called the endometrium.

At the base of the body of the uterus is the cervix, a muscular organ that acts as a sphincter to close the uterus except during mating and parturition.

The round ligament runs from the ovary towards and through the inguinal ring, where it terminates in a pad of fat known as the vaginal process. The round ligament is the female homologue of the gubernaculum, which in the male draws the gonad (the testis) through the inguinal ring and into the scrotum. The round ligament lies in a fold of the broad ligament.

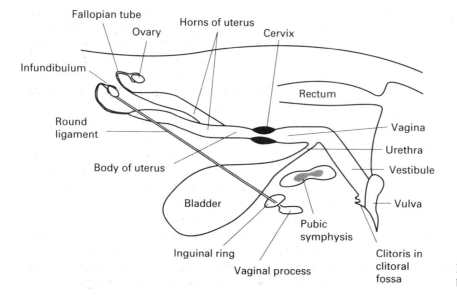

Fig. 14.46. Reproductive tract of the bitch (lateral view).

The Vagina and the Vestibule

The vagina extends from the cervix to the external urethral orifice, and lies entirely within the pelvis. After the vagina, the genital tract has a sharp bend downwards as the tract passes into the vestibule, which is that part of the tract that is used by both the genital and urinary systems. The muscles in the wall of the vestibule are very strong, and in the bitch they contribute to the 'tie' between bitch and dog during mating.

The Vulva and Clitoris

The vulval lips form the boundaries of the vertical slit that is the external opening of the female urogenital tract. The clitoris, the small knob of erectile tissue that is the female homologue of the penis, lies in the clitoral fossa—a small cavity just inside the base of the vulva. The vulval lips are normally soft, but become enlarged and turgid when a bitch is in season.

Reproductive Patterns

Most animal species have particular breeding seasons during the year. The time of the year when an animal chooses to have its young is usually based on there being a plentiful food source at that time. The onset of the breeding season may be triggered by external factors such as increasing or decreasing day length (changes in photoperiod) or the beginning of a wet season, or a rise or fall in temperature.

The domestic dog has two breeding seasons during the year, but these may fall at any time—although more bitches come 'on heat' during the spring and autumn than at other times. The timing of their seasons may be influenced not only by photoperiod but also by other bitches: bitches living in groups all tend to have their 'seasons' at about the same time.

The queen has a breeding season that is dictated by increasing then decreasing day length and runs from early spring until autumn (late August or September).

The Oestrous Cycle

Oestrus is the period during the oestrous cycle when the female is prepared to accept a male, and it varies in length from species to species. Oestrus coincides with the release of ova by the ovary, and the female's willingness to mate at this time makes it likely that they will be fertilised soon after ovulation.

The general pattern of the oestrous cycle in the mammal is as follows:

- **Pro-oestrus** is the period in which the follicles in the ovary enlarge and become mature.
- **Oestrus** is when the follicles rupture and the ova are released.

- **Metoestrus** is the period when a corpus luteum starts to form at the site of the ruptured follicle.
- **Dioestrus** is the time when the corpus luteum is established or, if the ova have been fertilised, a pregnancy may be established.
- **Anoestrus** is a period when there is no ovarian activity.

If there is no pregnancy, then after a time the corpus luteum will degenerate and either there will be a period of anoestrus or the ovary will enter another phase of pro-oestrus as another batch of follicles start to mature. (This subject is covered in detail in Chapter 19, Obstetric and Paediatric Nursing of the Dog and Cat.)

The Oestrous Cycle in the Bitch

The bitch is **monoestrous**: she has only one oestrous cycle in each breeding season. Bitches may come into season for the first time at any time between 6 and 18 months old. Thereafter they usually come into season about every 6 months (although there are plenty of exceptions that have one or three breeding seasons a year.)

Pro-oestrus in the bitch lasts on average about 9 or 10 days. During this time the vulva swells and there is a blood-stained mucous discharge from the vulva. Internally, the ovarian follicles are maturing and the endometrium is thickening and producing the secretion that appears at the vulva. Pro-oestrus is initiated by secretion of **FSH (follicle stimulating hormone)** from the anterior pituitary, which stimulates the development of the mature **Graafian follicle**. **Oestradiol** is secreted from the wall of the developing follicle, and this causes the thickening of the endometrium and the changes in the external genitalia seen at this time.

Oestrus lasts on average 7 to 10 days, though it may be longer or shorter. During this period the discharge becomes less bloody and the follicles rupture. The follicular fluid contains oestradiol secreted by the cells lining the follicle, and as ovulation occurs there is a sudden surge of oestradiol in the bloodstream that depresses any further production of FSH and stimulates the production of LH or **luteinising hormone**, which in its turn stimulates the development of the corpus luteum at the site of the ruptured follicle.

The bitch ovulates whether or not she is mated, and so is termed a spontaneous ovulator.

Corpora lutea form during the period of **metoestrus** whether or not the bitch has been mated, and produce **progesterone**, which maintains the pregnancy if it exists, and may produce the symptoms of **pseudopregnancy** (false pregnancy or pseudocyesis) if the ova have not been fertilised. Some bitches show signs of false pregnancy, such as mammary gland enlargement, milk production, and then nest-making; others show little or no signs.

After the period of **dioestrus**, when the corpora lutea are established and maintaining a pseudo-pregnancy, or at the end of the true pregnancy, the corpora lutea regress and the bitch goes into **anoestrus** until the next breeding season.

The total length of the 'season' in the bitch is usually quoted as 21 days—but many take much longer than that, and some will still be willing to stand for a dog on the 21st day or even later.

The Oestrous Cycle in the Queen

The oestrous cycle in the queen is different to that of the bitch: she is **seasonally polyoestrous**, and is an **induced ovulator**.

Seasonally polyoestrous means that after one oestrous cycle, instead of going into a period of anoestrus, the cat will return to pro-oestrus and have another oestrous cycle for as long as the breeding season lasts, or until she becomes pregnant.

Induced ovulation means that if the queen is not mated, she will not ovulate. Instead, after a period of oestrus, the unruptured follicles will regress, there will be no corpus luteum development, and another batch of follicles will develop between 1 and 3 weeks later.

Young queens become mature between 6 and 12 months of age, and first come into oestrus in the first spring following their maturity.

Pro-oestrus in cats lasts from 1 to 3 days, and oestrus up to about 10 days.

Mating

As a bitch comes into oestrus, she exhibits a number of signs that show her readiness to mate. As part of the pre-mating ritual, the dog will lick round the bitch's vulva and clitoris, and if she is ready to mate the bitch will exhibit 'lordosis'—arching the back downwards so that the vulva is presented to the dog, while stretching her tail to one side so that it is out of the way. She will also **stand** still to receive the dog's attentions (hence 'standing oestrus'), whereas before she reaches oestrus she will swing round to face him as he attempts to lick her vulva and to mount.

When the bitch is ready she will permit the dog to mount and mate. His erect penis enters her vagina, and with a series of thrusting movements he ejaculates. As he ejaculates, the strong vestibular muscles of the bitch tighten behind the erect bulb of the penis, so firmly holding the two animals firmly together in a '**tie**'. After ejaculation the dog will dismount by swinging one hind leg over the bitch's back so they are standing tail-to-tail. They remain in this position for the duration of the tie, which may be anything from a few minutes to more than an hour.

The dog and bitch should not (and indeed cannot) be forced apart during the tie. It is possible to have fertile mating without a tie.

Female cats in oestrus exhibit lordosis by crouching with dipped back and thrusting their perineal area into the air. Stroking down the cat's back at this stage will make the arch even more pronounced, and elicit vigorous trampling with the hind feet. They are also very vocal at this time. When cats mate, the procedure is much swifter than in dogs, and as the tom cat withdraws, the backward-pointing barbs on the glans irritate the female to the extent that she will usually turn round and take a swipe at the male.

Pregnancy

Pregnancy in bitches and queens may be diagnosed in a number of ways. Many owners will swear that they know a week or so after mating whether their pet is gravid (pregnant), by a change in attitude and behaviour.

Pregnancy diagnosis by abdominal palpation of the developing embryo can be performed, usually between 21 and 28 days (veterinary surgeons may have different preferred timings).

By 5 weeks there is a degree of abdominal enlargement, and the teats start to enlarge.

When an animal is pregnant for the first time she is said to be primagravid, or to be a primigravida. In later pregnancies she is known as multigravid. An animal that usually has only one offspring at a time is said to be uniparous, but the bitch and queen, with their larger litters, are said to be multiparous.

Early Embryological Development

Fertilisation

The ovum that is released from the ovary is surrounded by a double protective layer (Fig. 14.47). The inner layer, or **zona pellucida**, is glycoprotein: the outer layer, or **corona radiata**, is of small follicular cells.

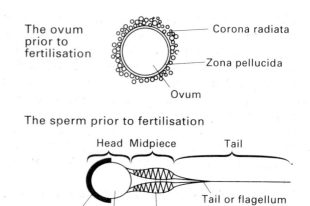

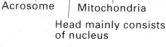

(Not to same scale)

Fig. 14.47. Structure of ovum and sperm.

Fertilisation takes place within the Fallopian tube. The first sperm to burrow through the corona radiata and penetrate the zona pellucida sets up the **fertilisation reaction**, which stops any other sperm entering the ovum.

The fertilised ovum is then called a **zygote**.

The lifespan of sperm within the reproductive tract of the female is very variable. In the cow it is less than a day, whereas in the dog is may be up to a week. Fertilisation occurs about 2–3 days after ovulation.

The zygote

After fertilisation the zygote continues to travel down the Fallopian tube, and as it does so the cells start to divide—first into two, then four, then eight, and then irregularly to form a solid ball of cells called a **morula** (Fig. 14.49).

Formation of Germ Cell Layers

The morula then develops a cavity, with a mass of cells towards one end of the structure. The mass of cells is called the **inner cell mass**, and the cells lining the cavity are the **trophoblast**. The inner cell mass will eventually form the embryo.

The next stage is the development of three **germ cell layers** (Fig. 14.48) that will eventually form recognisable parts of the body.

- The **ectoderm**, or outer layer, of the inner cell mass forms the skin and nervous system.
- The **mesoderm**, or middle layer, forms the musculoskeletal system and other internal organs.
- The **endoderm**, or inner layer, forms the lining of the gastrointestinal tract and other visceral structures.

The **mesoderm** forms as two longitudinal blocks of tissue, beneath which the endodermal cells spread round to line the trophoblast and form the yolk sac (Fig. 14.49). In the mammal there is no yolk within the yolk sac, but in reptiles and birds the yolk sac encloses the yolk of the egg that provides nourishment for the growing embryo.

Mesodermal cells then migrate to lie in two layers—one adjacent to the ectoderm and one to the endoderm—and a cavity starts to develop between them.

The inner cell mass starts to curl round to enclose the mesodermal and endodermal cells that will form its internal organs, leaving the yolk sac and the trophoblast to form **extra-embryonic membranes** which become the placenta and the membranes that we see covering the foetus at birth. (In this context 'extra' means 'outside'.)

Implantation

At about this stage the developing embryos reach the uterine horns, where they tend to distribute themselves evenly between the two horns, and then settle against the wall of the uterus to implant.

Implantation takes place in the cat between 11 and 16 days, and in the dog between 14 and 20 days after ovulation. During implantation the zygote invades and partly destroys an area of hypertrophied endometrium so that it can lie within it, well attached to the wall of the uterus.

Formation of the Extra-embryonic Membranes

The extra-embryonic membranes are:

- The **yolk sac**
- The **chorion**
- The **amnion**
- The **allantois**.

As the early embryo starts to curl up on itself, the top of the yolk sac becomes narrower and narrower as the top part of the endoderm is pinched off to become the primitive gut tube—though at this stage without openings at either end of the body. Then another diverticulum starts to develop from the primitive gut tube, and push its way out beside the yolk sac. This is the **allantois**; it will form the **allantoic sac**, which receives urine from the foetal kidneys via the **urachus**, which is the tube that carries the foetal urine from the bladder of the embryo out of the body.

As the embryo continues to develop, the yolk sac contracts and the allantois increases in size and starts to push its way into the mesodermal cavity between the two mesodermal layers.

While the allantois is developing, the trophoblast continues to expand, reaching round the developing embryo so that it forms a double layer of membrane that completely surrounds the embryo. The outer membrane is called the **chorion**, and the inner layer membrane the **amnion** (Fig. 14.50), each consists of two layers—ectoderm and mesoderm.

The allantois continues to expand as foetal urine is produced, and soon the whole cavity between the chorion and amnion is filled with the allantois and its contents. The membrane of the allantois then fuses with that of the chorion above it and the amnion below it and the basic plan of the extra-embryonic membranes is complete. The outer membrane is now called the **chorioallantois** and the inner is correctly known as the **allanto-amnion**.

During birth the chorioallantois is recognised as the '**water bag**' that ruptures as the foetus starts to move down the uterine horn and into the birth canal. The allanto-amnion (often just called the amnion) is the '**slime bag**' that closely surrounds the fetus and contains the slippery lubricant fluid that eases its passage along the birth canal.

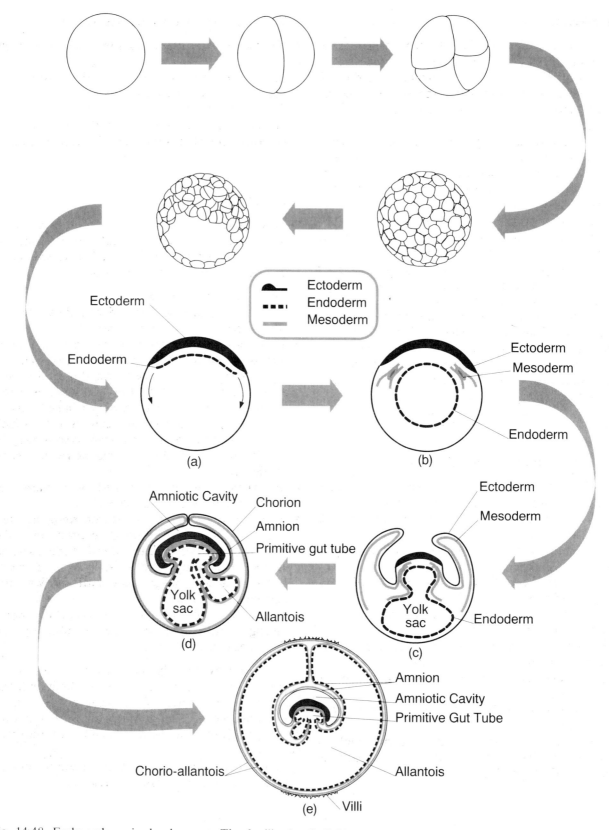

Fig. 14.48. Early embryonic development. The fertilised cell divides to form a ball of cells—a morula; a cavity then develops—this is now a trophoblast. (a) A layer of endodermal cells starts to line the trophoblast; (b) the endoderm forms the primitive yolk sac; (c) blocks of mesoderm start to form as the inner cell mass starts to be pinched off to form the embryo mesoderm; (d) another diverticulum forms from the primitive gut tube—this is the allantois; the yolk sac starts to regress. Early embryonic development. Developing villi forming a band around the extra-embryonic membranes.

The Placenta

The placenta is the thickened area of the extra-embryonic membranes by which the mammalian foetus is attached to the endometrium. It is through the placental blood supply that the embryo receives oxygen and foodstuffs, and gets rid of waste products.

The structure and shape of the placenta varies a great deal in the different mammal species. That of the dog and cat is called a **zonary placenta**, as the placental tissue forms a broad belt round the extra-embryonic membranes.

In the area of placenta formation the chorioallantois develops folds that form villi, which increase the area of contact with the maternal tissue.

At the edges of the placenta are the **marginal haematomas**, where there is degeneration of maternal endothelium, with bleeding into the spaces so formed. Substances secreted by the chorion prevent the clotting of this blood, which is broken down to form (it is thought) a source of iron for the embryo.

It is this marginal haematoma—coloured green in bitches and brown in queens—that gives the colour to the vaginal discharge at parturition.

Later Development of the Embryo

The following applies to a medium-sized dog. Kittens are slightly in advance of pups at each stage.

At 3 weeks: the amnion and allantois have formed; the embryo is 5 mm long.

At 4 weeks; 'limb buds' are visible; the embryo is 20 mm long.

At 5 weeks; eyelids and pinna are visible; the embryo is 35 mm long.

At 6 weeks; digits and external genitalia are well developed; the embryo is 60 mm long.

At 7 weeks; colour markings and hair are starting to develop; the embryo is 100 mm long.

At 8 weeks; the embryo is 150 mm long and has hair and pads.

At 9 weeks (approximately); the pup is born, with eyes and ears closed.

The actual process of birth (**parturition**) is described in Chapter 19, Obstetric and Paediatric Nursing of the Dog and Cat.

The Nervous System

The nervous system is made up of two parts:

- The **central nervous system**—consisting of the brain and the spinal cord.
- The **peripheral nervous system**—consisting of all the other motor and sensory nerves throughout the body.

The functions of the nervous system are:

- To receive information about the external environment.
- To receive information about the tissues and organs of the animal's own body.
- To interpret the information received.
- To send impulses throughout the body via the nervous system to stimulate activity of some kind.

Nervous Tissue

Nervous tissue is made up of nerve cells (**neurons**) that are able to conduct electrical impulses, and the connective tissue that runs between them (**neuroglia**).

The neuron (Fig. 14.49) consists of:

- a cell body with a nucleus
- several short processes called **dendrites**, through which nervous impulses enter the cell
- a long process, the axon, along which the nerve impulse travels. This may or may not be myelinated (i.e. surrounded by a sheath of a fatty substance called myelin). Nervous impulses travel faster in myelinated than in unmyelinated nerves. The myelin is produced by Schwann cells, which wrap themselves round the axon. Axons vary in length from less than a millimetre to many centimetres.
- the whole axon is surrounded by a sheath of connective tissue, the **neurilemma**.
- there are gaps in the myelin sheath along the axon where the axon is in direct contact with the neurilemma. These points are called the **nodes of Ranvier**. It is thought that at these points the nerve cell can take in oxygen and nutrients from the surrounding tissues.
- At the end of the axon are branching **nerve endings**, which transmit the impulse to the dendrites of the next axon.

Neurons may be unipolar, bipolar or multipolar, depending on the position of the cell body and the number of dendrites. One neuron may have connections with only one other nerve cell, or it may exchange information with a number of different nerve cells.

A nerve is made up of many neurons bound together in a connective tissue sheath.

The Nervous Impulse

The nervous impulse starts at the dendrites of a nerve cell and is passed down the axon to the nerve endings. From there, it must either pass to another nerve fibre or to a muscle fibre. The junction between two nerve fibres is a **synapse**, and that between a nerve fibre and a muscle fibre is a **neuro-muscular junction**.

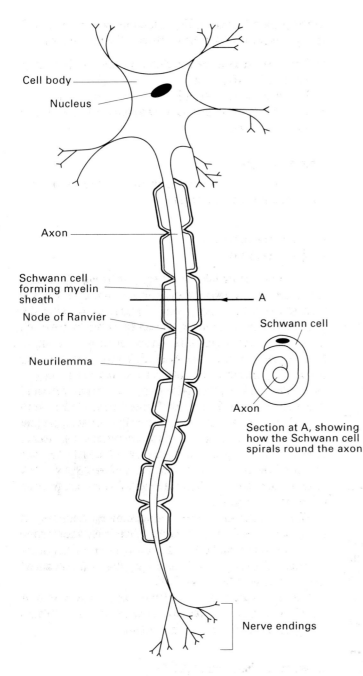

Cell body

Nucleus

Axon

Schwann cell
forming myelin
sheath

Node of Ranvier

Neurilemma

A

Schwann cell

Axon

Section at A, showing
how the Schwann cell
spirals round the axon

Nerve endings

Fig. 14.49. The structure of a neuron.

The movement of the impulse across the synapse or neuro-muscular junction is not by electrical conduction but by the release of chemical transmitters that diffuse across the gap to stimulate the next nerve or the muscle fibre.

The propagation of the electrical impulse is an 'all or nothing' phenomenon. Either a nerve cell is stimulated or it is not—there is no half-way house of a little bit of stimulation. The varying effects that the nervous system has depend on some neurons being inhibitory rather than stimulatory, and also on the number of nerve fibres involved.

The Brain

The division of the brain into **forebrain**, **midbrain** and **hindbrain** is a matter for descriptive convenience, and gives no indication as to the evolutionary age of the different parts of the brain (Fig. 14.50). The divisions are made from observing embryological development, where the brain develops at the anterior end of a hollow tube. It develops three and then five vesicles that elaborate into the complete structure of the brain.

When examining the different parts of the brain, and the brains of lower vertebrates, for clues as to how the brains of the higher mammals developed, the 'oldest' parts of the brain are found to be partly within the forebrain, partly in the midbrain and partly in the hindbrain. For instance, the brains of fish feature very large olfactory lobes (because smell is important under water) and these are part of the forebrain.

Among the higher vertebrates (birds and mammals) other parts of the forebrain become more

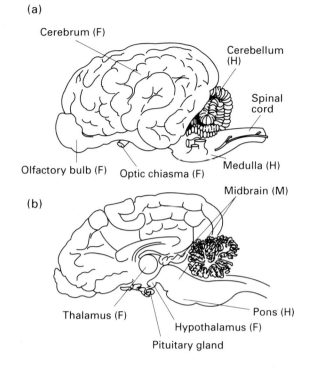

Fig. 14.50. The dog's brain, showing main features and division into forebrain, midbrain and hindbrain: (a) lateral view; (b) longitudinal section.

important—notably the cerebral hemispheres, which are the most obvious and largest part of the brain.

The forebrain includes of:

- The **cerebrum**, or **cerebral hemispheres**, which receive and process information from all over the body. The hemispheres are divided by a deep groove, the longitudinal sulcus.
- The **thalamus**, deep within the brain tissue at the base of the cerebral hemispheres; it relays impulses to and from the cerebral cortex.
- The **hypothalamus**, which lies just above the pituitary gland. It has an important role in regulating the autonomic nervous system and the pituitary gland.

The **midbrain** passes on impulses from the hindbrain and the senses of sight and hearing to the forebrain.

The **hindbrain** includes:

- The **pons**.
- The **medulla oblongata**, which contains centres that control the heart and respiration.
- The **cerebellum**, which coordinates muscular activity within the body.

The ventricles

The ventricular system of the brain originates from the canal down the middle of the primitive neural tube from which the brain was formed in the embryo. There are four ventricles, all of which contain cerebrospinal fluid (CSF), and are continuous with the spinal canal down the middle of the spinal cord.

- The **two lateral ventricles** lie one within each cerebral hemisphere.
- The **third ventricle** lies just above the thalamus.
- The **fourth ventricle** lies beneath and in front of the cerebellum.

The meninges

The meninges are the three layers of membrane that cover and protect the brain:

- The **dura mater**.
- The **arachnoid layer**.
- The **pia mater**.

The **dura mater** is the tough, fibrous membrane that lines the cranial cavity in the skull. It is formed from two layers: the outer is continuous with the periosteum, and the inner is mainly in contact with it, though at certain points it folds inwards to make a fold of membrane between different parts of the brain—for example the falx cerebri between the two cerebral hemispheres and the tentorium cerebelli between the cerebrum and cerebellum. The dura extends all the way down the central nervous system to the end of the spinal column. Within the spinal column it is not so closely attached to the surrounding bone, but leaves an **epidural space** that is used as a site for the injection of local anaesthetic in epidural analgesia.

The **arachnoid layer** (so named because it resembles a spider's web) is a delicate membrane that is closely attached to the inner layer of the dura. Beneath the arachnoid layer is the subarachnoid space, which is filled with CSF.

The **pia mater** is a delicate and very vascular membrane that is closely attached to and follows every contour of the brain beneath it.

Cerebro-Spinal Fluid (CSF)

Cerebro-spinal fluid fills the ventricles, the spinal canal and the subarachnoid space. It is secreted by structures called **choroid plexuses**, which are found within each ventricle. CSF is a clear liquid, very like plasma but with rather less protein in it.

The function of CSF is to protect the brain against sudden movement and trauma, and to provide a cushion between it and the skull. Samples of CSF for diagnostic purposes can be withdrawn from the **cerebromedullary cistern** (cisterna magna), which lies between the cerebellum and the medulla and, conveniently, can be reached with a needle via the atlanto-occipital space.

The Spinal Cord

The **spinal cord** (Fig. 14.51) runs from the medulla oblongata to the lumbar region, where it terminates

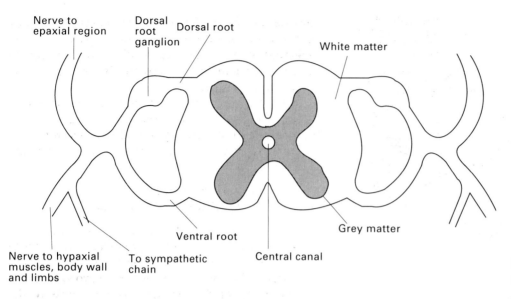

Fig. 14.51. Cross-section of the spinal cord.

in the **cauda equina**—a group of nerves running together that is supposed to look like a horse's tail.

Throughout its length, the spinal cord gives off pairs of nerves—one pair for each segment, or intervertebral space.

The nerve on each side of the cord is divided into two roots:

- the **dorsal root**, carrying sensory fibres into the cord.
- the **ventral root**, carrying motor fibres away from the cord.

Each dorsal root has a **ganglion**, where the cell bodies of the sensory nerves are found.

The spinal nerves supply the whole of the musculoskeletal system. At the levels of the pectoral and pelvic girdles the spinal nerves are thicker than elsewhere as they have to supply the limbs as well as the trunk.

The spinal nerves are named according to the vertebra in front of where they leave the central nervous system (CNS). The cervical (Ce) region, however, is the exception to this rule, because the first spinal nerve leaves in front of the first cervical vertebra and there are eight cervical nerves (Ce7 in front of the seventh cervical vertebra and Ce 8 behind it, then T1 behind the first thoracic vertebra).

The front limb is supplied by nerves from spinal nerves Ce6 to T2, and the hind limb by nerves from spinal nerves L4 to S2 (the fourth lumbar to the second sacral nerve).

Motor and Sensory; Visceral and Somatic

Motor nerves are **efferent nerves**—they take impulses away from the CNS to the periphery. Sensory nerves are **afferent nerves**—they carry impulses towards the CNS, taking information to the brain.

There can be a sensory nerve without a motor nerve (nerves from the eye or ear, or the skin) taking information to the brain, but there cannot be a motor nerve without a sensory nerve running with it and carrying information about its effect back to the CNS.

A somatic motor nerve takes instructions to the voluntary muscle of the body, and a somatic sensory nerve reports back on its action.

Visceral motor nerves take instructions to the smooth or cardiac muscle (i.e. the involuntary muscle of the body), and the visceral sensory nerves report back on their action.

Reflex Arcs

Reflex arcs are fixed, involuntary responses to certain stimuli. For example, if an animal stands on a sharp thorn the foot is withdrawn suddenly. If a person accidentally touches the hotplate of a cooker, they will withdraw their hand almost before they can register the fact of pain or burning, let alone say 'Ow!'. This is because both of these automatic withdrawals involve spinal reflexes, or local reflex arcs, that involve only the spinal cord and would still work even if the cord were cut through. The 'Ow!' and the consciousness of pain follow after the sensory information has been transmitted to the brain.

The spinal reflex arc works as follows (Fig. 14.52):

(1) The pin-prick pain or heat receptors initiate an impulse in the sensory nerve.
(2) The impulse travels up the nerve and enters the spinal cord through the dorsal root of the nerve.
(3) There is often (but not always) one extra neuron, called an intercalating neuron, between the sensory and the motor neuron.
(4) An impulse is initiated in the motor nerve, which leaves the spinal cord in the ventral root, and instructs the relevant muscles to withdraw the affected paw.
(5) Meanwhile, the information about the assault on the body is carried to the CNS.

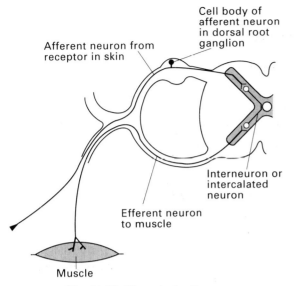

Fig. 14.52. The spinal reflex arc.

The Cranial Nerves

The cranial nerves all originate or end within the brain. Some are purely sensory, while others are mixed nerves (motor and sensory). They are numbered in roman figures I to XII.

A few important facts about the cranial nerves:

Three are purely sensory, and supply the special sense organs:

—I   **olfactory**—the sense of smell.
—II   **optic**—sight.
—VIII   **vestibulocochlear** (also called auditory)—the senses of hearing and balance.

Three supply motor fibres to the muscles of the eye:

—III   **oculomotor**
—IV   **trochlear**
—VI   **abducens**

Of the other six (all mixed nerves):

—V   **trigeminal** is sensory to the skin of the face and motor to the jaw muscles.
—VII   **facial** is motor to the muscles of facial expression.
—IX   **glossopharyngeal** carries sensory taste fibres from the tongue and carries motor fibres to the pharynx.
—X   **vagus** carries motor fibres to the larynx, and to the thoracic and abdominal viscera including the whole of the gastrointestinal tract, right down to the descending colon.
—XI   **accessory** carries motor fibres to the muscles of the neck.
—XII   **hypoglossal** carries motor fibres to the tongue.

The Autonomic Nervous System

The **autonomic nervous system** is the name given to the visceral motor system of the body (Fig. 14.53). It supplies nerves to all the internal organs of the body and also the blood vessels—all the organs not under voluntary control. The nerve fibres run to smooth and cardiac muscle and also to glands such as the liver and the pancreas.

Very often the term 'autonomic nervous system' is taken to include the sensory fibres carrying information from these organs to the CNS as well.

The autonomic nervous system can be divided into two parts:

• the **sympathetic nervous system**.
• the **parasympathetic nervous system**.

The two systems tend to have opposite effects, and most organs have both sympathetic and parasympathetic supplies. The control of the organ's function is a balancing act between the two systems.

The sympathetic nervous system quickens the heart and respiration and dilates the bronchi and bronchioles, so increasing the diameter of the airway. It slows the movement of the bowel and stops the secretion of digestive juices. It also dilates the blood vessels in skeletal muscle, so increasing their blood supply, and constricts the vessels supplying the bowel.

The parasympathetic nervous system has the opposite effect—it slows the heart and respiratory rate, and increases the peristaltic movement of the gut and the secretion of digestive juices.

The sympathetic system helps the body respond to stressful situations (the 'fight, flight and frolic' responses) whereas the parasympathetic system dominates when the animal is relaxed and not fearful or anxious.

The sympathetic fibres leave the spinal cord in spinal nerves T1 to L4 or L5. They synapse in the sympathetic chain or in ganglia close to it, then the long post-ganglionic fibres supply the various organs, mainly by taking a route that follows the blood vessels supplying the organs. The sympathetic chain is a nerve trunk that runs along the dorsal body wall and from which the sympathetic nerves arise.

The parasympathetic fibres leave the CNS in cranial nerves III, VII, IX and X. The first three supply structures within the head, but the vagus supplies all the viscera of the thorax and abdomen. The pelvic viscera are supplied by parasympathetic nerves from S1 and S2. Parasympathetic fibres synapse near their target organ, so have only very short postganglionic fibres.

The Special Senses

The special senses are:

• Smell
• Sight
• Hearing and balance
• Taste

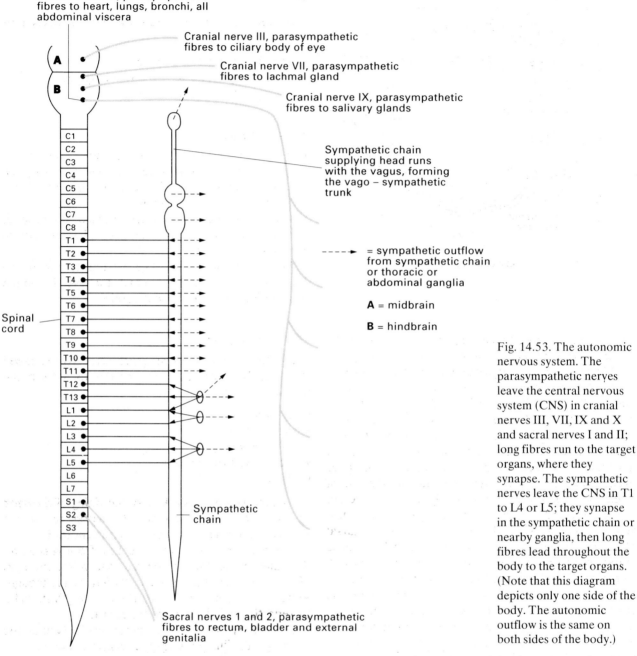

Fig. 14.53. The autonomic nervous system. The parasympathetic nerves leave the central nervous system (CNS) in cranial nerves III, VII, IX and X and sacral nerves I and II; long fibres run to the target organs, where they synapse. The sympathetic nerves leave the CNS in T1 to L4 or L5; they synapse in the sympathetic chain or nearby ganglia, then long fibres lead throughout the body to the target organs. (Note that this diagram depicts only one side of the body. The autonomic outflow is the same on both sides of the body.)

All these special senses have specialised receptors to receive stimuli from the external environment before they are passed on to the central nervous system.

Smell

The bipolar receptor cells of the olfactory system lie within the mucous epithelium covering the **ethmo-turbinate bones**, at the back of the nasal cavity. From there the fibres pass through the **mesethmoid bone** into the olfactory lobe of the brain in cranial nerve I (**olfactory nerve**).

Sight

The eye, the organ of sight, is situated within the orbit, where it is to some degree protected from injury by the zygomatic arch of the skull. The eyes are also protected by the the **eyelids** and the **lacrimal apparatus** (Fig. 14.54).

The eyelids

The eyelids consist of a layer of fibrous tissue (the **tarsal plate**) covered by skin on the outer surface and lined with mucous membrane. At the **medial canthus** (the angle where the upper and lower lids meet) the

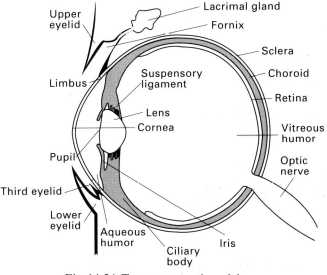

Fig. 14.54. Transverse section of the eye.

Upper eyelid
Lacrimal gland
Fornix
Sclera
Suspensory ligament
Choroid
Limbus
Retina
Lens
Cornea
Vitreous humor
Pupil
Optic nerve
Third eyelid
Lower eyelid
Aqueous humor
Ciliary body
Iris

The eye

The globe of the eye itself can be considered as having three layers:

- a fibrous, protective outer layer
- a middle layer that is vascular and pigmented
- an inner layer of receptor cells.

The outer layer

The outer layer of the eyeball can be divided into a posterior part, the **sclera**, and an anterior part, the transparent **cornea**. The junction between the sclera and cornea is termed the **limbus**.

The sclera has a white outer surface, which gives the colour of the 'white of the eye'. The conjunctiva is attached to the sclera.

The cornea bulges out slightly from the rest of the globe, and allows light to enter the eye. Its shape starts to focus the light onto the retina.

The middle layer

The whole of this vascular, pigmented layer is called the uvea but different parts of the **uvea** form the following structures:

- the **choroid**
- the **tapetum**
- the **ciliary body**
- the **suspensory ligament**
- the **iris**.

The **choroid** is the dark coloured lining of the back of the eye. The blood vessels supplying all the internal structures of the eye are in the choroid

The **tapetum** is the area of light-reflecting cells on the inner surface of the choroid that makes the eyes of dogs and cats shine at night. Its function is thought to be to improve vision when there is very little light, by reflecting light back on to the retina.

The **ciliary body** is the inward projection of the uvea from the lining towards the centre of the eye.

From the ciliary body is given off the **suspensory ligament**, a circular structure that supports the lens and, with the lens, divides the eye into two regions, and the **iris** which contains two layers of muscular tissue. The hole in the centre of the iris is the **pupil**. Opening and closing the iris varies the amount of light that reaches the retina. Dogs have a circular iris, but the pupil of the cat, when fully closed, is a vertical slit.

The inner layer

The inner layer of the eyeball is the retina, which is made up of three layers:

- a layer of **pigmented cells**, closest to the choroid;
- a middle layer of **light-sensitive cells**—the **rods**, concerned with night vision (black-and-white) and the **cones**, with day vision (colour).

eyelids are closely attached to the bone, but at the **lateral canthus** they can be moved relatively freely.

Opening on to the edge of the eyelids are the ducts of the **tarsal glands**, which secrete a fatty material that makes up about 10% of the tear film that moistens the eye. Eyelashes, or **cilia**, are thick hairs growing out of the edge of the eyelid that help to protect the eye from dust etc. The carnivores do not have true eyelashes (although the hairs on the upper eyelids may in some cases give the impression of 'eyelashes' where they are relatively long and overlap the edge of the eyelid) but there may be a few 'ectopic cilia' growing from the edge of the tarsal plate. Sometimes these 'ingrowing eyelashes' cause irritation to the cornea and have to be removed. Occasionally either eyelid may be curled inwards on to the eye so that the hairs of the skin irritate the cornea (**entropion**); or the lower lid may be too large for the eye and droop, exposing the conjunctiva and making the eye more prone to infection (ectropion). Both conditions may have to be corrected surgically.

The **third eyelid** lies below the true eyelids, on the medial side of the eye. It is supported by a piece of cartilage, but unlike the true eyelids it is covered with mucous membrane on both sides.

The lacrimal apparatus

This consists of the lacrimal glands and the lacrimal ducts.

The main **lacrimal gland** lies between the eyeball and the dorso-lateral wall of the orbit. There is also glandular tissue on the underside of the third eyelid.

Lacrimal fluid is distributed over the surface of the eye by the eyelids, and is then collected by the **lacrimal punctae**, near the medial canthus in the upper and lower lids, where it then drains via the **nasolacrimal duct** into the nasal cavity.

- an innermost layer of **bipolar receptor cells** and the neurones that carry the information into the **optic nerve** (cranial nerve II).

The end of the optic nerve lies within the retina, where it appears as the **optic disc**. It is an area where there are no receptor cells.

Lens and humors

Within the substance of the eye are:

- the **lens**
- the **aqueous**
- the **vitreous**.

The **lens** is held in place by the suspensory ligament, and the muscular ciliary body that it can pull on the lens to change its shape and so the focus of the eye.

The **aqueous** is the watery fluid that fills the space between the lens and the cornea. It provides nourishment for the lens and cornea and helps to maintain the shape of the relatively fragile cornea.

The **vitreous** is a transparent jelly-like substance that fills the space between the lens and the back of the eye.

How the eye works

- Light enters the eye through the cornea, which starts to focus it on to the retina.
- The iris controls the size of the pupil and so the amount of light allowed into the eye.
- The lens, its curvature altered by the ciliary muscle, focuses the light on to the retina.
- The light passes through the retinal layers to the light-receptive cells, where it produces an image upside down.
- Light that missed the receptor cells on the way through the retina is reflected back on to the retinal layers by the tapetum.
- The bipolar receptor cells then transmit the image through the optic nerve to the brain's optic chiasma, where the two optic nerves join, and some of the fibres cross over from one nerve to the other before continuing on into the midbrain and up to the cerebral cortex.

Hearing and Balance

The organ of hearing and balance is, of course, the ear, which can be divided into three parts (Fig. 14.55):

- the external ear
- the middle ear
- the inner ear.

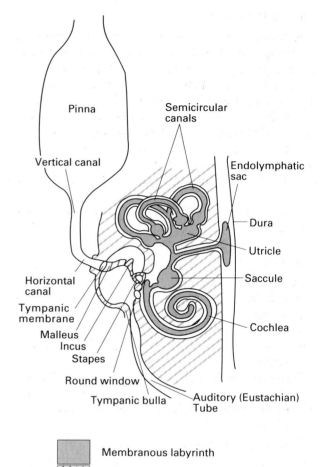

Fig. 14.55. The ear.

The external ear

The external ear is made up of three parts:

- The pinna
- The vertical canal
- The horizontal canal.

The **pinna**, or ear flap, varies a great deal in size and shape amongst dogs of different breeds. The 'wild type' of dog ear is upright: it acts to funnel sound towards the ear, and also as a means of expression between dogs (ears up, ears back, ears flat etc.).

The ear canal, or external auditory meatus, runs from the base of the pinna to the tympanic membrane or eardrum.

The shape of both the pinna and the ear canal are maintained by cartilage—a sheet of cartilage in the pinna and a tube surrounding the ear canal.

The **external auditory meatus** is lined with modified skin, which contains very few hair follicles (except in some hairy-eared breeds such as miniature and toy poodles), but a large number of modified sebaceous glands (**ceruminous glands**) that secrete wax. There is a bend part way down the ear canal that divides it into vertical and horizontal canals.

The middle ear

The middle ear lies within the **tympanic bulla** of the temporal bone. It is an air-filled space, connected to the pharynx by the **auditory (Eustachian) tube**.

A chain of three tiny bones (**ossicles**) lie across the middle ear, and they transmit vibrations from the tympanic membrane to the inner ear. The ossicles are called the **malleus**, the **incus** and the **stapes**.

The malleus is attached to the **tympanic membrane**, and the base of the stapes fills what is called the **oval window**, which leads into the inner ear.

Just below the oval window is a membrane called the **round window**.

The inner ear

The inner ear also lies within the temporal bone, inside a **bony labyrinth**—a cavity within the bone carved out to fit the organs of hearing and balance. Within the bony labyrinth is the **membranous labyrinth**, and between the two is a fluid known as **perilymph**.

Nervous impulses are carried to the brain from the inner ear in the two branches of the VIIIth cranial nerve—the **vestibulocochlear** or **auditory nerve**.

The membranous labyrinth

The membranous labyrinth contains a fluid called **endolymph**, and consists of:

- The utricle
- The saccule
- The semicircular canals
- The cochlear duct.

The **semicircular canals** are three tubes that lie within a cavity of exactly their shape within the bony labyrinth. At their base are two more open cavities, the **utricle** and the **saccule**. The semicircular canals lie in different directions: one is vertical, one is horizontal and the third is transverse.

At the base of each semicircular canal is a bulge—the **ampulla**. With each **ampulla** is a sensary **crista** with hair cells embedded in a jelly like cupula which swings to and fro under the influence of endolymph in the canals, pulling the hair cells whose combined outputs along the **auditory nerve** register turning movements in all spatial planes. Within the utricle and saccule are two further receptor areas, **maculae**, that respond to the position of the head with respect to gravity. Thus the semicircular canals sense the movements of the head, and the maculae sense the position of the head.

The **cochlea**, is concerned with hearing. It is in the form of a spiral, like a snail shell, and the internal canal of the spiral is divided into three channels. Within the cochlea is the **spiral organ**, or **organ of Corti**, which reacts to different frequencies as a sound travels through the endolymph up the spiral of the cochlea.

Taste

Taste buds are found on the tongue and there are also scattered patches of them on the palate, pharynx and epiglottis. Stimuli from the taste buds pass to the brain in cranial nerves VII (facial), IX (glossopharyngeal) and X (vagus).

The Endocrine System

The endocrine system is part of the regulatory system of the body. It consists of a number of ductless glands which produce chemical substances (hormones) that are carried round the body in the bloodstream. The target organ for a hormone is often a considerable distance from the gland.

Not all hormones are produced by the endocrine glands. For example, **secretin** (which stimulates the secretion of pancreatic and intestinal juice) is produced by the wall of the small intestine, in response to the presence of food in the duodenum. **Gastrin** (which stimulates the secretion of hydrochloric acid from the oxyntic cells) is secreted by the stomach wall in response to the stimulus of food entering the stomach. **Chorionic gonadotrophin** is secreted by the ectodermal layer of the chorion during pregnancy, and helps maintain the corpus luteum throughout the gestation period.

The Thyroid Glands

The thyroid glands lie on either side of the midline on the ventral aspect of the first few tracheal rings. Hormones produced by the thyroid glands are:

- **Thyroxin**
- **Tri-iodothyronine**
- **Thyrocalcitonin**

Thyroxin and **tri-iodothyronine** have a similar effect in the regulation of metabolism. Undersecretion of these hormones will produce the condition called **myxoedema**, in which the animal is fat and sluggish, with poor skin and coat, all due to a lowered metabolic rate. Oversecretion causes an increase in metabolic rate, with weight loss, increased heart rate and often overactivity and increased irritability.

Thyrocalcitonin decreases the level of plasma calcium by slowing the resorption of the mineral from bone.

Parathyroid Glands

The parathyroid glands lie on either side and very close to the thyroid glands. The hormone produced is **parathormone**, which regulates the metabolism and distribution of calcium in the body. Secretion of the hormone increases as the plasma level of calcium decreases. Parathormone increases the absorption of calcium from the digestive tract and increases the reabsorption of calcium from bone and in the kidney.

Hyperparathyroidism may occur in three ways:

- **Neoplasia** of the glands may result in over-production of parathormone, which may lead to demineralisation of bone.
- **Chronic renal failure** may result in secondary indirect hyperparathyroidism as calcium is lost in the urine and the body tries to compensate by absorbing more from the bone. In this case there is often preferential reabsorption from maxillae and mandibles, producing the condition **rubber jaw**.
- **Secondary nutritional hyperparathyroidism** occurs as a result of a diet so low in calcium that the daily requirement cannot be met. This is most common in young animals fed entirely on butcher's meat.

The Pancreas

The pancreas lies in the mesentery of the duodenum. It is a mixed gland: most of its substance is the lobulated exocrine gland that secretes digestive enzymes, but within its substance is the endocrine part of the gland, the **Islets of Langerhans**, which secrete three hormones:

- Insulin
- Glucagon
- Somatostatin.

Insulin is secreted by the beta cells, which make up about three-quarters of the cells in the Islets. It is secreted in response to a rise in blood glucose (e.g. after a meal) and lowers the blood level by increasing the uptake of glucose into cells, and its storage in the form of glycogen. A shortage of insulin, such as occurs in diabetes mellitus, results in the urinary excretion of glucose and the body using fats and protein for energy.

Glucagon is secreted by the Islets' alpha cells, in response to a fall in blood sugar. It stimulates the conversion of glycogen to glucose, so raising the blood sugar level again.

Somatostatin is secreted by the Islets' delta cells. It mildly inhibits the secretion of both insulin and glucagon, thus eliminating large swings in blood glucose caused by a sudden overwhelming effect of one or other hormone. It also decreases the motility of the gut and reduces the secretion of the digestive juices.

The Ovary

Hormones produced in the ovary are:

- Progesterone
- Oestradiol
- Relaxin.

Oestradiol is one of a group of compounds called oestrogens. The function of oestradiol is to prepare the genital tract and external genitalia for coitus and the reception of fertilised eggs. It is produced by the cells of the wall of the developing ovarian follicle, and passes from there into both the bloodstream and the follicular fluid.

Progesterone is essential for the maintenance of pregnancy. It is produced by the corpus luteum that develops in the place of the ruptured follicle after ovulation, and acts on the lining of the uterus and on the mammary tissue.

Relaxin is produced by the corpus luteum in the late stages of pregnancy, and causes relaxation of the sacrosciatic and other ligaments round the birth canal, to ease the passage of the foetus.

The Testis

Hormones produced in the testes are:

- **Testosterone**
- **Oestrogens**.

Testosterone is produced by the **interstitial cells** of the testis (**cells of Leydig**) and is responsible for the development and maintenance of male secondary sexual characteristics.

Oestrogens are also produced by the testis, from the **Sertoli cells**. Tumours of the Sertoli cells of the testis may result in an increase in oestrogen output, and the feminisation of the dog so that it develops a soft, pendulous prepuce, increased nipple size, and often coat changes resulting in a soft 'puppy' type of coat.

Adrenal Glands

The adrenal glands lie close to the anterior pole of each kidney. Each has an outer region, the **cortex**, and an inner region, the **medulla**. The cortex and medulla act independently, and can be considered as two different endocrine glands.

Adrenal medulla

The hormones secreted by the adrenal medulla are:

- **Adrenaline (epinephrine)**
- **Noradrenaline (norepinephrine)**.

They act on the body in a similar way to the sympathetic nervous system, preparing the body to meet emergencies, and are controlled by fibres of the sympathetic nervous system. They increase heart rate, and they increase blood glucose level by increasing glycogen breakdown. They also increase the rate and depth of respiration and dilate the arteries supplying skeletal and voluntary muscle.

Adrenal Cortex

The adrenal cortex produces three groups of hormones, each from a different layer of tissue:

(a) **Glucocorticoids**
  - cortisol (hydrocortisone)
  - corticosterone
(b) **Mineralocorticoids**
  - aldosterone
(c) **Adrenal sex steroids**

All of these are **steroids** and have a similar structure based on lipid.

The **glucocorticoids**, although present at all times in the bloodstream, are secreted in increased quantities as a response to stress within the body. They increase the blood sugar level by decreasing the use of glucose by cells, stimulating the conversion of amino acids to glucose in the liver (**gluconeogenesis**), and mobilising fatty acids from adipose tissue. In large quantities they depress the inflammatory and so the healing or repair mechanisms of the body.

The **mineralocorticoid aldosterone** regulates the level of electrolytes in the body, particularly sodium and potassium. It stimulates the resorption of sodium in the kidney tubule, and increases the excretion of potassium. The reabsorption of sodium is linked to that of chloride and water.

The adrenal sex steroids and male and female sex hormones are produced by both sexes in the adrenal cortex. They are not generally of great importance, although they may have a significant effect in the spayed or castrated animal.

The Pituitary Gland

The pituitary gland can be considered as two different glands: the anterior pituitary (or adeno-hypophysis) and the posterior pituitary (neuro-hypophysis).

The adenohypophysis

The anterior pituitary produces the following:

- **Thyrotropic**, or **thyroid stimulating hormone** (TSH)
- **Somatotrophin**, or **growth hormone**.
- **Adrenocorticotropic hormone** (ACTH)
- **Prolactin**

- **Follicle stimulating hormone** (FSH)—a gonado-trophin
- **Luteinising hormone** (LH)—a gonadotrophin
- **Interstitial cell stimulating hormone** (ICSH)—a gonadotrophin—the male equivalent of LH

Thyroid stimulating hormone (TSH) regulates the uptake of iodine by the thyroid gland, thyroid hormone manufacture, and the release of the thyroid hormones into the circulation.

Growth hormone, or **somatotrophin**, controls the rate of growth in the young animal. It acts mainly on the bones, controlling the rate of growth of the epiphyses. It is also involved in the production of proteins from amino acids and the regulation of energy use within the body during periods of poor food supply, conserving glucose for use by the nervous system and stimulating the breakdown of fat for use by the rest of the body.

Adrenocorticotropic hormone (ACTH) regulates the secretion of adreno-cortical hormones.

Prolactin stimulates milk production in late pregnancy and lactation.

Follicle stimulating hormone (FSH) stimulates the maturation of ovarian follicles in the ovary.

Interstitial cell stimulating hormone (ICSH) is the male equivalent of FSH and stimulates the production of sperm.

Luteinising hormone (LH) stimulates the development of the corpus luteum in the female after ovulation. In the male it controls the secretion of testosterone.

The neurohypophysis (the posterior pituitary)

The hormones listed as coming from the posterior pituitary are in fact manufactured higher up in the brain by secretory nerve cells, and stored in the posterior pituitary prior to release:

- **Anti-diuretic hormone** (ADH or vasopressin)
- **Oxytocin**

Anti-diuretic hormone (ADH), also known as vasopressin, increases the absorption of water by the kidney tubules, so reducing the amount of urine excreted and increasing the water retained by the body.

Oxytocin acts during pregnancy and parturition. It causes contraction of the smooth muscle of the uterus and of the ducts in the mammary glands.

Index